THE
EAT
THIS
NOT
THAT!®
DIET

NO DIET!

The World's Easiest Weight-Loss Plan!

BY DAVID ZINCZENKO
WITH MATT GOULDING

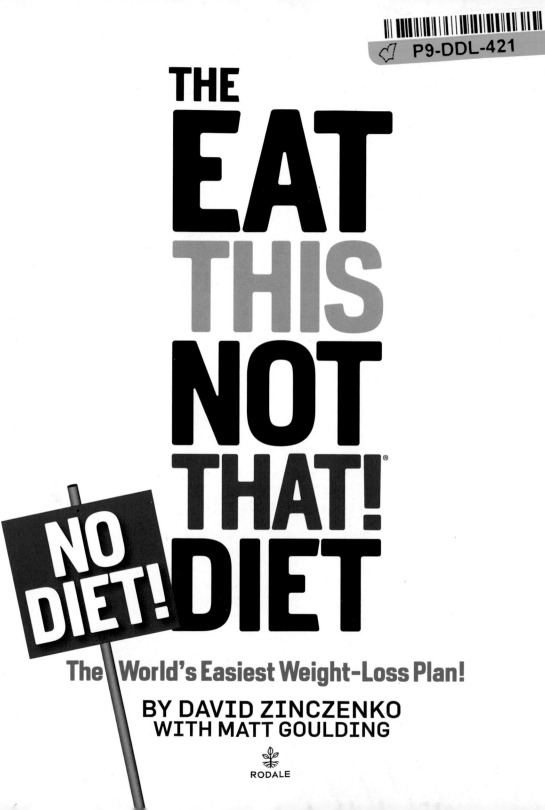

RODALE

Rodale books may be purchased for business or promotional use or for special sales. For information,
please write to: Special Markets Department, Rodale Inc., 733 Third Avenue, New York, NY 10017

Printed in the United States of America

Rodale Inc. makes every effort to use acid-free ∞, recycled paper ♺

Book design by George Karabotsos

Photo direction by Tara Long

All interior photos by Mitch Mandel and Thomas MacDonald/Rodale Images,
with the exception of the following: 98, © Orly Catz; 271, © Lisa Adams

Rodale Images food styling by Melissa Reiss

Library of Congress Cataloging-in-Publication Data is on file with the publisher
ISBN-13: 978-1-60961-249-8   paperback

Distributed to the trade by Macmillan
4   6   8   10   9   7   5   3   paperback

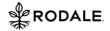

www.rodalebooks.com

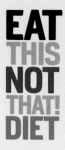

DEDICATION

To anyone who's tired of being told
what they can't eat, shouldn't eat,
or aren't allowed to eat:
It's time to put the freedom—and
the fun—back into food!

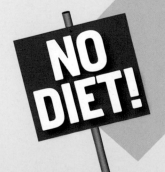

ACKNOWLEDGMENTS

This book is the product of thousands of meals, hundreds of conversations with nutritionists and industry experts, and the collective smarts, dedication, and raw talent of dozens of individuals. Our undying thanks to all of you who have inspired this project in any way. In particular:

To Maria Rodale and the Rodale family, whose dedication to improving the lives of their readers is apparent in every book and magazine they put their name on.

To Clint Carter, whose creativity and dedication to the *Eat This, Not That!* brand has made this book, and so many more of our efforts, possible.

To George Karabotsos and his crew of immensely talented designers, including Laura White, Mark Michaelson, Elizabeth Neal, Courtney Eltringham, and Rob Campos. Thanks for working through the holidays to make 2011 a healthier, happier year for millions of Americans.

To Carolyn Kylstra, Theresa Dougherty, Adam Campbell, and Andrew Del-Colle: Your willingness to take on any and all tasks—no matter how bizarre—has been vital to this project.

To Tara Long, who spends more time in the drive-thru and the supermarket aisles than anyone on the planet, all in the name of making us look good.

To Debbie McHugh, whose ability to keep us sane and focused under the most impossible circumstances cannot be overstated.

To Ken Citron, whose oversight has helped give *Eat This, Not That!* room to grow.

To Elaine Kaufman. Thanks for everything. We'll never forget you.

To the Rodale books team: Steve Perrine, Karen Rinaldi, Chris Krogermeier, Erin Williams, Ruth Davis Konigsberg, Sara Cox, Nancy Elgin, Sonya Maynard, Mitch Mandel, Tom MacDonald, Troy Schnyder, Melissa Reiss, Nikki Weber, Jennifer Giandomenico, Wendy Gable, Keith Biery, Liz Krenos, Brooke Myers, Sean Sabo, and Caroline McCall. You continue to do whatever it takes to get these books done. As always, we appreciate your heroic efforts.

—Dave and Matt

Check out the other books in the EAT THIS, NOT THAT!® and COOK THIS, NOT THAT!® series:

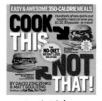

Cook This,
Not That!
Easy & Awesome
350-Calorie
Meals

Eat This,
Not That!
2011

Drink This,
Not That!

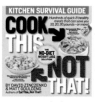

Cook This,
Not That!
Kitchen
Survival Guide

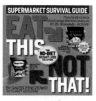

Eat This,
Not That!
Supermarket
Survival Guide

CONTENTS

Introduction
The No-Diet Weight-Loss Solution.................. viii
*Millions of people have discovered how easy it is to shed 10, 20, 30 pounds
or more the Eat This, Not That! way. Now, for the first time, the principles
of Eat This, Not That! have been condensed into a complete nutrition plan—The
No-Diet Diet! Get ready to eat more—and get ready to weigh less!*
PLUS: *Meet just some of the millions of Americans who've already dropped
those unwanted pounds, and discover their easy-to-use secrets!*

Chapter 1
How to Use this Book to Lose Weight.................. 1
*The No-Diet Diet isn't about restricting calories, cutting out the things you love,
or going hungry. Instead, it's about creating balanced meals using all your
favorite fast foods, supermarket products, and restaurant fare. It's so easy,
it ought to be illegal!*

Chapter 2
Four Ways The No-Diet Diet Will Change
Your Life—Starting Today!............................ 11
*Lose fat, build lean muscle, boost your energy, enjoy better sex, beat
depression, live longer and healthier—what, that's not good enough for you?
Okay, we'll show you how The No-Diet Diet will also save you tons of time
and money—and never leave you feeling hungry or deprived!*

Special Report
Know Thy Enemies....................................... 20
*What exactly is diabetes? What causes heart disease? What is high blood
pressure anyways? A quick overview of your greatest health risks, and how
The No-Diet Diet can help to overcome them.*

Chapter 3
Choose Your Weapons!................................. 35
*Discover The No-Diet Diet Snack Matrix, and learn how to quickly whip up the
most delicious, nutritious bites ever designed! Make hunger a thing of the past!*

Chapter 4
Breakfasts 55
*Forty perfect ways to start your day. You'll be amazed at how easy they
are—and how quickly they'll start burning off the pounds!*

Chapter 5

Lunch 103

Beat the 3 p.m. slump with high-energy midday meals that will keep your body burning fat all day long!

Chapter 6

Dinner 179

Eat like royalty at your favorite restaurants, or whip up easy comfort foods at home. The No-Diet Diet will help you make every day a nutritional masterpiece.

Chapter 7

Snacks 253

Discipline? Who needs it? Eat what you want, when you want, using this simple and effective snacking guide.

Chapter 8

Dessert 267

No indulgence is off limits on The No-Diet Diet! Discover why sweet, creamy desserts are an essential weight-loss weapon!

Chapter 9

Sweat This, Not That! 297

Discover how to turbocharge the effects of The No-Diet Diet with this complete workout that anyone can do—and an eye-opening exposé of some common workouts you should never try!

Special Report

The World's Most Dangerous Activity 310

It's not cave diving, it's not swimming with sharks, it's not dating Lady Gaga. It's something you do every single day, often for hours at a time, and chances are, you might be doing it right now. It's....

Appendix 316

Index 324

Sarah Palin is on a diet.
So too are Rand Paul, Rush Limbaugh, and even wiry, wily Bill O'Reilly.
In fact, every right-wing politician and conservative commentator in America is on a diet right now.

But don't worry, liberals. The Obamas are on a diet too—Barack, Michelle, Sasha, even little Malia. Nancy Pelosi, Joe Biden, Rachel Maddow, the entire editorial board of the *New York Times*? On a diet, every day. In fact, if you're one of the 6 billion human beings currently populating the planet Earth, you're on a diet, too. (And if you are not, please contact us immediately—we have a unique condo offering in Roswell, New Mexico, that you might be interested in.)

Now, at first thought, you might be wondering: I don't remember going on a diet—how can this be true? And how can everyone else also be on a diet at the same time? And where would Osama bin Laden find a copy of a diet book, anyway? At the Pakistani Borders?

Well, the fact is that anything you partake of on a regular basis is considered your "diet." If you eat mostly rice, tofu, and bean sprouts, that's your diet. Beer, battered chicken, and barbecued ribs? Also a diet. What if you dine exclusively on fried eel, toffee ice cream, and stuff you find stuck between sofa cushions? Yep, that counts as well. If you eat it, it's your diet.

The problem is that most of us have been taught to equate the word "diet" with a temporary, extreme, often terrible-tasting assortment of bland foods, coupled with bouts of hunger pangs, long stretches of self-denial, and desperate moments spent standing outside the window of Pepe's Pepperoni Palace, wondering why everyone else gets to go inside but we don't.

Worse, "going on a diet" is just about the biggest mistake you can make when it comes to fighting fat. According to several studies, the number-one indicator that you'll weigh more a year from now is: being "on a diet." That's why we created the no-diet weight loss solution. Because, plain and simple, traditional diet plans don't work.

So whether you're one of the 6 million Americans who has already discovered how easy it is to drop 10, 20, 30 pounds or more using

Eat This, Not That! or you're a newcomer to our unique take on weight loss, you probably took one look at the cover of *The Eat This, Not That! No-Diet Diet* and had the same reaction that many of our friends, colleagues, and fans have already expressed to us:

What the $&*#)@ are you talking about?

Really, what is a "no-diet diet"?

Well, it's simple. As we said above, the word "diet" has become corrupted to the point where it now means a short-term, unappealing, restrictive, and utterly futile way of eating. As a result, our own diets have become corrupted as well. Today, a shocking two out of three American women and nearly three-quarters of American men are either overweight or obese.

That makes for some rather unlovely viewing at ye olde community swimming hole. But it's also making for something worse—a health crisis that's hunting us down relentlessly.

Why Fat Hates You More Than You Hate Fat

Double chin, spare tire, muffin top, potbelly, cankle—we have more words for body fat than Eskimos have for snow. But in reality, most of us don't know that much about fat—how it gets there, why it stays there, or what it's doing to us during its visit. So let's do a deep dive into your belly fat (look out for the lint!) and take a look around.

You see, body fat—especially belly fat—doesn't just sit there, globlike and idle. Fat actually functions like a great big gland, churning out hormones and other substances that are essential to many bodily functions. And to that end, fat plays a key role in keeping us alive and thinking: In fact, if you were to look closely at a human brain—for example, by cracking open a zombie's head with a battle-ax—you'd discover that 60 percent of the gloopy gray matter inside is fat.

Basically, fat is just stored energy. When you eat, your body transforms your Trix, Twix, and Twinkies into fatty acids, blood sugar, and amino acids. These provide energy that you either burn up right

The Making of The Eat This, Not That! No-Diet Diet

The following transcript offers a unique look into the collaborative efforts of David Zinczenko and coauthor Matt Goulding as they discuss initial plans for *The Eat This, Not That! No-Diet Diet*.

[BRRIINGGG! BRRIINGGG!]

MATT: Hello?

DAVE: Matt, it's DZ. I have an awesome idea!

MATT: Shoot!

DAVE: Why does your phone sound like it's 1957? What's with the BRRIINGGG, BRRIINGGG? They have cell phones now. They're cheap.

MATT: Dave, I'm busy. What's the idea?

DAVE: Seriously, it's like I'm talking to the cast of *Mad Men*.

MATT: Dave, I'm busy! I'm slaving over a hot stove in the freezing-cold Pennsylvania winter, trying to whip up some exciting new recipes for our readers. What's the idea?

DAVE: What's the one thing all 6 million *Eat This, Not That!* readers want?

MATT: To draw and quarter a Wall Street banker and fertilize their gardens with the extruded viscera?

DAVE: No, besides that. It's this: the *Eat This, Not That!* diet! We've taught people how to lose weight just by making smart swaps at the grocery store and at their favorite restaurants. We've taught them how to cook their favorite indulgent foods and cut thousands of calories. We've gotten testimonials from people who've lost 50, 60, 70 pounds just making these swaps. But what we haven't done is give them a complete eating guide—a day-by-day, meal-by-meal strategy for putting it all together!

[PAUSE]

DAVE: Why do I hear seagulls?

MATT: Those are pigeons. So you're saying we'd create a complete diet plan using the principles of *Eat This, Not That!*?

DAVE: Exactly! The *Eat This, Not That!* diet!

MATT: But the whole idea of *Eat This, Not That!* is that you can lose weight without dieting. It's the no-diet weight loss solution.

DAVE: Yes, but we make a diet out of the idea of no diet! We teach people to use smart swaps so they can eat their favorite foods, from burgers to pizzas to ice cream, either from the grocery store or at their favorite restaurants, and they eat them anytime they want! We take them through breakfast, lunch, and dinner, and that's the *Eat This, Not That!* diet!

[PAUSE]

DAVE: Is there typically the sound of crashing surf in the middle of Pennsylvania?

MATT: Lots of pots and pans boiling here, Dave. But seriously, diets are boring, painful, and restrictive. This is a plan that lets people eat whatever they want, whenever they want. That doesn't sound like a diet.

DAVE: It's the *Eat This, Not That!* diet.

MATT: It's no diet!

DAVE: It's the *Eat This, Not That!* . . .

MATT: NO-DIET! . . .

DAVE: DIET!

MATT: Whoa, I think we're on to something! *THE EAT THIS, NOT THAT! NO-DIET DIET!*

DAVE: Genius! Wait . . . I distinctly hear distant strains of Hawaiian musician Israel Kamakawiwo'ole's ukulele version of "Somewhere over the Rainbow." Matt . . .

MATT: *THE EAT THIS, NOT THAT! NO-DIET DIET!* Great idea! Gotta go!

[CLICK]

away—like if you're battling zombies, for example—or that your body will save and store, in case of future battles with zombies. If you couldn't store fat, you'd have to eat all the time just to keep your body functioning. And while that sounds like fun, 24/7 feasting would get old pretty fast. A little shuteye, or maybe some romance, helps break up the day, doesn't it?

Fat that isn't used right away gets stored in your fat cells. If you looked at a fat cell under a microscope, you'd see the standard cell stuff you remember from sixth grade—the nucleus, the mitochondria, that sort of thing—dwarfed by a big fat droplet that makes up about 85 percent of the cell's volume. As you burn off this stored energy, the cell gets smaller, then plumps up when you once again eat more energy than you expend. Burn more calories on a regular basis than you eat, and your fat cells shrivel up like David Spade in a cage match. Eat more calories than you burn over and over again, however, and those cells will stretch and stretch until they're the size of the period at the end of this sentence. And when they can't stretch any more? They go all Agent Smith on you, duplicating themselves just like the bad guy from the Matrix movies. Bam, new fat cell, ready for duty.

And once you create a new fat cell, guess what? It's there to stay. No amount of dieting or exercise will make it go away. While an adult of "normal" size might have roughly 30 billion to 40 billion fat cells, someone who's very obese might have as many as 100 billion.

But as I said earlier, fat doesn't just hang out there, bouncing around a bit whenever you Hula-Hoop. While you know that being overweight is bad for your health, you might not realize exactly why.

In just the past decade, scientists have uncovered more than 100 biochemical substances, called adipokines, that are created by our fat. Many of these substances cause inflammation in tissues and blood vessels, raising the risks of heart attack and stroke, increasing our blood pressure, even interfering with our ability to process food and turn it into energy. Today, nearly one in three of us will develop type 2 diabetes in our lifetime—a horrible disease closely linked to obesity whose side effects include stroke, heart attack, blindness, sexual dysfunction, and more.

So fat is like a parasite that's actively trying to kill its host. In this case, that host is you.

"I lost 180 pounds with minimal exercising."

Strange as it seems to him now, **Raul Guerrero** used to take pride in being overweight. "I knew I was a big guy—I played into it by priding myself on looking intimidating." Raul had grown up on a diet of battered and fried homemade foods, and eventually he graduated to fast-food value menus and other cheap fills. "I figured, 'If it only costs a dollar, how bad could it be?'" he says. He thought it was crazy when he'd see a coworker cutting off a piece of doughnut. He'd think: "It's free, grab as much as you can!"

Dangerous Gains.

At a free health screening at his company, Raul was told that his blood pressure was nearing dangerous levels. At his checkup a mere 12 days later, he had added an additional 15 pounds to his 370-pound frame. Raul knew something had to change. He picked up a copy of *Eat This, Not That!* and was shocked by what he saw. "I brought it home and showed my wife right away: 'Look at how we eat!'" *Eat This, Not That!* had pulled back the curtain on some of his standby restaurants. "Whoever looks at the labels at a fast-food place? They're hidden by the bathroom!" Horrified by the saturated fat levels, Raul cut fast food out of his diet entirely and began cooking at home. Raul lost 20 pounds in his first month "without even trying," he says. But he was still drastically overweight. "It's kinda sad, but it took 100 pounds before people started to notice." Simply by learning to make better choices, Raul eventually lost all the weight he wanted to—180 pounds before stabilizing at a 175-pound loss. "I tell everybody—just eat the right amount of food and you'll be amazed. I run now, but I lost 180 pounds with minimal, if any, exercising." But what may have been the biggest surprise was that Raul discovered he could eat well without giving up his hunt for value. "I learned that it's a myth that healthy living is expensive," he says. "I still eat like a big man, but before I only wanted the best bang for my buck. That's still true, but now I also get the best bang for my calories."

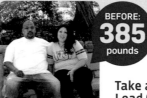

BEFORE: 385 pounds

VITALS:
Raul Guerrero, 40
Los Angeles, CA

HEIGHT: 6'2"

TOTAL WEIGHT LOST: 175 lbs

TIME IT TOOK TO LOSE THE WEIGHT: 11 months

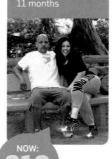

NOW: 210 pounds

Take a Load Off.

Raul knew he had beaten his old habits when they became impossible to revisit. "The first time I cheated and grabbed an In-N-Out burger, I felt physically awful afterward. I realized my body had really changed." A weight loss of nearly 200 pounds is significant, to say the least, but the biggest change Raul has experienced is mental. "I'm happy, I just feel really good deep down," he says. "When life threw me a curveball, I used to binge. Now I know everything can work itself out. It's how I feel, in my head and my heart."

"I still eat like a big man, but now I get the best bang for my calories."

More than two out three of us are overweight or obese. One in three will develop diabetes. How did this happen?

How Did We All Get So Darn Fat?
Attack of the Frankenfoods

Consider this: In 1971, the average American male consumed about 2,450 calories a day; the average woman, 1,542. But by the year 2008, American men were averaging about 2,507 daily calories, while women were eating 1,766 calories (up a whopping 14.5 percent, or 224 additional calories every day!).

Let's run the math on this one: It takes 3,500 calories to create an extra pound of body weight. That means that every 61 days, the average guy eats enough extra calories to outweigh his 1971 contemporary by a pound. That's 6 extra pounds of heft every year. For the average woman, the picture is even bleaker: She's eating enough to gain an extra pound every 16 days, or 23 pounds per year, over her 1971 version!

So what the heck happened here? Did all that medical marijuana just give the country an enormous case of the munchies?

No. The truth is that the food we consume today is simply different from the food our parents and grandparents ate. And the reasons are as simple as they are sneaky:

We've added extra calories to traditional foods.

In the early 1970s, food manufacturers, looking for a cheaper ingredient to replace sugar, came up with a substance called high-fructose corn syrup (HFCS). Today, HFCS is in an unbelievable array of foods—from breakfast cereals to bread, from ketchup to pasta sauce, from juice boxes to iced tea. According to the FDA, the average American consumes 115 grams of added sugars every day, which contribute an empty 418 calories to his or her diet. Though our bodies technically metabolize HFCS the same way they do plain old table sugar, it no doubt shares some of the blame; as a cheap by-product with a long shelf life, it's an easy way for food manufacturers to appeal to our

"My pants were literally falling off me. I had to buy all new clothes."

Dave Boyd grew up in a household many of us would recognize, which is to say one loaded with candy, snacks, and frozen TV dinners. "I had no handle on what I should eat," he says. Dave was an active guy—he hiked and played baseball—but he still found himself growing softer with age. "Tasks that used to be no sweat, like helping a friend move, had lasting physical repercussions." The lifelong habit of eating nutritionally empty foods was finally catching up with him. When he went in for a physical, Dave was not only heavier, but his HDL cholesterol—the good one—was also 10 points below the healthy range.

A Healthier Way.

Dave read about *Eat This, Not That!* in *Men's Health* and realized that the book could help him turn things around. He started jogging and making smart food swaps. Dave's job requires a lot of travel, so he particularly relied on *Eat This, Not That!* to find healthy meals on the road. "I had no idea that some of the things I thought were healthy are so awful," he says. "And I'd never even thought about all the mayo restaurants and gas stations slather on a chicken sandwich."

Sharing Success.

Dave realized his efforts were paying off when his belt became the only thing keeping him clothed. "My pants were literally falling off me," he says. "I had to buy all new clothes, and I'm still wearing them." As he closed in on a healthy weight, he set a goal to run a 5-K on his 35th birthday. Dave completed the race and went on to run five half-marathons. Now he's training for his first full marathon. "Literally every day is different now," he says. "I don't think, 'I can't do that'; I think, 'How do I make it work.'" Dave's resting heart rate is down from 85 to the 50-to-60 range, and his lifestyle improvements have motivated his children to start forming their own healthy habits. They cheered him on at his first half-marathon, and within a month, his oldest son had run a mile for school. "He told me he pushed himself because I inspired him," he says. "That's beyond words." When people ask what his secret is, he enjoys sharing it: "I tell them about *Eat This, Not That!* It feels great to set an example."

> "I had no idea some of the things I thought were healthy are so awful."

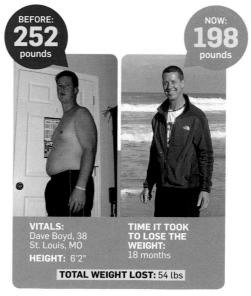

BEFORE:
252 pounds

NOW:
198 pounds

VITALS:
Dave Boyd, 38
St. Louis, MO
HEIGHT: 6'2"

TIME IT TOOK TO LOSE THE WEIGHT:
18 months

TOTAL WEIGHT LOST: 54 lbs

sweet tooths, even in products (like bread or ketchup) that shouldn't be sweet at all. So Grandma's sauce now comes in a jar, and it doesn't just stick to your ribs—it sticks over your belt!

We've been trained to supersize it.

It seems like Economics 101: If you can get a lot more food for just a few cents more, then it makes all the sense in the world to upgrade to the "value meal." And because food is so inexpensive for manufacturers to produce on a large scale, your average fast-food emporium makes a hefty profit when you do supersize your meal— even though you're getting an average of 73 percent more calories for only about 17 percent more money. But that's actually dummy economics—you wouldn't buy a new Blu-ray Disc and then pay the guy at the electronics store extra money to throw in some old, worn-out videotapes, would you? Well, that's essentially what you're doing when you supersize it. We should be paying more money to get the meals with the fewest calories, not the most!

We've laced our food with time bombs.

A generation ago, it was hard for food manufacturers to create baked goods that would last on store shelves. Most baked goods require oils, and oil leaks at room temperature. But since the 1960s, manufacturers have been baking with—and restaurateurs have been frying with—something called trans fats. Trans fats are cheap and effective: They make potato chips crispier and Oreo cookies tastier, and they let fry cooks make pound after pound of fries without smoking up their kitchens. Only one problem: Trans fats increase your bad cholesterol, lower your good choles-terol, and greatly increase your risk of heart disease.

We're drinking more calories than ever.

Studies show that Americans now drink—drink!—an average of 458 calories every day, or more than 21 percent of our daily calorie intake. Sound like a lot? It is: In 1965, we drank just 236 calories daily. So how did we all become two-fisted drinkers? Many of those additional calories come from our old archenemy, HFCS. Indeed, just about every nonalcoholic beverage in your fridge right now, unless it's milk or diet soda, contains HFCS. Go ahead, read the label!

"I feel sexy again. It's an amazing feeling."

Growing up, **Allison Holden** had always been one of those naturally thin people whom others envied. She knew little about diet and exercise, but it didn't matter. Once she hit her twenties, however, her youthful metabolism could no longer keep her thin. All of a sudden, she had morphed into an oversize version of her former self. It wasn't until the day she went clothes shopping and could not find anything that fit her that she realized how bad it had gotten. "I hadn't realized how much weight I'd gained," she says. "I had always been a cute girl—now no one was looking at me."

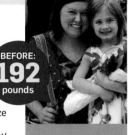

One Little Book.

Allison now had the same problem that faces 64 percent of all American women. "I knew I needed to change something, but I didn't know how," she recalls. "It was overwhelming. All I could think was, 'How do I get this weight off?'" Allison began exercising and eating healthier foods, but after the first month, she still hadn't seen much progress. Sensing Allison's unhappiness, her mom gave her a copy of *Eat This, Not That!* for Christmas. Allison thought, "This is a sign." As soon as she began paying closer attention to the number of calories in her food, Allison suddenly began to shrink. "I saw a 5-pound loss in 1 week, and it's been

continuous weight loss since. Everyone I worked with was astonished—they had always known me as overweight, and to them the change seemed to happen overnight."

How *Eat This, Not That!* Helped.

With the book's help, she was able to cut hidden calories out of her diet and learned to indulge responsibly, and now she's as fit and happy as she was growing up. "I feel sexy and cute and little again," she says. "It's an amazing feeling." She even got a pro-motion at work, which she attributes to her boost in confidence. "When you get healthier, you exude something. I have that confidence now, and that definitely helped me get the job." And before, Allison didn't

exercise; now she's training for her first half-marathon.

Allison's New Life.

Today, Allison continues to scrutinize food labels and car-ries *Eat This, Not That!* with her to the grocery store. "There is so much hidden, weird stuff in some food," she says. "Now I know when the big restaurants and food companies are lying to me." When it came to turning her weight problem around, all she needed, in the end, was *Eat This, Not That!* (and her own determination). "Not everyone can afford a personal trainer or food guru," she says. "No one can do it but you."

BEFORE:
192 pounds

VITALS:
Allison Holden, 26
Memphis, TN
HEIGHT: 5'4"
TOTAL WEIGHT LOST: 58 lbs
TIME IT TOOK TO LOSE THE WEIGHT: 11 months

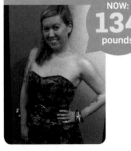

NOW:
134 pounds

"I saw a 5-pound loss in 1 week, and it's been continuous weight loss since."

We've socked ourselves with corn and soy.

You'd be shocked to learn where else corn and its similarly cheap sister, soy, show up. When researchers from the University of Hawaii analyzed 480 servings of food (hamburgers, chicken sandwiches, and fries) from some of the most popular chain restaurants in the United States (McDonald's, Burger King, and Wendy's), they found that out of the 480 samples, only 12 burgers—bought at a Burger King on the West Coast—did not show traces of corn. Corn was present in the fat in the fries and in all chicken samples. And they didn't even bother to test the soft drinks, which are basically HFCS and food coloring, or the buns, which are sweetened with HFCS and chock-full of soy. The problem with all of that corn and soy is that it means we're eating too much of what's called omega-6 fatty acids—fats that come from seeds like corn kernels and soybeans. (Heart- and brain-healthy omega-3 fatty acids, on the other hand, come from things like seafood, leafy vegetables, and nuts.) And recent research indicates that an out-of-balance omega-6—to—omega-3 ratio leads to adipogenesis—the creation of fat cells! In one study published in the *British Journal of Nutrition*, mice fed an omega-6—to—omega-3 ratio of 6:1 gained significantly more fat than mice on a 1:1.2 omega-6—to—omega-3 ratio. Another study, in the journal *Progress in Lipid Research*, determined that consuming more omega-6s than omega-3s leads to an increased risk of fat development. Now, we need omega-6s in our diets. They're essential for heart and brain function. But, thanks to corn and soy, our foodscape has an omega-6—to—omega-3 ratio of about 20:1. Ideally, that ratio should be 1:1.

No matter how much time or money we spend on trying to jog, bike, lift, kickbox, or Zumba away our additional calorie loads, we're in a losing battle. Like Lucy at the chocolate factory, our bodies can't possibly handle the deluge of sweet, fatty, carb-loaded stuff; all we can do is store it. And then, desperate for a change, hoping to rediscover our former skinny selves, we "go on a diet." (See above for the success quotient of that idea.)

So if diets don't work, what will?

Welcome to a revolution in weight loss. Welcome to the No-Diet Diet!

The No-Diet Diet
At a Glance

This revolutionary plan teaches you how to lose weight while eating all your favorite foods, simply by making swaps or additions that boost nutritional content and trim calories. By eating six times a day, you'll ensure a constant infusion of energy to keep your fat burners fired up, and by smartly selecting the right foods you can achieve super-fast weight loss even while enjoying your favorite fast foods, packaged goods, and comfort meals.

NUMBER OF MEALS:
3 meals and 3 snacks a day, spaced relatively evenly throughout the day.

Breakdown of meals*
Breakfast: 400–600 calories **Snack:** 150–250 calories
Lunch: 300–600 calories **Snack:** 150–250 calories
Dinner: 250–450 calories **Dessert:** 150–250 calories

TYPE OF FOOD ALLOWED:
Fast food, sit-down or family-style restaurant,
packaged supermarket food, home-cooked food, take-out and delivery food,
and pretty much anything else your heart desires.

NUTRITIONAL INGREDIENTS TO EMPHASIZE:
Lean proteins, healthy fats, good-for-you (whole grain) carbs, fiber.
These will power up your natural fat burners, protect you from illness and
injury, and keep you lean and healthy for life!

NUTRIONAL INGREDIENTS TO LIMIT:
Refined carbs, saturated fats, trans fats, excess salt and sugar.

TYPE OF FOOD NOT ALLOWED:
Monkey brains, haggis, chocolate-covered ants. (That's about all we could think of.)

PORTION SIZE:
The No-Diet Diet is designed to be self-controlling.
By eating nutritious foods your body will tell you when it's time
to eat—and when it's time to stop.

ALCOHOL:
Limit yourself to a few drinks a week to maximize the benefits of The No-Diet Diet!

EXERCISE PROGRAM:
Optional but highly recommended to boost your health, increase your energy,
and turbocharge your weight loss! See Chapter 9 for details.

*****Note:** These caloric values are an estimate of where you'll want your meals and snacks to fall, calorie-wise. Eating significantly more calories than this on a regular basis may lead to weight gain. But eating significantly fewer calories may reduce muscle mass, which will slow your metabolism—and that too can lead to weight gain.

How Eat This, Not That! Changed The World (Kind Of)

Dec '07 | Jan '08 | Feb '08 | Mar '08 | Apr '08 | May '08 | Jun '08 | Jul '08 | Aug '08 | Sep '08 | Oct '08 | Nov '08 | Dec '08 | Jan '09 | Feb '09 | Mar '09 | Apr '09 | May '09 | Jun '09

DECEMBER '07

>> *Eat This, Not That!* is released, detailing the worst (and best!) options in restaurants and supermarkets across America. At the time, some of the biggest restaurant chains in America were refusing to disclose nutrition information, and the book's dedication page addresses them specifically: "We hope this book plays some part, small or large, in compelling you to provide what every diner in America deserves: full disclosure."

>> We publish a Restaurant Report Card story on the front page of Yahoo! grading every major restaurant chain in America and providing the phone numbers and e-mail addresses of restaurants still refusing to release nutrition information. Soon after, Red Lobster, Olive Garden, and Quiznos go public with their nutrition information.

>> Also contained within the first book is the first-ever 20 Worst Foods in America list, which prompts restaurant chains to begin ditching their unfit fare. Among the purged items are 1,000-plus calorie offerings like Chili's Awesome Blossom, Ruby Tuesday's The Colossal Burger, Romano's Macaroni Grill's Double Macaroni 'n' Cheese, On the Border's Stacked Border Nachos, and Pepperidge Farm's Roasted Chicken Pot Pie.

>> Nestlé sends a cease-and-desist letter. We do neither. Kraft protests against *Eat This, Not That!* after we accuse them of selling sugar water to children with one of their core products, Capri Sun. A few months later they announce that they're dropping the sugar content of their entire Capri Sun drink line by 25 percent.

JANUARY '08

>> Taco Bell launches its healthy Fresco menu, which they later begin calling the Drive-Thru Diet.

APRIL '08

>> An *Eat This, Not That!* blog post titled "The Worst Drink on the Planet" exposes Baskin-Robbins for producing a 2,310-calorie Heath Bar milk shake. The company eventually pulls the shake, and later scraps its entire line of "premium" milk shakes.

>> KFC begins serving grilled chicken.

MAY '08

>> In a story on Yahoo!'s home page, *Eat This, Not That!* names Jamba Juice's Chocolate Moo'd Power Smoothie the Worst Drink in America. The company removes the Power size of that smoothie from the menu, and in a letter to *Eat This, Not That!* company spokesman Tom Suiter declares the company is setting out to become "the healthiest restaurant chain in America."

DECEMBER '08

>> *Eat This, Not That! Supermarket Survival Guide* is released. The book runs a series of Label Decoders to expose misleading label claims. A year later, the FDA sends a flurry of warning letters to food processors to crack down on inflated label claims. Then the FDA joins forces with the Institute of Medicine to try to develop new guidelines for acceptable front-of-package labeling.

APRIL '09

>> VitaminWater, which had protested an earlier report calling its sugar-laden line of waters the Worst "Healthy" Drink in America, introduces VitaminWater Zero. The product quickly becomes a best-seller; VitaminWater thanks us for our efforts.

Since we launched the original *Eat This, Not That!* in 2007, more than 7 million Americans have joined the battle against unhealthy food and discovered that they could strip away pounds—fast—simply by making smart swaps and selecting healthier versions of their favorite foods. And food manufacturers have taken notice. Here's what we witnessed on the way to the revolution.

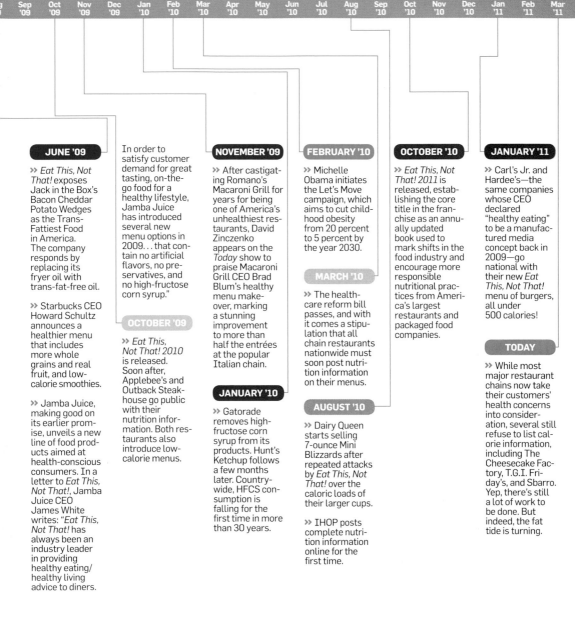

Sep '09 | Oct '09 | Nov '09 | Dec '09 | Jan '10 | Feb '10 | Mar '10 | Apr '10 | May '10 | Jun '10 | Jul '10 | Aug '10 | Sep '10 | Oct '10 | Nov '10 | Dec '10 | Jan '11 | Feb '11 | Mar '11

JUNE '09

>> *Eat This, Not That!* exposes Jack in the Box's Bacon Cheddar Potato Wedges as the Trans-Fattiest Food in America. The company responds by replacing its fryer oil with trans-fat-free oil.

>> Starbucks CEO Howard Schultz announces a healthier menu that includes more whole grains and real fruit, and low-calorie smoothies.

>> Jamba Juice, making good on its earlier promise, unveils a new line of food products aimed at health-conscious consumers. In a letter to *Eat This, Not That!*, Jamba Juice CEO James White writes: "*Eat This, Not That!* has always been an industry leader in providing healthy eating/healthy living advice to diners.

In order to satisfy customer demand for great tasting, on-the-go food for a healthy lifestyle, Jamba Juice has introduced several new menu options in 2009...that contain no artificial flavors, no preservatives, and no high-fructose corn syrup."

OCTOBER '09

>> *Eat This, Not That! 2010* is released. Soon after, Applebee's and Outback Steakhouse go public with their nutrition information. Both restaurants also introduce low-calorie menus.

NOVEMBER '09

>> After castigating Romano's Macaroni Grill for years for being one of America's unhealthiest restaurants, David Zinczenko appears on the *Today* show to praise Macaroni Grill CEO Brad Blum's healthy menu makeover, marking a stunning improvement to more than half the entrées at the popular Italian chain.

JANUARY '10

>> Gatorade removes high-fructose corn syrup from its products. Hunt's Ketchup follows a few months later. Countrywide, HFCS consumption is falling for the first time in more than 30 years.

FEBRUARY '10

>> Michelle Obama initiates the Let's Move campaign, which aims to cut childhood obesity from 20 percent to 5 percent by the year 2030.

MARCH '10

>> The healthcare reform bill passes, and with it comes a stipulation that all chain restaurants nationwide must soon post nutrition information on their menus.

AUGUST '10

>> Dairy Queen starts selling 7-ounce Mini Blizzards after repeated attacks by *Eat This, Not That!* over the caloric loads of their larger cups.

>> IHOP posts complete nutrition information online for the first time.

OCTOBER '10

>> *Eat This, Not That! 2011* is released, establishing the core title in the franchise as an annually updated book used to mark shifts in the food industry and encourage more responsible nutritional practices from America's largest restaurants and packaged food companies.

JANUARY '11

>> Carl's Jr. and Hardee's—the same companies whose CEO declared "healthy eating" to be a manufactured media concept back in 2009—go national with their new *Eat This, Not That!* menu of burgers, all under 500 calories!

TODAY

>> While most major restaurant chains now take their customers' health concerns into consideration, several still refuse to list calorie information, including The Cheesecake Factory, T.G.I. Friday's, and Sbarro. Yep, there's still a lot of work to be done. But indeed, the fat tide is turning.

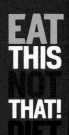
EAT
THIS
NOT
THAT!
DIET

CHAPTER 1

How to Use this Book to

NO DIET!

Lose Weight

The Eat This, Not That! No-Diet Diet

is a low-calorie, high-fiber, fat-free product made with no trans fats or added sugars.

It's designed to strip pounds from your body like magic! Simply tear any chapter from the book for each meal (or any 5- to 7-page section at snack time), place in a microwave-safe container, add ¼ cup water per page, and microwave on high for 60 to 90 seconds. Add salt and ground black pepper to taste, and serve with a side of steamed kale. By eating only pages from *The Eat This, Not That! No-Diet Diet* (and some kale) five or six times per day, you'll shed 5, 10, even 20 pounds per week!

What could be easier?

Okay, we're kidding. But the claims and strategies outlined in the above paragraph aren't really that different from what most traditional diet books try to sell you. Perhaps you're not physically eating their books, but you are often eating a rigid, unappealing, and, in the end, temporary "diet" that's seldom any more realistic than the plan outlined above. And that's why, in the long run, most diets fail. A recent study in the *New England Journal of Medicine* found that regardless of the type of diet plan you choose, any diet you go on will lead to weight loss if it includes a calorie deficit. This finding is echoed by recent studies published in the journals *Diabetes Care*, the *American Journal of Clinical Nutrition*, and the *Archives of Internal Medicine*. And typically people on diets lose 5 to 10 percent of their starting weight in the first 6 months. But according to researchers at UCLA, most people who go on these diets gain that weight back, and then some, within 1 year.

That's because most diet plans require you to do one of five things:

Eat only meals that fall within the narrow confines of a particular "zone" or food ratio or point system. This was the classic Weight Watchers plan, a concept that used to assign the same value to a couple of apples as it did to a mini packet of Oreos. In fact, Weight Watchers revamped its point value system right after Thanksgiving 2010 because it had become apparent that you could live entirely on nutrition-free junk food and still be on their program. Worse, you can eat up all of your points at one meal and starve yourself for the rest of the day—the worst thing you can do for your metabolism (the internal calorie-combustion system you read about in the last chapter).

Eat only foods containing one particular ingredient. You've heard of these: the Cheesecake Diet, the Peanut Butter Diet, the Grapefruit Diet. They all work—until they don't work. People fall off of restrictive diets for the same reason dogs eat Christmas wrapping paper—because after days and weeks of the same food, day in and day out, you'll put any piece of garbage in your gullet just to break up the boredom.

Eat only foods that don't contain one particular ingredient. Think of the Atkins diet, in which you have to give up carbohydrates—even severely restricting fruits and vegetables. You miss out not only on vitamins, minerals, fiber, and other things necessary to make life possible, but also on the flavors and textures that make life bearable. In the long run? Not sustainable.

Eat only foods you've cooked at home. There are plenty of "diet books" out there that are composed of only the culinary musings of some faltering celebrity chef who's desperate to cash in on his fading status. Sure, you'll lose weight eating low-cal foods at home—and cooking for yourself is by far the best way to control your calorie and nutrition intake. But unlike former celebrity chefs, most of us have day jobs. It's not like we can whip up Acorn Squash with Porcini Mushroom Stuffing in the break room at the office, you know?

Eat only extremely expensive foods delivered to your home by the company that came up with the diet. Hey, we applaud Dan Marino, Marie Osmond, Don Shula, and all the other folks who got rich and fat in the latter part of the last century and who are now touting home-delivery weight-loss plans. But seriously: Unless you're a Howard Hughes–type billionaire shut-in, shelling out big bucks for the privilege of waiting for dinner to arrive night after night isn't that viable a way to live. It's rare, but sometimes even we get invited to work functions, birthday parties, holiday gatherings, dates, that sort of thing. And then there are those pesky day jobs that so many of us have.

What's needed is an eating strategy that's not so much a traditional "diet," but rather a completely new approach to food and weight loss. We need a plan that takes into consideration the simple fact that we eat in different ways, at different times, and in different settings. Sometimes we do cook at home. Sometimes we have meals at nice restaurants. Sometimes lunch or dinner arrives at our doorsteps, or comes at us through our car windows. And sometimes we just nosh on ready-to-eat food that's been prepared in a supermarket and stored on its shelves. Any "diet" or eating plan that forces you to focus on only one of these sources of food—or forces you to eliminate one or more foods—just isn't going to work in today's world.

Plus, we have a variety of cravings. Sometimes we want sweets, sometimes we want meats. Sometimes we feel like a nut, sometimes we don't. Sometimes we hunger for an exotic culinary adventure (new sushi restaurant? Cool!). Other times we just want to curl up with comfort food and some bad TV (a bowl of Campbell's Chicken & Stars makes a nice accompaniment to *Dancing with the Stars*, by the way).

And that's where *The Eat This, Not That! No-Diet Diet* comes in. For years, we've been showing you how to make smarter choices in the grocery store, at your favorite restaurants, even in your own kitchen. But for the first time, we're putting it all together in a way that allows you to plan a full day of healthy eating, packing in all the nutrients your body craves while cutting calories and shedding unwanted pounds, effortlessly.

The premise of this food plan is simple: You need to eat a lot, and you need to eat often. We've based this plan on the ideal of eating three meals,

Make the Most of The Eat This, Not That! No-Diet Diet

If *Eat This, Not That!* teaches you anything, it's that knowledge is power. You can lose weight by knowing calorie counts, sure, but mastering your meal plan can help you do a lot more than just manage your waistline: Once you understand the power of certain nutrients, you can select food products that'll make you stronger, lower your cholesterol, reduce your risk of diabetes, battle depression, and even improve your sex life! *Eat This, Not That!* can help you harness that power.

Here's the really cool part. Most diet books are just that—books. But *Eat This, Not That!* is everywhere—on your bookshelf, sure, but also on your smart phone, on your computer, and even in your e-mail inbox. The *Eat This, Not That!* team never stops testing, analyzing, researching, and, yes, eating the best and worst foods in America—and we're constantly updating our information to make sure you're always in the know. Here's how to maximize your 360-degree, 24/7 support system, so you're looking, feeling, and functioning at your personal best.

PREMIUM ONLINE WEIGHT-LOSS TOOL

Sign up for our premium *Eat This, Not That!* Web experience for a personalized tool that'll help you keep track of your caloric intake, exercise output, and all the weight you're losing—every day! Our premium Web experience also gives you full access to nutrition information from more than 80 national chain restaurants (from Applebee's to White Castle and everything in between), as well as more than 200 articles that show you top swaps and smart food picks in every possible category. For just $19.99 a year, you'll have a round-the-clock weight-loss coach at your fingertips. Go to www.EatThis.com for more details.

E-MAIL NEWSLETTERS

Signing up for e-mails that contain weight-loss advice can help you drop pounds, a new study reveals. When researchers in Canada sent diet and exercise advice to more than 1,000 working adults weekly, they discovered that the recipients boosted their levels of physical activity and ate smarter. People who didn't receive the reminders didn't change. Because e-mail is so convenient, people are more likely to read and act on the tips, the scientists say. Luckily for you, we publish the best diet tips and tricks every single weekday. Sign up for our free newsletter, which comes straight to your inbox every morning. Learn more at www.EatThis.com.

WEB SITE

Not yet ready to spring for a premium membership? You can still check out our Web site, where you'll be able to read our daily blog, watch *Eat This, Not That!* top-swap videos, and read scores of articles offering swaps and picks for every type of food on the planet. Check out www.EatThis.com to see what all the hype is about.

SMART PHONE APPS

Look—we love our books and don't plan to stop making them. That said, it's a little awkward to whip out a copy of *Eat This, Not That!* when the waiter is standing at your table, tapping his toe. To help you (discreetly) outsmart America's chain restaurants, we've expanded into the smart phone app arena! The next time you're standing in line at McDonald's, or mulling over what to order at Chili's, simply tap into our brand-new *Eat This, Not That! Restaurant Survival Guide* app. It comes with hundreds of top swaps, a calorie tracker, a weight logger, complete nutritional information for thousands of restaurant items, and a custom comparison tool.

CHAPTER 1

two snacks, and even dessert, each and every day. Each of these meals and snacks has an ideal ratio of fats, carbs, and protein—but don't sweat it, they're just guidelines! And each meal or snack is designed to pack in the most nutrients (and flavor) possible, for a sensible number of calories.

And what makes this plan really unique is that no matter where you are, or what you crave, or what your stress level might be, we've given you a plan for high-nutrition, low-calorie eating. We've assessed every food in the supermarket, we've analyzed every item on every chain restaurant's menu, and we've broken down the nutritional content of every whole food in your fridge. If you can put it in your mouth, we've ranked it and rated it. And we've used these rankings to create complete meals that will make weight loss effortless, no matter where you are.

For example, studies show that eating a calorie-dense, high-protein meal to start your day is one of the hallmarks of weight loss. And adding high-fiber carbohydrates such as whole grains and fruits to your morning meal will help keep hunger at bay for hours. In a 2008 study, researchers at Virginia Commonwealth University found that people who regularly ate a protein-rich, 600-calorie breakfast lost significantly more weight in 8 months than those who consumed only 300 calories and a quarter of the protein. The big-breakfast eaters lost an average of

40 pounds and had an easier time sticking with the diet, even though both groups were prescribed about the same number of total daily calories.

Pretty convincing, right? So with that in mind, to reap the maximum benefits of the latest nutritional science we're recommending a breakfast of between 400 and 600 calories, at least 25 grams of protein, and as much fiber as you can pile on.

But of course, you don't always have the time to study the labels, measure the portions, and ensure that you're getting the exact right kind of food at the exact right time. And life doesn't always conspire to give us control of our breakfast plans. Fortunately, we've done the work for you. Consider these four Monday morning breakfast scenarios to see how *The Eat This, Not That! No-Diet Diet* has you covered, no matter what your day looks like.

Scenario #1

You woke up early. You've got 15 minutes or so to cook up a leisurely meal! Terrific, we've provided plenty of great recipes that will fill you up and power you through your day. Take, for example, our French Toast Stuffed with Strawberries. By sneakily using low-fat ricotta cheese and fat-free milk, we've created a simple high-protein, high-fiber recipe that you can make, and eat, in less than a quarter hour. (Check out page 92.) Add a couple of chicken

"This book rescued my wardrobe. I look the way I want to look."

As a lanky motocross enthusiast, **Michael Clark** never expected to face a weight problem. Then he hit his forties, and his fast-food lifestyle started to catch up with his belly. "I remember traveling a little farther to a different Carl's Jr. for my Western Bacon Cheeseburger," he says. "I was embarrassed that my usual restaurant would start my order as soon as they saw my car pull in."

Midlife Midsection.

Michael had a habit of avoiding photos by always offering to take the pictures. Then one night when he went out to eat with his fiancée and a friend, their waiter insisted on taking camera duty. "When I saw the picture, I was startled," he says. He didn't see the Michael he knew; "I looked 8 months' pregnant," he says. When he told his fiancée that he was unhappy about his appearance, she picked him up a copy of *Eat This, Not That!* "It was her way of saying, 'How about doing something about it?'" he now says. Michael accepted the challenge.

Eat This, Not That! became Michael's bible. "I took it everywhere," he says. "I had been so naïve," he says. "I'd just literally never given a thought to the nutritional consequences

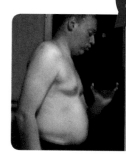

BEFORE: 199 pounds

NOW: 165 pounds

VITALS:
Michael Clark, 43
Bakersfield, CA

HEIGHT: 5'9"

TOTAL WEIGHT LOST: 34 lbs

TIME IT TOOK TO LOSE THE WEIGHT: 6 months

of my food choices." With *Eat This, Not That!* Michael learned how to scrutinize the fat and sugar content of his food. He started making smart swaps, and he quickly dropped below 190. Then, he says, "It just kept going." He felt successful when his co-workers pointed out that his face was slimmer, and shortly after that he ran into an ex-girlfriend. "She wanted to know why I didn't lose weight while I was with her." Now he's back to the weight where he wants to be, and still enjoying the foods he loves.

Say Cheese!

This year, while swimming with his fiancée, Michael let someone photograph him in his swimming trunks. It was his first shirtless photo since high school. His boost in confidence has been further helped along by an unexpected uptick in his health. "I've had asthma all my life, and it's gotten far more manageable," he says. "I've gone from using my rescue inhaler every day to using it only once a month."

Before *Eat This, Not That!* Michael was barely squeezing into his clothes and resorted to buying pants with elastic waistbands. "The book rescued my wardrobe: All of my clothes fit again. I look the way I want to look!"

"I've gone from using my rescue inhaler every day to using it only once a month."

sausage links and some milk and you've got a hearty, fat-melting breakfast of 580 calories, 39 grams of protein, and 6 grams of fiber.

Scenario #2

You meant to wake up early, but you hit the snooze button three times. Now you've got only 5 minutes, and the best you can do is to grab some cereal, or maybe reheat something from the fridge. No problem: We've given you the best possible cereals and instant breakfasts to start your day with maximum nutrition. All you have to do, for example, is pull a Jimmy Dean D-Lights Canadian Bacon Honey Wheat Muffin out of the freezer, nuke it, and pour a cup of milk and have yourself a banana while you're counting down the seconds. The combo of these three ready-to-snarf foods will give you 445 calories, 24.5 grams of protein, and 5 grams of fiber.

Scenario #3

You meant to wake up early, but you hit the snooze button three times and then you threw the alarm clock out the window. You don't even have 5 minutes—you're going to have to hit the drive-thru on the way to work (while simultaneously trying to button your shirt). No problem, we'll show you how to build a nutritious fast-food breakfast. For example, swing by Burger King. Order a Ham, Egg & Cheese Croissan'wich, pair it with some Apple Fries and fat-free milk, and your breakfast is complete. Even though you ate it while driving, you still got 455 calories, 28 grams of protein, and even a gram of fiber (tough to do at a fast-food joint).

Scenario #4

It doesn't matter how early you woke up, because your kids are screaming for you to take them to breakfast at Denny's/IHOP/Bob Evans. You name the restaurant, and we've armed you with the information you need to build a low-calorie, high-nutrition, high-flavor meal. For example, at Denny's, combining their Grilled Honey Ham with a side of oatmeal and a handful of grapes will give you 29 grams of protein and 8 grams of fiber for just 465 calories.

Four entirely different food situations, four entirely different meals—and one great weight-loss plan. You'll find the same assortment of strategies for lunch, for dinner, for snacks, and for dessert. Stress free or stressed out, on the road or safe at home, we've got you covered.

And you won't even have to eat microwaved copies of our pages!*

* Which would be silly. Everyone knows paperback books taste better lightly sautéed with grapeseed oil and paprika!

"When my wife saw me lose the weight, she knew she could do it too."

In his youth and early twenties, **James Cuartero** was thin and athletic, so he didn't worry much about what he put in his mouth day to day. He worked several jobs to support his growing musical career, and convenience was the driving factor in most of his food decisions. "I ate like I was still a kid—whatever, whenever," he says. "If I was sitting around the house bored, I'd think, 'Hey, I'll just get a pizza!'"

Meatloaf Moment.

Then one day, a videographer documenting one of James's concerts asked a kid at the show what he knew about the group. His response: "That's the band with some fat guy for a singer!" That fat guy was James, and when he saw the clip, his jaw hit the floor. He'd never thought of himself as overweight, but with the insult still fresh, he decided to do something about it. He picked up *Eat This, Not That! Restaurant Survival Guide* and *Eat This, Not That! Supermarket Survival Guide* and began replacing his junk calories with more nutritious foods. "I realized how many empty calories I used to take in every day."

James was happy to discover that losing weight isn't about self-denial, so he didn't have to give up things like ice cream and cheese. What's more, he learned that not all "healthy" foods are as good as they sound. "I figured all salads were good for me," he says. "But with *Eat This, Not That!* I learned that often you'd be better off with a burger—that sometimes the salad's twice as bad!"

> "I learned that often you'd be better off with a burger—that sometimes the salad's twice as bad!"

BEFORE:
185 pounds

NOW:
135 pounds

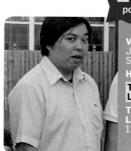

VITALS:
James Cuartero, 37
Sicklerville, NJ

HEIGHT: 5'6"

TOTAL WEIGHT LOST: 50 lbs

TIME IT TOOK TO LOSE THE WEIGHT: 12 months

Rock Solid.

Soon, James was able to get back into slim-fitting clothes. "The results were so quick—within 2 weeks I was losing 2 or 3 pounds a week," he says. Inspired by his success, his wife decided to join him in eating the *Eat This, Not That!* way. "When she saw me, she knew she could do it too," says James. "*Eat This, Not That!* completely changed my life. I have tons more energy. Eating well and exercise are just normal now."

When James's friends come to him for nutrition advice, his message is simple: Pay attention to your food. "It's not a struggle at all. It's actually easy."

CHAPTER 2

Four Ways The No-Diet Diet Will Change Your Life— Starting Today!

NO DIET!

There's never been a weight-loss plan like

The Eat This, Not That! No-Diet Diet

Simply put, there's never been a plan that allowed you to lose weight while eating fast food. Or one that allowed you to lose weight while eating at your favorite family restaurants, or ordering your favorite take-out, or reheating your favorite frozen dinners, or mixing up your favorite packaged treats, or cooking delicious dishes that taste just like restaurant foods.

And there really, really, really hasn't been a plan that would allow you to do any and all of these things, whenever you feel like it.

The secret of *The Eat This, Not That! No-Diet Diet* is to help you create perfectly nutritious meals and snacks —and even desserts!—simply by making a few smart substitutions and by ordering, purchasing, or, if you feel like it, cooking the right foods in the right combinations.

The goal of this plan is to help you create a "balanced diet"—a term that sounds musty and clichéd, but one that's a critical component of any sensible, long-term weight-loss strategy. The balanced mix of protein, carbohydrates, fats, fiber, and other nutrients found in every *Eat This, Not That! No-Diet Diet* meal will help you fight fat in three unique ways:

✱ It will end overeating.

When you overload your system with a giant calorie rush, it causes your body to store flab. Our plan will give you a consistent intake of calories—plenty of food—spread throughout the day, so you never overeat.

✱ It will stop sugar crashes.

Overdosing on simple carbohydrates leads to sugar rushes and crashes that mess with your blood glucose level. When your blood glucose level gets out of whack, it causes your body to store flab.

✱ It will prevent you from feeling hungry.

And believe it or not, feeling hungry is a sure sign that your body is storing flab!

Just look at all you stand to gain from this program—the easiest (no diet!) diet plan ever!

You'll Eat More Than Ever—And Never Feel Hungry Again

To understand why eating more is the key to losing weight, think of these two diet-related terms: "calories" and "nutrients." You sorta know what they are, right? Calories are the units of energy stored in food, and they are either burned off by your body or turned into body tissue—usually fat.

Nutrients are all the good things inside the food—vitamins and minerals, protein and fiber, fats and complex carbohydrates—that your body uses to build muscle, fight disease, and keep the general works humming along.

Now, imagine that calories are money: You're looking to spend around 2,000 or so a day. You might spend a little less if you're a petite woman (or looking to become one), maybe a little more if you're a husky guy (or looking to become one). But on average, that's about where you're going to be. You have a dietary allowance of 2,000 calories a day. (By the way, you can earn more caloric income by exercising—think of it as working overtime. You'll read more about that in Chapter 9.)

Now, imagine that nutrients are the things you buy with your calories —the flashy car, the nice home, the designer duds, the cool electronics. It's a simple economic exchange: When you go to the mall or the car dealership, your goal is to buy as much cool, useful stuff for as little money as possible. Your goal in the super-market or restaurant is just the same: You want to buy more nutrients for fewer calories.

Problem is, most of what's out there in the food world is overpriced junk. Can of soda? It'll cost you 150 calories—that's 7.5 percent of your daily calorie allowance! And what did you buy for that 7.5 percent?

Absolutely nothing: There are no nutrients whatsoever in a can of soda. (That's why people who drink a can of soda a day are nearly 30 percent more likely to be obese; people who drink two cans are 47 percent more likely!)

And that, in the end, is the reason we're all suffering from so much weight gain. Just as you don't want to have to spend valuable cash on junk you don't need, neither do you want to spend valuable calories on junk that's just going to sit around your waistline, giving you nothing in return for your hard-earned calories. And we waste a lot of our calories on junk. Indeed, a study in the *Journal of Food Composition and Analysis* determined that nearly one-third of the calories we consume are pure junk, coming from sweets, soft drinks, and salty snacks. And there's no nutrition in there: no protein, no fiber, no vitamins or minerals. It's like you spent 30 percent of your monthly income on broken TVs, cars without engines, and clothes that are too small to wear.

Well, *The Eat This, Not That! No-Diet Diet* is like a bargain hunter's guide to buying more nutrients for fewer calories. It's not about eating less, it's about getting more out of the food you do eat. Protein, fiber, vitamins and minerals, even healthy fats all play a role in helping us stay slim. So that's where you want to spend your hard-earned calories. It's about being a savvy food insider who knows how

The Eat This, Not That! No-Diet Diet Checklist

If you can answer yes to these four questions, then your meal, snack, or dessert earns the highly coveted approval stamp of The Eat This, Not That! No-Diet Diet.

Breakfast
- [ ] Am I eating within the first hour of waking, so I prime my metabolism for the day?
- [ ] Can at least half the foods in this meal be described as sources of protein?
- [ ] If there's bread, a muffin, or cereal, is it made from whole grains?
- [ ] Does this meal make up about a quarter of my day's calories? (That's 450 for a 1,800-calorie diet.)

Lunch
- [ ] Am I eating this meal within 2 hours of my last snack?
- [ ] Can I identify at least one source of protein and one source of fiber?
- [ ] Can I point to the produce in this meal?
- [ ] Is this meal slightly smaller than the meal I had for breakfast?

Dinner
- [ ] Am I eating this meal at least 2 hours before I go to sleep?
- [ ] Can I identify at least one source of protein and one source of fiber?
- [ ] Can I point to the produce in this meal?
- [ ] Is this the smallest of my three main meals of the day?

Snacks
- [ ] Does this snack break up one of the two long stretches between proper meals?
- [ ] Does this snack provide nutrients that I've missed in the other meals I've eaten— and plan to eat—today?
- [ ] Can I identify a source of protein, fiber, or both?
- [ ] Am I limiting my snack to a snack-size portion of about 150 to 200 calories?

Dessert
- [ ] Have I met my nutritional goals for the day, so I can afford the indulgence?
- [ ] Am I eating this dessert within 2 hours of dinner to blunt the potential blood sugar spike?
- [ ] Can I point to at least one nutritionally beneficial ingredient, such as fruit, nuts, or dairy?
- [ ] Is this dessert portion about the same size as a snack?

to get the plasma TV for a low price—and can weasel him- or herself a free Blu-ray in the deal.

You'll Lose Belly Fat—And Build Muscle!

You've heard the term "yo-yo dieting" before, but you probably don't know why such a phenomenon happens. It's pretty simple, really, and it starts with our bodies' survival instinct. When ancient man had trouble finding food, his body needed to be able to weather the hard times by using its store of body mass to keep its vital organs functioning. And guess what kind of tissue a hungry body burns first?

Muscle.

FIRE UP YOUR METABOLISM

Metabolism is the rate at which your body burns its way through calories just to keep you alive—to keep your heart beating, your lungs breathing, your blood pumping, and your mind fantasizing about the Caribbean while crunching accounting figures. Your body is burning calories all the time, even while you're reading this sentence. The average woman burns about 10 calories per pound of body weight every day; the average man, 11 per pound. But that number can vary wildly, and the key to managing your weight over the long haul is to maximize that calorie burn in every way possible.

To that end, you can use the three main types of calorie burn that happen throughout your day. Understand how they work, and you'll understand exactly why simply changing the way you think about the food you eat and how much you move each day will help turn your body into a fat-burning machine.

CALORIE BURN #1: THE THERMIC EFFECT OF EATING

Roughly 10 percent of the calories you burn each day get burned by the act of digesting your food. But not all foods are created equal: Your body uses more calories to digest protein (20 to 35 calories burned for every 100 calories consumed) than it does to digest fats and carbohydrates (5 to 15 calories burned for every 100 calories consumed). That's why adding lean, healthy protein to each meal and snack will help you burn more calories. Even better, protein can dull hunger and protect against obesity, diabetes, and heart disease.

Here's why: Muscle burns up a lot of calories—about 5 calories a day, per pound, just to maintain itself. Fat, on the other hand, burns only 2. So if your body is in starvation mode and needs to burn something to keep going, what tissue will it burn first? Right: muscle tissue, because it costs more for your body to maintain it than fat. Sure, when you restrict calories you'll lose fat, but you'll lose muscle too. And with it, you'll lose muscle's fat-burning power.

And that's exactly what happens when we follow a traditional diet plan. Once we stop "dieting," we go back to the same way of eating, but this time without that valuable calorie burn we get from muscle, so we gain everything—and more—back. That's why

CALORIE BURN #2: EXERCISE AND MOVEMENT

Lifting weights in the gym, running to catch the bus, twiddling your thumbs during a meeting, and winking at attractive attendees across a crowded room all fall into this category. It's a common misconception that fit people burn off the majority of their calories at the gym. Even superhero athletes like Tom Brady and Serena Williams only smoke about 10 to 15 percent of their calories by moving their muscles while exercising. That doesn't mean that exercise isn't important, however—it's just not important in the way you think. What exercise really does is to help with Burn #3.

CALORIE BURN #3: BASAL METABOLISM

This one's the biggie. Your basal, or resting, metabolism refers to the calories you burn when you're doing nothing at all. Sleeping, watching TV, sitting through yet another mind-numbing presentation on corporate profit-and-loss statements—you're burning calories all the while. In fact, between 60 and 80 percent of your daily calories are burned up just doing nothing. That's because your body is constantly in motion: Your heart is beating, your lungs are breathing, and your cells are dividing, all the time, even when you are asleep.

Now, those people who seem to keep weight off effortlessly? They do it not by focusing on the 10 to 15 percent of calories burned in the gym, but by maximizing the 60 to 80 percent of calories burned by their resting metabolisms. That's why the food choices we outline for you in this book are designed to maximize the number of calories you burn while eating and digesting, and to help boost your resting metabolism as well. So, focus less on the calories you're burning during those 30 minutes at the gym and concentrate on the calories you're burning the other 23½ hours a day.

we created our no-diet diet—because going on a diet is a sure way to boost fat and lose muscle.

Well, not on our watch! By keeping you eating plenty of food, we'll help you shed pure fat and retain lean muscle—which means that you'll then shed even more fat!

You'll Have More Energy, Better Health, and a Better Outlook on Life

Vitamins, minerals, healthy fats, and other nutrients are key to keeping not only our bodies in balance, but our minds as well. But most of what's on offer both in restaurants and in the supermarkets is anything but "balanced." As you read in the introductory chapter, eating a typical fast-food meal is like eating soy, with a side of corn and soy, and washing it down with a big glass of corn. You're missing out on all the many nutrients that are so critical not only for fighting disease, but for balancing your emotional health as well.

Folate, for example, is a B vitamin that's found in green vegetables and beans, and it's crucial for proper brain and body functioning, according to Harvard researchers. Low levels of folate are linked to obesity, heart disease, depression, low energy level, and even memory loss. And that's just one example of the importance of a balanced diet: Vitamins A, C, D, E, and K have all been linked to a lower risk of obesity, as have minerals like calcium, magnesium, and selenium. When you're not eating them, you're inviting fat to build a condo complex in your belly.

Whether you cook at home, dine at restaurants, or simply nosh whatever came through your car window, we'll show you how to boost its nutritional content so you can keep obesity, depression, and health risks at bay.

You'll Cut the Cost of Eating Dramatically

How often do you get home at night, empty your pockets, and find much less in them than you expected to? One of the reasons money gets hoovered out of our pockets like lint from a sofa cushion is that we're always hungry, so we're constantly wringing those last quarters out of our coat pockets for the vending machine, or anteing up for supersized versions of our meals, or digging into our wallets to hit the drive-thru one more time before heading home.

By keeping you always full and satisfied, *The Eat This, Not That! No-Diet Diet* will stop your cravings in their tracks and make you more aware of what you're eating, and why. Sure, you'll still be eating a lot, but not eating on impulse—instead, you'll be constantly topping off your tank with filling, nutrition-rich foods that beat back hunger and fatigue.

"Eat This, Not That! *has affected my life dramatically. It's literally a second chance.*"

Every year, like so many other Americans, **Del Phillips** made a New Year's resolution to lose weight. But every year came and went and his weight continued to climb, until his health and mobility were in serious danger. At more than 450 pounds, Del couldn't even fit into an airplane seat, and his career started to suffer. "I work in real estate, and when you're showing a property, your appearance matters," he says.

New Curb Appeal.

Finally, after being disgusted by a photo of himself that a friend had posted on Facebook, he knew he needed to do something. He'd seen a copy of *Eat This, Not That!* lying around the office, and he decided to give it a shot. "I'd been on every single diet in the world," he says. "*Eat This, Not That!* is so easy—more a lifestyle change than a diet. I can eat just about anything." Del used the book, Web site, and iPhone app to help him make smart choices, and the initial gains came so quickly that his coworkers were incredulous. "Everyone wanted to hear what the miracle was," he says. So he told them the truth: He'd learned to eat better.

Smooth Takeoff.

Several months later, when Del went out to eat at a sit-down restaurant, he realized how much progress he'd made. "I couldn't remember the last time I wasn't too big for a booth at a restaurant," he says. "Suddenly I was the right size—because I was making the right decisions on the menus in those booths." Del started to feel like a normal person again, and this year he even flew to Disneyland. He fit not only in his plane seat, but also on the rides at the park. Before discovering *Eat This, Not That!* he had been seriously considering Lap-Band surgery. And now? He's decided to stick with what's working. "*Eat This, Not That!* has affected my life dramatically," he says. "It's literally a second chance. It's a new beginning."

BEFORE: 461 pounds

VITALS:
Del Phillips, 44
San Diego, CA
HEIGHT: 6'2"
TOTAL WEIGHT LOST: 152 lbs
TIME IT TOOK TO LOSE THE WEIGHT: 11 months

NOW: 309 pounds

"Everyone wanted to hear what the miracle was."

Know Thy Enemies

FOOD IS YOUR FIRST LINE OF DEFENSE IN THE BATTLE AGAINST THREE OF THE MOST SERIOUS HEALTH PROBLEMS AFFECTING AMERICANS TODAY.

When it comes to protecting your health and well-being, the most powerfulperson in the world is—you. But to wield that power in the battle for well-being, you need to understand your top health threats—and the incredible tools at hand to defeat them.

You might think that, when it comes to your health, certain things are writ in stone: Men in your family have their first heart attack before age 60, for example. Or diabetes is an epidemic on your mom's side. Or you'll somehow follow the exact same pattern of decline as your grandparents. But family history and genetic disposition are not the same as destiny. The power to shape your health future is in your hands, and the tools you'll use are simple: They're food.

Eating a smart, balanced diet—one with the right kinds of fats, carbs and protein; plenty of fiber, vitamins, and minerals; and fewer unhealthy additives like sugar, trans fats, and sodium—can change the course of your life as effectively as a magic lamp or a bite from a radioactive spider. In this Special Report, we're going to explain the causes of the Big Three health threats—the man killers whose risks can be diminished or even avoided altogether by making smart tweaks to your daily diet.

You see, heart disease, stroke, and diabetes combined kill one in three Americans. And these three diseases, these Titans of Terrible, are very closely related—diabetes is a top cause of heart attacks, for example, and heart attacks are very similar in nature to strokes. In fact, they're so closely related that some doctors say all three should be lumped into one single health issue called metabolic syndrome.

Sounds ominous at first—it's as if Freddy Krueger, Predator, and that creepy Jason guy in the hockey mask had all joined forces to form some sort of Injustice League, and we're powerless to stop them. But as any good field general knows, if all three of your enemies are in the same room, just one smart bomb can wipe them right out. And that smart bomb? It's your diet. The eating plan outlined in *The Eat This, Not That! No-Diet Diet* will dramatically reduce your risk of all three Titans of Terrible, while also giving you a lean, flat belly (which, by the way, is like a badge of immunity against metabolic syndrome).

Consider, for example, what an enormous life-changing difference a handful of almonds could make: When researchers at Loma Linda University tracked the eating habits of 34,000 Seventh-Day Adventists—a population famous for its longevity—they discovered that those who ate nuts 5 days a week tended to outlive by 3 years those who didn't eat nuts. (Three years of life! That's 1,095 additional days of stalking your exes on Facebook!) Scientists believe the monounsaturated fat and fiber in the nuts make the difference by improving heart health and keeping weight in check. What's more, Harvard researchers found that men who replaced 127 calories of carbohydrates—that's about 14 Baked

CHAPTER 2

Lay's potato chips—with 1 ounce of nuts decreased their risk of heart disease by 30 percent.

And that's just the tiniest of tweaks! Imagine what more you could achieve if you actually put a little effort into it! That's what *The Eat This, Not That! No-Diet Diet* can help you achieve.

Of course, when it comes to battling serious health risks like heart disease, diabetes, and stroke, diet is only part of the equation. Having a good working partnership with a top-notch family physician is another crucial component. Going for regular checkups at least once a year, and more often if your doctor suggests it, is the very first step in taking control of your health. So before we begin this special report on nutrition-related health risks and explain how following *The Eat This, Not That! No-Diet Diet* can dramatically reduce your chances of developing these three man killers, we'd like to pause and take a moment to address the health-care professionals in the audience whose job it is to watch over our well-being.

Dear Health-Care Professionals:

What the hell?
Seriously, why do you have to make coming to your office suck so bad? We know, we know: Being a doctor isn't an easy job—lots of training, lots of bureaucracy, lots of paperwork. It's tough, we get it. But jeez, no wonder 30 percent of American women—and up to 50 percent of American men—skip their annual checkups. Ever read Dante's Inferno? That's what the average waiting room is like, except that in Hell, nobody's waiting to stick a finger up your bum. (That only happens in alien abductions.)

So, some suggestions: First off, ditch the gowns. Why can't we have a nice, comfy robe instead? And how about some updated magazines in the waiting room for a change? It's like a time capsule from the Clinton Library in there. And the decor: There are colors in the world other than gray and beige, you know. And if you want to make a nervous patient more comfortable, how about piping in a little Coltrane, or even acoustic Nirvana? Because when you're waiting to hear whether the mysterious mole on your groin is benign or malignant, the Muzak version of "Superfreak" is just not going to cut it.

Thanks for listening,
Dave and Matt

P.S.: And would it kill you to warm up the stethoscope a little? Yeesh!

Okay, with that out of the way, we've put together a quick overview of three of the main health threats to American adults, threats that can be reduced and in some cases even reversed, with proper diet and nutrition, and by working in close cooperation with your doctor. After all, you can't conquer an enemy until you understand it. So, to that end . . .

What The Heck Is...
High Blood Pressure?

When most people think of blood pressure, they think in terms of a garden hose: Too much pressure and the hose bursts, unless you open the valve. But that model is too simplistic. Instead, think of your circulatory system as more like the Erie Canal—a series of gates that help move blood around to where it's needed.

You need a certain amount of blood pressure, because without it, gravity would do the same thing to your blood that it does to the rain: pull it toward the earth. So imagine yourself hopping out of bed tomorrow morning and standing up. Gravity wants to take all that blood that's distributed throughout your body and pull it down into your feet. You, on the other hand, would like that blood to be pumped to your brain, where it can help you figure out where the hell your keys are.

On cue, arteries in the lower body constrict while the heart dramatically increases output. The instant result: Blood pressure rises, and blood flows to the brain. Ahh, there they are—in the dog's water dish, right where you left them. It's really pretty amazing, when you think about it.

But no matter how ingenious your circulatory system is, it's also incredibly easy to throw it out of whack. Here are four ways you can crank up your blood pressure:

Pack on extra pounds. That means your heart has to pump harder to force blood into all that new fatty tissue, which means more stress on your heart and more stress on your arteries.

Nosh on high-sodium foods. When you do, your body has to retain water in order to dilute the excess sodium, increasing overall blood volume—and putting added stress on your arteries.

Eat too many fatty meals, especially meals containing trans fats. That boosts the cholesterol level in the blood, which results in fatty deposits, or plaque, forming in the walls of your arteries. Now your heart has to work harder to squeeze that blood through newly narrowed arteries.

Let the pressures of the day haunt you into the night. When you're under stress, your brain pumps out stress hormones that keep your body in a perpetual state of fight-or-flight anxiousness, also forcing your heart to pump harder. That again puts your heart and your arteries under duress.

When the pressure remains high for years on end, thin-walled vessels in the brain can burst under extreme pressure, killing brain cells in what's known as a hemorrhagic stroke. Or hypertension can cause plaque buildup in one of the brain's arteries, eventually cutting off bloodflow. (High blood pressure damages the smooth artery walls, creating anchor points for plaque to latch onto.) Kidney failure or a heart attack can also result from dangerous plaque accumulation.

Then there's the plain old wear and tear that high blood pressure causes

your ticker. Over time, the extra work brought on by high blood pressure causes the walls of the heart to stiffen and thicken. The heart becomes a less efficient pump, unable to push out as much blood as it takes in. Blood backs up, the heart gives out, and the coroner scribbles "congestive heart failure" on your death certificate.

Blood pressure numbers, decoded

Ideally, your blood pressure should be lower than 120/80 mmHg. The top number, called the systolic pressure,

Ways You Can Cut the Pressure

LOAD UP ON POTASSIUM	EAT MORE SEAFOOD	DE-STRESS YOUR DISTRESS	LIFT TO LIGHTEN YOUR LOAD	TURN YOUR NOOKIE UP A NOTCH
One of the most common contributors to elevated blood pressure is an imbalance of minerals in the body—too much sodium (salt) and not enough potassium. A study at Loyola University showed that cardiovascular disease increased by 50 percent for participants with a high sodium-to-potassium ratio in their blood. Potassium helps sweep excess sodium from the circulatory system, causing the blood vessels to dilate. Studies show that not getting at least 2,000 milligrams of potassium daily can set you up for high blood pressure.	Omega-3 fats in tuna and other fish as well as flaxseed help strengthen the heart muscle, lower blood pressure, prevent overclotting, and reduce the level of potentially deadly inflammation in the body. And favor fruits high in vitamin C, like oranges and pineapple: According to research from England, people with the most vitamin C in their bloodstreams are 40 percent less likely to die of heart disease.	It could be an after-dinner massage, an hour of quiet reading, or a little more sexual healing, but make sure to adopt a ritual of de-stressing before bedtime. It will not only help you sleep, but also help your arteries relax.	Researchers at the University of Michigan found that people who performed three total-body-weight workouts per week for 2 months decreased their diastolic pressure (the bottom number) by an average of 8 points—that's enough to lower your risk of stroke by 40 percent, and your risk of heart attack by 15 percent. And a Medical College of Georgia study found that, compared to those who had the least muscle, the blood pressure levels of the people with the most muscle returned to normal the fastest after a stressful situation.	Speaking of sexual healing, one study found that people who had sex regularly showed lower levels of stress hormones and more stable blood pressures when faced with a stressful situation like public speaking.

is the pressure generated when the heart beats. The bottom number is the diastolic pressure, the pressure in your blood vessels when the heart rests between beats. Higher readings are broken out into three categories.

PREHYPERTENSION: 120 to 139 systolic and 80 to 89 diastolic.

Prehypertensives should start worrying about their blood pressure, and focusing on diet and exercise tips like those found in this book. You may not see the flashing lights in your mirror right now, but your radar detector just went off. Time to slow down.

STAGE 1 HYPERTENSION: 140 to 159 systolic and 90 to 99 diastolic.

For people who fall in this range, drug therapy is usually recommended in addition to lifestyle changes. Their risk of heart attack or stroke is elevated, and they need to be under a doctor's care.

STAGE 2 HYPERTENSION: 160 or higher systolic and 100 or higher diastolic.

Advanced drug therapy is often a must for people at this level, who face a serious risk of being injured or killed by their condition. Cholesterol is a soft, gooey substance—sort of like earwax—that's one of the lipids (fats) in your bloodstream and in all of your body's cells.

By the Numbers

Overweight people are:

- **50 percent more likely to develop heart disease** (obese: up to 100 percent)
- **Up to 360 percent more likely to develop diabetes** (obese: up to 1,020 percent)
- **16 percent more likely to die of a first heart attack** (obese: 49 percent)
- **Roughly 50 percent more likely to have total cholesterol above 250** (obese: up to 122 percent)
- **14 percent less attractive to the opposite sex** (obese: 43 percent)
- **Likely to spend 37 percent more a year at the pharmacy** (obese: 105 percent)
- **Likely to stay 19 percent longer in the hospital** (obese: 49 percent)
- **20 percent more likely to have asthma** (obese: 50 percent)
- **Up to 31 percent more likely to die of any cause** (obese: 62 percent)
- **19 percent more likely to die in a car crash** (obese: 37 percent)
- **120 percent more likely to develop stomach cancer** (obese: 330 percent)
- **Up to 90 percent more likely to develop gallstones** (obese: up to 150 percent)
- **590 percent more likely to develop esophageal cancer** (obese: 1,520 percent)
- **35 percent more likely to develop kidney cancer** (obese: 70 percent)
- **14 percent more likely to have osteoarthritis** (obese: 34 percent)
- **70 percent more likely to develop high blood pressure** (obese: up to 170 percent)

What The Heck Is...
High Cholesterol?

For all the bad press it gets, the fact is that you need cholesterol, just as you need earwax. Your body uses cholesterol to form cell membranes, create hormones, and perform several other crucial maintenance operations. But a high level of cholesterol in the blood—hypercholesterolemia—is a major risk factor for coronary heart disease, which can lead to a heart attack.

You get cholesterol in two ways. The body—mainly the liver—produces varying amounts, usually about 1,000 milligrams a day. But when you consume foods that are high in certain fats—particularly trans fats—your body goes cholesterol crazy, pumping out more than you can use. (Some foods also contain cholesterol, especially egg yolks, meats, fish, and whole-milk dairy products. But cholesterol in food isn't really an issue; the majority of it, and the stuff you should focus on, is made by your body in reaction to certain fats.)

Some of the excess cholesterol in your bloodstream is removed from the body through the liver. But some of the excess winds up exactly where you don't want it—along the walls of your arteries, where it combines with other substances to form plaque. Plaque raises blood pressure by making your heart work harder to get blood through your suddenly narrower vessels, which can eventually wear out your ticker. Plaque can also break off one of its little perches and form a clot that can lead to a heart attack or stroke, which can cause paralysis, death, and other annoyances.

Cholesterol numbers, decoded

Inside your body, a war is raging right now between two factions of specialized sherpas called lipoproteins that move cholesterol around your insides according to their own specialized agendas. There are several kinds—good cholesterol, bad cholesterol, non-partisan cholesterol, stupid-but-well-meaning cholesterol, and hooker-with-a-heart-of-gold cholesterol. But the ones to focus on are the Jekyll and Hyde of health, HDL (high-density or "helpful" lipoprotein) and LDL (low-density or "lazy" lipoprotein) cholesterol.

The good guy: HDL cholesterol.
Nearly one-third of blood cholesterol is carried by helpful HDL. HDL wants to help you out by picking up cholesterol and getting it out of your bloodstream by carrying it back to the liver, where it's passed from the body. A high HDL level—above 60 milligrams per

deciliter (mg/dl)—seems to protect against heart attack. The opposite is also true: A low HDL level—less than 40 mg/dl—indicates a greater risk. A low HDL cholesterol level may also raise stroke risk.

The bad guy: LDL cholesterol.

Lazy LDL just wants to stick cholesterol in the most convenient place it can find, meaning your artery walls. LDL doesn't care that having too much cholesterol lining your arteries forms a buildup of plaque, a condition known as atherosclerosis. A high level of LDL cholesterol (160 mg/dl or above) reflects an increased risk of heart disease.

A lower level of LDL cholesterol indicates a lower risk of heart disease.

The other bad guy: Triglycerides.

These are a kind of fat in your blood that your body uses for energy. You need them, but when you have too much, you increase your risks of high blood pressure, diabetes, and stroke. A triglyceride check should be part of your regular cholesterol blood work. Ask for it if it isn't. A good triglyceride level is below 150 mg/dl. Triglycerides rise when you eat more calories than you burn off, drink a lot of alcohol, or consume trans fats, which are typically found in baked goods and chips.

Ways to Improve Your Stats

CRAM IN THE CRANBERRY	GAIN WITH GRAINS	BE A SPONGE	BURN 900	LAUGH A LOT
Researchers at the University of Scranton in Pennsylvania found that men who drank 3 cups of cranberry juice daily raised their HDL (the good kind) cholesterol levels by 10 percent, which in turn lowered their risk of heart disease by 40 percent. Plant compounds called polyphenols are believed to be responsible for the effect. (Note: Cranberry juice often comes diluted, so make sure the label says that it contains at least 27 percent cranberry juice.)	In a study at Tulane University, researchers found that people who ate 4 or more servings of foods like whole grains, nuts, and beans a week had a 22 percent lower risk of developing heart disease (and 75 percent fewer camping companions) than those who ate the foods once a week or less.	Loma Linda University researchers found that drinking 5 or more 8-ounce glasses of water a day could help lower the risk of heart disease by up to 60 percent—exactly the same drop you get from stopping smoking, lowering your LDL cholesterol number, exercising, or losing a little weight.	To raise HDL cholesterol, you need to burn at least 900 calories a week through exercise—roughly 120 minutes per week. Side benefit: According to the *Journal of the American College of Cardiology*, when researchers analyzed 24 studies of 145,000 people, they discovered that as the HDL cholesterol level increased, the cancer rate dropped significantly. The exact connection isn't clear, but one theory is that HDL cholesterol possesses powerful anti-inflammatory properties that may help tame tumors.	In one study reported by the American Physiological Society, researchers divided 20 patients with type 2 diabetes, high blood pressure, and high cholesterol into two groups: control and laughter. Both groups took standard medications for their illnesses, but the laughter group also watched 30 minutes of self-selected humorous content per day. At the end of the study, people in the laughter group had lower levels of stress hormones and inflammation markers plus higher HDL levels than people in the control group did.

What The Heck Is...
High Blood Sugar?

An elevated blood glucose level, or high blood sugar, has another, creepier name: diabetes. Twenty-four million Americans are living with diabetes, and up to 57 million may have prediabetes. It's a leading cause of heart disease, kidney disease, and stroke, and its other complications include blindness, amputation, sexual dysfunction, and nerve damage. Fortunately, type 2 diabetes is also highly preventable (and even reversible).

Diabetes works like this: Your digestive system turns food into glucose—the form of sugar your body uses for energy—and sends it into the bloodstream. When the glucose hits, your pancreas—a large gland located near your stomach—produces insulin, a hormone, and sends that into the bloodstream as well. Insulin is your body's air traffic controller: It takes command of all your glucose and directs it into your cells, where it can be used for energy to rebuild muscle, keep your heart pumping and your brain thinking, and do just about everything else your body does.

But our bodies aren't built to handle massive infusions of sugar—they didn't have Dunkin' Donuts on the African savanna half a million years ago. So when you overeat, particularly high-glycemic-index foods (foods that have a lot of sugar and very little fiber, like candy, sodas, and baked goods made with refined flour), your body gets flooded with massive amounts of glucose. Insulin goes crazy, screaming at your cells to process because too much sugar has hit your bloodstream all at once. Your body works overtime to clear the sugar away, in most cases storing it as fat around your midsection.

But over time, insulin starts to get treated like the boy who cried wolf. After years of insulin sounding the alarm, your cells—specifically, their insulin receptors—get burned out. "Yeah, yeah, again with the 'toxic levels of sugar'!" Your cells don't respond to insulin's pleas as readily, and sugar winds up spending more time in your bloodstream than it should. This is what's known as insulin resistance. After several years, the pancreas gets fed up with producing all that ineffective insulin and begins to produce less than you need. This is called type 2 diabetes. (Type 1 is caused by a defect in or damage to the pancreas.) Glucose builds up in the blood, overflows into the urine, and passes out of the body. Thus, the body loses its main source of fuel even though the blood contains large amounts of glucose.

When you have diabetes, two bad things can happen: First, you start to lose energy. You feel fatigue and unusual thirst, and you begin losing weight for no apparent reason; you get sick more often and injuries are slow to heal because your body loses its ability to maintain itself. Second, the sugar that is hanging around in your blood begins to damage the tiny vessels and nerves throughout your body, particularly in your extremities and vital organs. Blindness, impotence, numbness, and heart damage may ensue.

Blood sugar numbers, decoded

Monitoring your blood sugar from year to year might be the most important thing your doctor can do for you. He or she will likely perform two blood tests that check for type 2 diabetes. The fasting glucose test requires you to give blood in the morning, before you've had breakfast. It's often paired with the A1C test, which reveals your average blood glucose level over several months.

Score high on either one, and your doctor should order an oral glucose tolerance test. This one requires about 4 hours of your time and multiple donations of your blood, but it could save your eyesight, your toes, your sex life, and, well, just your life in general. You drink a sweetened beverage and then a blood sample is taken at intervals to measure how efficiently insulin is working within your body.

If you have not had a doctor test your blood glucose level in the last year, put this book down and dial up a physician, today. Seriously: A government report found that one in three of us will end up with diabetes, yet the disease is almost entirely preventable.

Ways to Cut the Sweet Stuff

GET MUSHY	CRUISE THE MEDITERRANEAN	STEAL FROM THE TEACHER	MAXIMIZE YOUR MUSCLES	MOVE MORE
Oatmeal is high in soluble fiber, which may decrease your risk of heart disease, some cancers, diverticulitis, and diabetes. Mix it up: Eat oatmeal with berries and nuts one day, and have eggs and meat another.	Eating a Mediterranean-style diet—that is, whole grains, fresh vegetables, and fish—slashes diabetes risk. A 2008 study of 13,380 people reported in the *British Medical Journal* showed that those who adhered closely to a Mediterranean diet had a 35 percent lower risk of diabetes than those who did not consistently follow that eating style.	Researchers at the National Public Health Institute in Finland studied the diets of 60,000 men and women over the course of a year and found that individuals who ate apples the most frequently were 12 percent less likely to die during the course of the study than were those who rarely bit into a McIntosh. They also cut their risk of diabetes by 27 percent.	In a 4-month study, Austrian scientists found that people with type 2 diabetes who started strength training significantly lowered their blood sugar levels, improving their condition. Lifting weights not only fights the fat that puts you at an increased risk for the disease, but also improves your sensitivity to insulin.	Research shows that the difference between normal-weight Americans and those considered to be overweight is a mere 100 calories a day. Some ways to burn off 100 calories today: Go for a brisk 23-minute walk, vacuum for 30 minutes, play Wii Tennis for 13 minutes, swim for 17 minutes, and drink 3 cups of green tea (which raises metabolism).

"My outlook on life improved instantly."

Marcus Thorpe is a former college football player and a lifelong fitness enthusiast, so he wasn't completely surprised when he started putting on weight. The problem wasn't his workout regimen, it was his eating habits, and things came to a head when Marcus took a job that required travel. "I was just grabbing things as quickly as I could. I didn't think about the fact that restaurants often avoid being forthright about nutritional information. I didn't know any better."

Pink-Slip Blues.

Then, in 2008, Marcus lost his job when his company downsized. Now he was jobless and overweight, and it was hard to decide which was making him unhappier. Marcus had always known how to maximize his body's potential through working out—he just didn't know how to feed it. He'd seen our "*Eat This, Not That!*" column in a friend's copy of *Men's Health*. He was intrigued, so he bought the book and put it to work. "With *Eat This, Not That!* I taught my body to adapt to less food. As a former athlete, I ate large portions out of habit—a footlong sub, or a footlong and a half. Now I'm satisfied with a 6-inch sub." Marcus now also enjoys fruits and vegetables every day, and he buys much of his food organic. "I learned to minimize the amount of unnecessary ingredients in the food I purchase," he says.

The Turnaround.

Marcus started losing weight, and instantly he started feeling better about his prospects. "My outlook on life improved despite everything I was going through personally," he says. He soon landed an interview for a job as a prosecutor outside of Atlanta. His personal success with his diet helped him nail the interview. "I came off more confident and better prepared than I would have otherwise," he says. With *Eat This, Not That!* he got the body, the job, and a new, smaller-size wardrobe. "I find that I enjoy shopping a lot more than I did before," he says. "And as I purchase new things, my fiancée and I are giving the old clothes to Goodwill."

BEFORE:
282
pounds

VITALS:
Marcus Thorpe, 31
Atlanta, GA

HEIGHT: 5'8"

TOTAL WEIGHT LOST: 105 lbs

TIME IT TOOK TO LOSE THE WEIGHT: 20 months

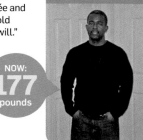

NOW:
177
pounds

"With *Eat This, Not That!* I learned to minimize the amount of unncesessary ingredients in the food I purchase."

"Eat This, Not That! *really does teach you how to eat.*"

Danielle Starn had been chubby as a kid, but when she hit her midtwenties, she eclipsed 200 pounds and became dangerously obese. "I was eating all the wrong things in all the wrong quantities," she said, and it was making her daily routine a struggle. "I would get home from work and want to go to sleep immediately. Who does that? I work in an office, so I really had no reason to be physically tired."

The Bikini Bulge.

Danielle made the decision to change her life when she was organizing her closet. She discovered a bikini she'd worn in high school, and she decided to try it on. "I looked at my back in the mirror— I was just shocked," she says. "There were rolls that could hold a pencil. It was depressing." Danielle was tired of being fat. Then she noticed *Eat This, Not That!* in a bookstore.

Danielle had tried Weight Watchers and other diets before, so it was a revelation to her that she didn't have to deprive herself to lose weight. "I swapped white bread for this great whole

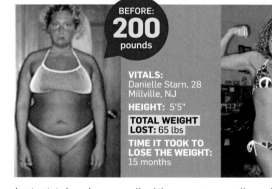

BEFORE:
200
pounds

VITALS:
Danielle Starn, 28
Millville, NJ
HEIGHT: 5'5"
TOTAL WEIGHT LOST: 65 lbs
TIME IT TOOK TO LOSE THE WEIGHT: 15 months

NOW:
135
pounds

wheat potato bread, which has fewer calories and tastes so much better," she says. "*Eat This, Not That!* taught me tons of tips like that." As the pounds started to melt away, even her ring size dropped, her feet grew thinner, and she could wear heels for the first time in years. "Something just clicked, and I

realized there were healthier options out there," says Danielle. "I feel so much better about myself and actually enjoy clothes shopping now."

Back to the Beach.

As the weight continued to peel off, Danielle noticed another change: She began looking forward to going out. "Before, if I went out, I would just feel down about all the pretty, 'in-shape' girls," she says. But as she

slimmed down, she gained more energy and shed her nervous fear of running into old friends from high school. And the successful conclusion of Danielle's journey recalled its beginning: She found herself at the beach in a new, better-fitting bikini and loving it. "*Eat This, Not That!* really does teach you how to eat," she says. She's kept the weight off for 2 years now, and she doesn't plan on gaining it back.

"I feel so much better about myself and actually enjoy clothes shopping now."

WHEN DOCTORS SAY...
"Your blood pressure's a little high."

THEY REALLY MEAN...
"You're at increased risk for heart disease and stroke, as well as sexual dysfunction."

THE EAT THIS, NOT THAT! DOCTOR DECODER

Use this guide to help you interpret some of the things you might hear a doctor say (often with a little bit of a "tsk, tsk" in his or her voice). Then adjust your diet accordingly.

When it comes to food advice, most doctors are pretty good at telling you what to cut down on. Eat less fat. Eat less salt. Eat less sugar. Etcetera, etcetera. But most doctors aren't experts in nutrition—ask a doctor what brand of peanut butter to buy and you might as well be asking Charlie Sheen for relationship advice. They've got no clue! (The answer, by the way, is "all-natural, full-fat, no sugar added.") So we're stepping in to fill the void. The next time your doctor raises a concern about the way your health statistics are trending and starts telling you what not to eat, use this handy cheat sheet to figure out what you should be eating.

So, Eat This!

BANANAS,
SWEET POTATOES,
SPINACH,
RAISINS,
PAPAYAS,
LIMA BEANS,
TOMATOES,
and trendy
COCONUT WATER
for potassium

MILK,
CHEESE,
YOGURT,
and other
DAIRY PRODUCTS

BROCCOLI,
and calcium-fortified
ORANGE JUICE
for calcium

TUNA,
SALMON,
MACKEREL,
SARDINES,
and other
FATTY FISH; and
FLAXSEEDS,
HEMP SEEDS,
PUMPKIN SEEDS, and
WALNUTS for omega-3
fatty acids

HERBS and
SPICES to put a
little salt-free kick
in your food

Not That!

Salty snacks like
CHIPS,
FRIES, and
PRETZELS

CURED SANDWICH
MEATS and
PIZZA-TOPPING
MEATS like
HAM,
HOT DOGS,
SAUSAGE, and
PEPPERONI

CANNED SOUPS

WHITE BREAD

AMERICAN
CHEESE and other
PROCESSED
CHEESES.

All of these foods are among our greatest dietary sources of sodium, according to the Grocery Manufacturers Association.

WHEN DOCTORS SAY...

"I'm worried about your cholesterol."

THEY REALLY MEAN...

"You're at increased risk for heart disease and stroke, as well as sexual dysfunction."

So, Eat This!

OATMEAL,
BROWN RICE,
QUINOA,
WHOLE GRAIN
BREADS,
RYE BREAD,
WHOLE GRAIN
CEREALS, and other
HIGH-FIBER
GRAINS

BEAN,
LENTIL, and
PEA SOUPS, and
anything else
that's chock-full of
one of these three
legumes, which also
provide cholesterol-
lowering fiber

ALL FRUITS and
VEGETABLES

UNSALTED NUTS and
ALL-NATURAL
PEANUT BUTTER
(no ingredients other
than peanuts and salt);
both contain fiber and
heart-healthy mono-
unsaturated fats

CRANBERRY JUICE
(at least 27 percent
cranberry) and at
least five 8-ounce
GLASSES OF WATER
per day

GUACAMOLE
containing real
avocado (make it at
home if you can),
OLIVE OIL, and
CANOLA OIL;
all contain mono-
unsaturated fats

GRASS-FED BEEF and
GAME MEATS, which
contain high levels of
CLA, a cholesterol-
lowering fatty acid

LOW-FAT DAIRY
FOODS

PLANT-BASED
SPREADS (like Benecol)
for breads, etc.

Not That!

COMMERCIAL BAKED
GOODS that contain
hydrogenated or
partially hydrogenated
oils (also known as
trans fats)

MARGARINES

ANYTHING MADE
WITH "SHORTENING"

Restaurant fried
foods like
FRENCH FRIES,
CHICKEN WINGS,
etc.; these foods
are typically fried in
trans fats

ANYTHING FROM
A FAST-FOOD CHAIN
THAT STILL
USES PRIMARILY
TRANS FATS
(we're talking to you,
Long John Silver's!)

WHEN DOCTORS SAY...

"You have elevated blood sugar."

THEY REALLY MEAN...

"You're at risk for diabetes, which can lead to heart disease, blindness, loss of limbs, and too many other horrible things to name."

So, Eat This!

OATMEAL,
BROWN RICE,
QUINOA,
WHOLE GRAIN
BREADS,
RYE BREAD,
WHOLE GRAIN
CEREALS, and other
HIGH-FIBER GRAINS;
fiber is digested
slowly, stabilizing
blood sugar

BEAN,
LENTIL, and
PEA SOUPS, and
anything else
that's chock-full of
one of these three
legumes, which also
provide fiber

ALL FRUITS and
VEGETABLES,
especially
APPLES, which are
high in fiber and have
been linked to lower
diabetes risk

UNSALTED NUTS and
ALL-NATURAL
PEANUT BUTTER
(no ingredients other
than peanuts and salt);
they contain fiber

TUNA,
SALMON,
MACKEREL,
SARDINES, and other
FATTY FISH; and
FLAXSEEDS,
HEMP SEEDS,
PUMPKIN SEEDS, and
WALNUTS for omega-3
fatty acids

DARK CHOCOLATE
(at least 70 percent
cacao), in small
quantities

PROTEIN-RICH
MEATS LIKE
LEAN BEEF and
CHICKEN

Not That!

Refined carbo-
hydrates such as
WHITE BREAD,
WHITE RICE, and
SUGARY CEREALS

Baked goods like
PIES,
COOKIES,
BROWNIES,
DOUGHNUTS, and
CAKES

MILK CHOCOLATE,
WHITE
CHOCOLATE, and
SUGARY CANDIES

SODAS,
SWEETENED
ICED TEAS,
ENERGY DRINKS,
and other
LIQUIDS THAT
CONTAIN SUGAR
(all rush glucose into
your bloodstream
and lead to insulin
problems)

FRUIT JUICES
and other fruit
products like sauces
that have all the sugar
and none of the fiber
of whole fruit

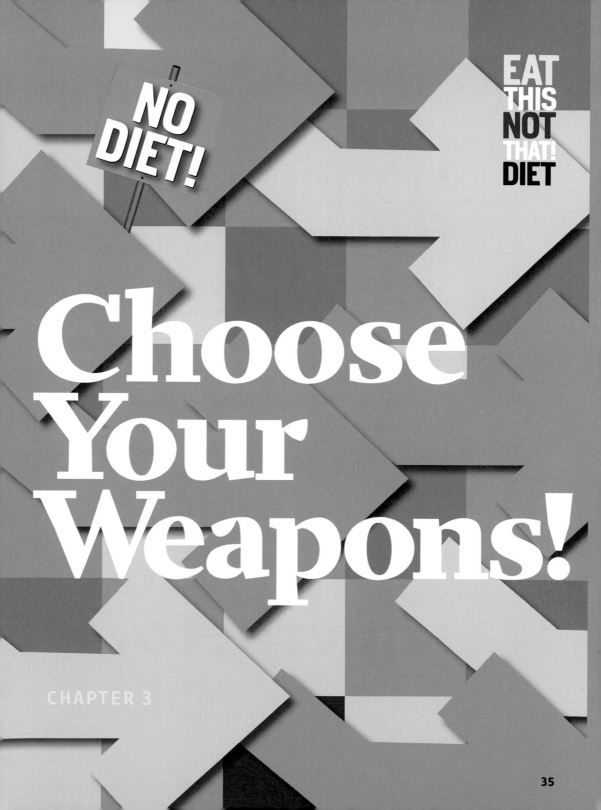

NO DIET!

Choose Your Weapons!

CHAPTER 3

Armed with the secrets contained in this book, you are well on your way to becoming a nutritional superhero,

one who can turn a drive-thru into a weight-loss spa and a pizza delivery into a bonafide fat-burning tactic.

But even a superhero needs a hand: Batman had his utility belt, the Green Hornet had his souped-up luxury car, even Spider-Man needed little packets of super glue hidden up his sleeve. So, too, will you need secret weapons to battle the Green Goblins of grease and the Catwomen of corpulence.

Those secret weapons are outlined in this chapter. Whenever you're faced with a nutritionally questionable meal or in need of an emergency snack, one of these simple concoctions can be **a)** whipped out of your pocket or purse, or **b)** whipped together in 3 minutes or less. They'll stabilize your blood sugar, quench your hunger, and provide vital nutrients that will keep your body burning fat all day and all night. With this chapter tucked into your utility belt, you'll never have to worry about looking like the Penguin.

TRAIL MIX MATRIX

You may be among the vast number of Americans who approach a bowl of nuts with some degree of trepidation.

Nuts are full of fat, after all, and the prevailing wisdom tells us to eat less fat. But remember when prevailing wisdom told us to take out big mortgages on beach homes, because real estate values could only go up? Yeah, turns out prevailing wisdom isn't all it's cracked up to be, and in the case of nuts, it couldn't be further off base.

So here's the truth about the fat found in almonds, walnuts, pecans, and other nuts: It's as healthy—or healthier—than anything else in your diet. It fills your belly better than any other snack on the planet while decreasing your risks of cardiovascular disease and diabetes, smoothing your skin, pumping you full of antioxidants, and helping you stay thin. In fact, a study from Georgia Southern University found that eating a high-protein, high-fat snack like nuts can increase your calorie burn for more than 3 hours. Think about that. It means that next time you go to the theater, if you replace your Mike and Ikes with macadamia nuts and your Whoppers with walnuts, you'll increase your calorie burn for the full duration of the movie. And that's true even if you're sitting through one of Cameron Crowe's 180-minute marathon movies.

To that end, we've provided the blueprint for incorporating nuts into your diet—along with seeds and flavor enhancers that boost their nutritional impact and make the less-palatable nuts easy to handle. A quarter cup of trail mix makes a perfect snack on its own, but it's also ideal for adding protein, fiber, and nutritional bang to any meal. Make it in big batches and scoop it into a sandwich bag before you head out for the day. Then you'll be prepared to fight hunger whenever it strikes.

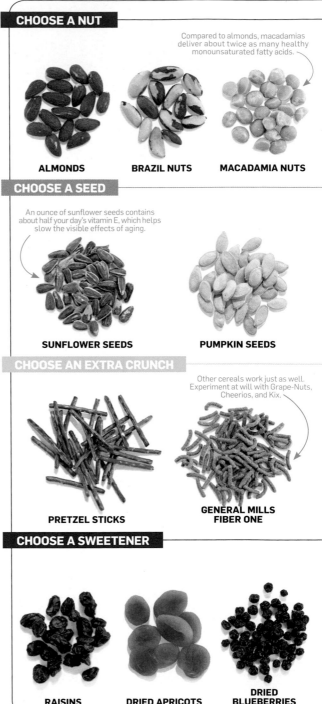

CHOOSE A NUT

Compared to almonds, macadamias deliver about twice as many healthy monounsaturated fatty acids.

ALMONDS   BRAZIL NUTS   MACADAMIA NUTS

CHOOSE A SEED

An ounce of sunflower seeds contains about half your day's vitamin E, which helps slow the visible effects of aging.

SUNFLOWER SEEDS   PUMPKIN SEEDS

CHOOSE AN EXTRA CRUNCH

Other cereals work just as well. Experiment at will with Grape-Nuts, Cheerios, and Kix.

PRETZEL STICKS   GENERAL MILLS FIBER ONE

CHOOSE A SWEETENER

RAISINS   DRIED APRICOTS   DRIED BLUEBERRIES

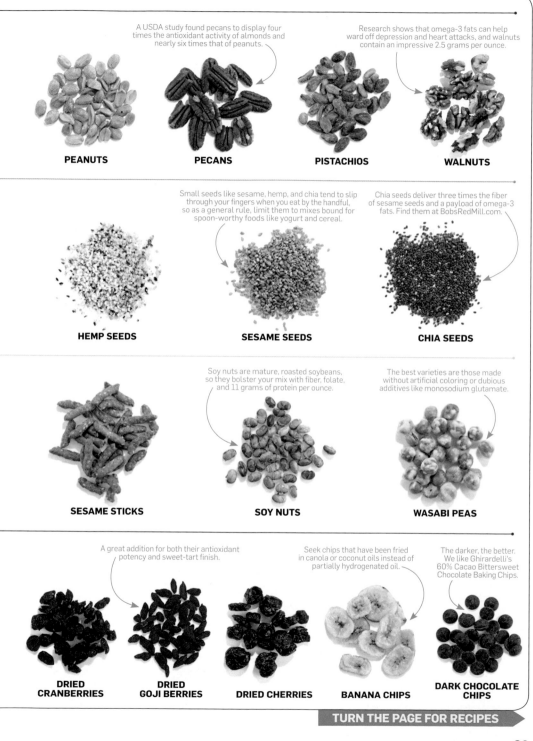

A USDA study found pecans to display four times the antioxidant activity of almonds and nearly six times that of peanuts.

Research shows that omega-3 fats can help ward off depression and heart attacks, and walnuts contain an impressive 2.5 grams per ounce.

PEANUTS

PECANS

PISTACHIOS

WALNUTS

Small seeds like sesame, hemp, and chia tend to slip through your fingers when you eat by the handful, so as a general rule, limit them to mixes bound for spoon-worthy foods like yogurt and cereal.

Chia seeds deliver three times the fiber of sesame seeds and a payload of omega-3 fats. Find them at BobsRedMill.com.

HEMP SEEDS

SESAME SEEDS

CHIA SEEDS

Soy nuts are mature, roasted soybeans, so they bolster your mix with fiber, folate, and 11 grams of protein per ounce.

The best varieties are those made without artificial coloring or dubious additives like monosodium glutamate.

SESAME STICKS

SOY NUTS

WASABI PEAS

A great addition for both their antioxidant potency and sweet-tart finish.

Seek chips that have been fried in canola or coconut oils instead of partially hydrogenated oil.

The darker, the better. We like Ghirardelli's 60% Cacao Bittersweet Chocolate Baking Chips.

DRIED CRANBERRIES

DRIED GOJI BERRIES

DRIED CHERRIES

BANANA CHIPS

DARK CHOCOLATE CHIPS

TURN THE PAGE FOR RECIPES

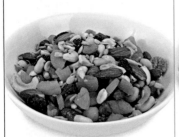

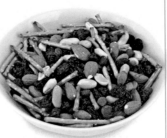

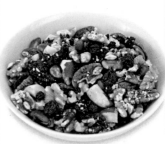

THE ULTIMATE *ETNT* TRAIL MIX*

2 cups mixed nuts
1 cup raisins
1 cup chopped dried apricots or other dried fruit
½ cup sunflower seeds

The bigger variety of nuts and fruits you include, the more expansive your nutritional arsenal will be. Mix these ingredients together in a large bowl and store in an airtight container.

155 calories
10 g fat (1 g saturated)
5 mg sodium
16 g carbohydrates
4 g protein
2.5 g fiber

All recipes make 18 servings, ¼ cup each.

THE TRAIL BLAZER

1½ cups raisins
1 cup almonds
1 cup pretzel sticks
½ cup peanuts
½ cup dark chocolate chips

The relatively high ratio of fast-digesting carbs makes this the ideal mix to eat before a big hike, jog, or workout. The added bonus is that the salt from the pretzels will help replace the sodium you lose to sweat.

150 calories
7 g fat (1 g saturated)
105 mg sodium
21 g carbohydrates
4 g protein
2 g fiber

THE BRAIN BOOSTER

1 cup pecans
1 cup chopped Brazil nuts
1 cup walnuts
1 cup dried blueberries
½ cup dried cherries
½ cup hemp or chia seeds (optional)

Every component of this mix champions at least one nutrient necessary for cognitive power. The collective impact is a head-healthy mix of fats, minerals, and antioxidants.

170 calories
15 g fat (2 g saturated)
0 mg sodium
7 g carbohydrates
4 g protein
2 g fiber

Spice Roasted Nuts

Toasting nuts awakens and deepens their natural flavors, plus it allows you to customize them with your own spices. Try these four recipes for a tastier trail mix and set them out in bowls when you have guests.

YOU'LL NEED

For Chili Almonds:
1 cup whole unpeeled almonds
⅛ tsp chili powder
⅛ tsp cayenne
Salt
Black pepper

For Curried Cashews:
1 cup unsalted cashews
1 tsp curry powder

For Five-Spice Peanuts:
1 cup salted peanuts
½ tsp Chinese five-spice powder

For Cocoa Pecans:
1 cup pecan halves
½ Tbsp cocoa powder
¼ tsp ground cinnamon
2 Tbsp sugar

HOW TO MAKE IT

Preheat the oven to 400°F. Heat 1 tablespoon of butter and the appropriate spices in a small saucepan. Stir in the nuts, then spread them on a baking sheet. Roast for 10 to 12 minutes, until very fragrant and warm, but not overly toasted.

The Ultimate Fruit Salad Matrix

The goal in making fruit salad should be to construct as colorful a creation as possible. Sure, it makes for a better-looking, more flavorful salad, but more importantly, using the full palette of nature's colors means you're taking advantage of a diversity of nutrients. That's because each color in the food rainbow represents a unique set of vitamins and antioxidants. A bowl of chopped watermelon may lend you a welcome dose of lycopene, but mix in cantaloupe, kiwifruit, and a handful of blueberries and you have a low-calorie snack with the potential to stave off cancer, reduce inflammation, increase circulation, bolster bone strength, sharpen cognitive function, and improve overall vision. In short, Mother Nature's multivitamin.

To maximize deliciousness, start by cutting all the fruits into similar-size pieces. A pinch of salt will heighten the flavors all the way around, and a generous squeeze of lime adds a welcome blast of tartness (plus the citric acid helps preserve the colors of the fruit). If you want to get real fancy, a handful of chopped fresh mint may just land your bowl in the fruit salad hall of fame.

Nutritional Average
(per ½ cup)
40 calories
0 g fat
0 mg sodium
10 g carbohydrates
0.5 g protein
2 g fiber

RED

WATERMELON, PERSIMMONS, GUAVA, PINK GRAPEFRUIT

Most rosy hues in the fruit and vegetable kingdom are the result of an important antioxidant called lycopene, a red-colored carotenoid associated with a long list of health benefits. Among the most notable are lycopene's role in protecting the skin from sun damage and decreasing the risks of heart disease and certain forms of cancer. Lycopene-rich foods have also been shown to decrease symptoms of wheezing, asthma, and shortness of breath in people when they exercise.

BLUE

BLUEBERRIES, BLACKBERRIES, PLUMS, GRAPES

Blue and purple foods get their colors from the presence of a unique set of flavonoids called anthocyanins. Flavonoids in general are known to improve cardiovascular health and prevent short-term memory loss, but the deeply pigmented anthocyanins go even further. Researchers at Tufts University have found that blueberries may make brain cells respond better to incoming messages and might even spur the growth of new nerve cells, providing a new meaning to "smart eating."

GREEN

GRAPES, KIWIS, HONEYDEW MELON, GRANNY SMITH APPLES

Not just potent vitamin vessels capable of strengthening bones, muscles, and brains, green foods are also among the most abundant sources of lutein and zeaxanthin, an antioxidant tag team that, among other things, promotes healthy vision. Green fruits and vegetables get their color from chlorophyll, which studies show plays an important role in stimulating the growth of new tissue and hindering the growth of bacteria. As a topical treatment, it can speed healing time by 25 percent.

YELLOW/ORANGE

CANTALOUPE, PINEAPPLE, PEACHES, APRICOTS, ORANGES, BANANAS

Orange- and yellow-colored foods are loaded with beta-carotene, the now-famous nutrient that contributes to immune health, improves communication between cells, and helps fight off cell-damaging free radicals. But beta-carotene has a lesser known, yet equally powerful, cousin called alpha-carotene. A recently published study found that those with the most alpha-carotene in their diets were 40 percent less likely to die from any cause during the 14-year study period.

THE SALAD MATRIX

In recent years, food marketers have seized upon a secret weapon, a magical word that, when uttered, makes any food seem healthy. Ham, cheese, bacon, and oily bread? Healthy, once you call it this. Fried chicken, ranch, and tortilla strips? Also healthy, once this special label is applied. Candied nuts, chunks of cheese, and mayonnaise? Healthy! It has to be, because we said the magic word.

That magic word? "Salad."

Say the word "salad" and you tend to imagine a bowl of greens with slivers of carrots and peppers and other healthy stuff nestled among the leaves. But that's not quite accurate. In reality, the word "salad" means nothing more than a collection of foods mixed together and usually served cold with dressing. You put heaps of fat, sugar, and salt together, add some liquefied blue cheese, and you've got a salad—a salad that's much cheaper, and hence more profitable, than one requiring really healthy greens and vegetables. That's why many restaurant salads can carry as much as 1,500 calories and more grease than an auto-body shop.

And that sucks, because by co-opting our salads, restaurateurs have robbed us of one of the easiest, healthiest ways of roping extra produce into our diets—and that's essential to the fight against flab. When researchers from the University of Florida tracked people's diets, they found that those who were the thinnest also ate the most produce, regardless of the number of overall calories consumed!

It's time to take back the salad. Use this matrix to build your own at home, and if you're out on the town and what you see on the menu doesn't look like something you could build from this list, don't be afraid to ask the kitchen to customize one for you.

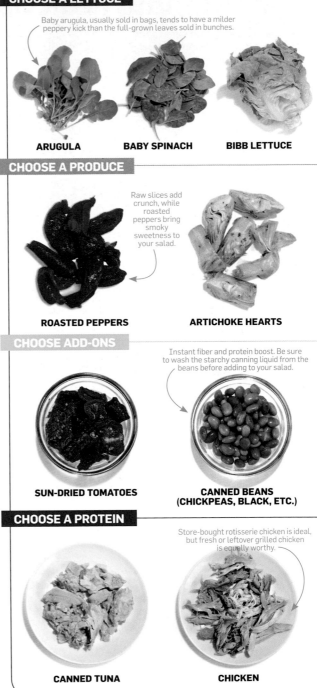

CHOOSE A LETTUCE

Baby arugula, usually sold in bags, tends to have a milder peppery kick than the full-grown leaves sold in bunches.

ARUGULA   BABY SPINACH   BIBB LETTUCE

CHOOSE A PRODUCE

Raw slices add crunch, while roasted peppers bring smoky sweetness to your salad.

ROASTED PEPPERS   ARTICHOKE HEARTS

CHOOSE ADD-ONS

Instant fiber and protein boost. Be sure to wash the starchy canning liquid from the beans before adding to your salad.

SUN-DRIED TOMATOES   CANNED BEANS (CHICKPEAS, BLACK, ETC.)

CHOOSE A PROTEIN

Store-bought rotisserie chicken is ideal, but fresh or leftover grilled chicken is equally worthy.

CANNED TUNA   CHICKEN

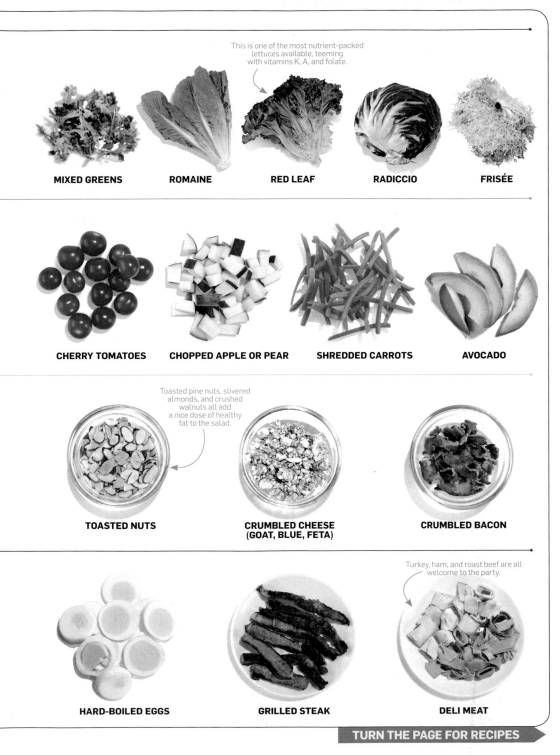

This is one of the most nutrient-packed lettuces available, teeming with vitamins K, A, and folate.

MIXED GREENS

ROMAINE

RED LEAF

RADICCIO

FRISÉE

CHERRY TOMATOES

CHOPPED APPLE OR PEAR

SHREDDED CARROTS

AVOCADO

Toasted pine nuts, slivered almonds, and crushed walnuts all add a nice dose of healthy fat to the salad.

TOASTED NUTS

**CRUMBLED CHEESE
(GOAT, BLUE, FETA)**

CRUMBLED BACON

Turkey, ham, and roast beef are all welcome to the party.

HARD-BOILED EGGS

GRILLED STEAK

DELI MEAT

TURN THE PAGE FOR RECIPES

4 SUPER SALADS

Each recipe makes 4 servings

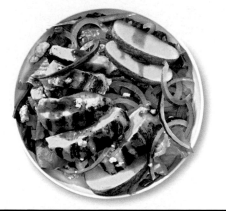

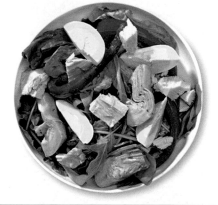

APPLE-BLUE

8 oz Bibb lettuce	8 oz cooked chicken
1 red onion, sliced	½ cup yogurt
1 apple, sliced	dressing
¼ cup blue cheese	

The sweet crunch of apple and the salty velvet of blue cheese form a yin and yang of flavor harmony.

210 calories / 6 g fat (3 g saturated)
180 mg sodium / 18 g carbohydrates
21 g protein / 3 g fiber

MEDITERRANEAN

8 oz arugula	¼ chopped olives
1 can tuna, drained	1 cup roasted
2 hard-boiled eggs,	peppers
quartered	½ cup balsamic
1 cup artichoke	vinaigrette

Several studies have linked Mediterranean diets to longer lifespans. Credit the antioxidant-rich foods in this bowl.

350 calories / 27 g fat (3.5 g saturated)
460 mg sodium / 8 g carbohydrates
19 g protein / 2 g fiber

Rules of the Salad

RULE #1:

KEEP IT CLEAN.
Lettuce needs to be thoroughly washed and dried; any water that remains on the leaves will prevent the dressing from adhering to the salad. Invest in a salad spinner today.

RULE #2:

MATCH YOUR TOPPINGS TO YOUR LETTUCE.
Sturdier leaves like iceberg and romaine are fit to hold bulkier ingredients and thicker dressings, while delicate lettuces like arugula and baby spinach tend to be best suited for vinaigrettes and lighter toppings.

RULE #3:

THINK BALANCE.
For a salad to be filling, it needs protein (chicken, eggs, deli meat) and fiber (beans, avocado). To maximize flavor, pair sweet (tomatoes, apples) with sharp (onions, olives) and savory (meat, cheese). Round it out with crunch from nuts or raw vegetables.

RULE #4:

DRESS FOR SUCCESS.
Bottled dressings are fine in a pinch, but nothing could be simpler (or better) than the

Ultimate Dijon Vinaigrette:
1 clove garlic, minced
¼ cup red wine or balsamic vinegar
½ Tbsp Dijon mustard
⅓ cup olive oil
Salt and black pepper

Combine garlic, vinegar, and Dijon. Drizzle in olive oil, whisking constantly. Season with salt and pepper.

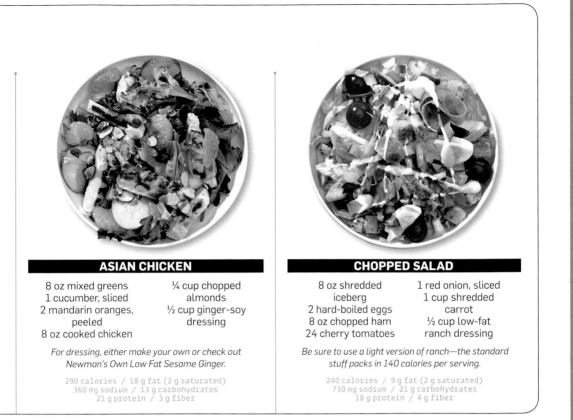

ASIAN CHICKEN

8 oz mixed greens
1 cucumber, sliced
2 mandarin oranges,
    peeled
8 oz cooked chicken

¼ cup chopped
    almonds
½ cup ginger-soy
    dressing

*For dressing, either make your own or check out
Newman's Own Low Fat Sesame Ginger.*

290 calories / 18 g fat (2 g saturated)
360 mg sodium / 13 g carbohydrates
21 g protein / 3 g fiber

CHOPPED SALAD

8 oz shredded
    iceberg
2 hard-boiled eggs
8 oz chopped ham
24 cherry tomatoes

1 red onion, sliced
1 cup shredded
    carrot
½ cup low-fat
    ranch dressing

*Be sure to use a light version of ranch—the standard
stuff packs in 140 calories per serving.*

240 calories / 9 g fat (2 g saturated)
730 mg sodium / 21 g carbohydrates
18 g protein / 4 g fiber

ETNT SIMPLE SIDE SALAD

Each lettuce pairs a signature texture and flavor with a unique package of nutrients, so the key to maximizing flavor and nutrition is to bring in as many different leaves as possible. Whatever combination you end up with, be sure your greens are dry; otherwise you'll end up with soupy salad. (A $15 salad spinner may be the best kitchen investment out there.)

8 oz (about 16 cups) leafy greens
½ cup roasted red peppers
1 cup shredded carrots
2 hard-boiled eggs, peeled and diced
1 apple or pear, peeled and thinly sliced
ETNT Ultimate Dijon Vinaigrette (see opposite page)

Combine the lettuce (and any other ingredients from the list) with the vinaigrette, adding the dressing a few tablespoons at a time and tossing thoroughly with tongs. Stop when you have a light layer of vinaigrette clinging to the leaves. Store any leftover dressing, covered, in the refrigerator for up to 1 week.

Makes 4 servings

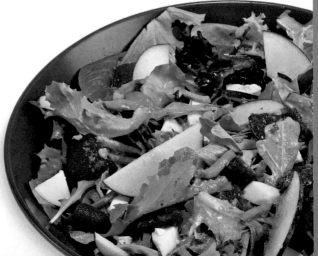

THE ULTIMATE DELI SALAD MATRIX

The importance of protein simply cannot be overstated, and intrinsically we've always known it. Think how we've labored through history to keep it on our plates. Before supermarkets and steakhouses popped up on every street in America, we earned protein by spearing it, hooking it, shooting it, trapping it, or otherwise arranging for its untimely demise. Then we dragged it back to our caves, igloos, teepees, or whatever we called home, and we grilled it up.

Today, however, we don't necessarily have time to stalk an elk across the plains. Nor do we have time to defrost a pork loin and roast it for hours. We need easy-to-make, easy-to-eat protein sources for our on-the-go lives.

Now, a lesser diet book might have you wolfing down palate-punishing fitness bars constructed from soy protein isolate and enrobed in chalky imitation chocolate. But where's the joy in that? The best way to get quick, flavorful, muscle-building protein—without all the junk—is to whip up a salad, one you can dip into for lunchtime again and again.

The problem with traditional recipes—chunks of tuna struggling to swim in a goopy sea of mayonnaise, for instance—is that they don't necessarily do our bodies any favors. To find the right ratio—one that will melt fat rather than pack it on—ditch the local deli and take to the comforts of your own kitchen. Simply pick your protein and binder, mix in a few base ingredients and flavor enhancers, and tinker with the seasoning as you go. Make a big batch on Sunday and divvy it out for lunches and snacks throughout the week.

CHOOSE A PROTEIN

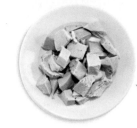

Leftover grilled or roasted chicken works great, as does a whole rotisserie chicken from the supermarket (sans skin).

CHICKEN

CHOOSE A BASE

DICED ONION

CHOPPED CELERY

CHOOSE A BINDER

More flavor and healthy fat for half the calories. What's not to love?

OLIVE OIL–BASED MAYONNAISE

CHOOSE A FLAVOR ENHANCER

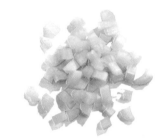

Mix a teaspoon with mayonnaise or yogurt for binder bliss.

Leafy herbs like parsley, dill, cilantro, and basil bring a hit of freshness to the mix.

CURRY POWDER

FRESH HERBS

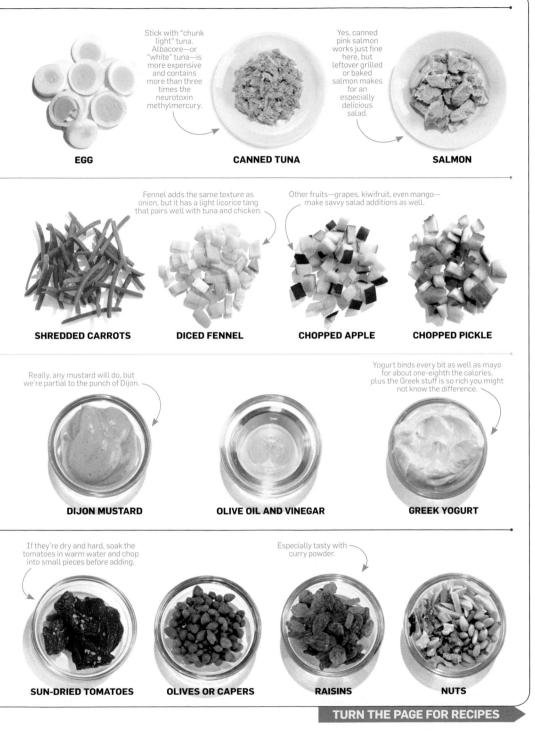

Stick with "chunk light" tuna. Albacore—or "white" tuna—is more expensive and contains more than three times the neurotoxin methylmercury.

Yes, canned pink salmon works just fine here, but leftover grilled or baked salmon makes for an especially delicious salad.

EGG

CANNED TUNA

SALMON

Fennel adds the same texture as onion, but it has a light licorice tang that pairs well with tuna and chicken.

Other fruits—grapes, kiwifruit, even mango—make savvy salad additions as well.

SHREDDED CARROTS

DICED FENNEL

CHOPPED APPLE

CHOPPED PICKLE

Really, any mustard will do, but we're partial to the punch of Dijon.

Yogurt binds every bit as well as mayo for about one-eighth the calories, plus the Greek stuff is so rich you might not know the difference.

DIJON MUSTARD

OLIVE OIL AND VINEGAR

GREEK YOGURT

If they're dry and hard, soak the tomatoes in warm water and chop into small pieces before adding.

Especially tasty with curry powder.

SUN-DRIED TOMATOES

OLIVES OR CAPERS

RAISINS

NUTS

TURN THE PAGE FOR RECIPES

47

STANDOUT SALADS

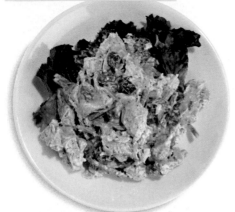

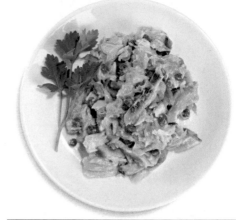

CURRIED CHICKEN*

4 cups chicken	¼ cup golden raisins
1 small diced onion	½ cup mayo
1 cup shredded carrot	1 tsp curry powder

Curry powder is perhaps the most under-utilized seasoning in your spice rack. Try this salad and you'll agree.

160 calories / 8 g fat (1 g saturated)
160 mg sodium / 10 g carbohydrates
11 g protein / 1 g fiber

RIVIERA SALMON

4 cups flaked salmon	1 Tbsp Dijon mustard
¼ cup olive oil	2 Tbsp capers
	Fresh parsley or dill

Scoop it over a halved English muffin for a healthy spin on a bagel with lox and cream cheese.

197 calories / 16 g fat (3.5 g saturated)
410 mg sodium / 1 g carbohydrates
11 g protein / 0 g fiber

* Each recipe makes 4 servings

Protein: The Only Weight-Loss Drug You Need

Why all the fuss about protein? Because it burns fat on two levels.

IT STOKES YOUR METABOLIC FURNACE

On average, about 10 percent of the calories you burn every day are smoked simply in the process of digestion, but that average climbs when you eat more protein. Here's why: For every 100 calories of protein you consume, 20 to 35 percent is burned off in digestion. By comparison, fat and carbs only burn between 5 and 15 percent of their caloric load. That means more calories get vaporized before they make a move on your body.

So it makes sense that when Arizona State University researchers compared a high-protein diet with a high-carbohydrate diet, they found that people who ate high-protein diets burned more than twice as many calories in the hours after their meals.

IT BUILDS MUSCLE

And that, in turn, burns calories. See, every pound of muscle on your body burns about 6 calories every 24 hours. Every pound of fat? Only about a third of that. And the best way to build and maintain muscle is to emphasize protein.

Here's the proof: Danish researchers put 65 subjects on a 12 percent protein diet, a 25 percent protein diet, or no diet. The low-protein dieters lost an average of more than 11 pounds, but the high-protein subjects lost an average of 20 pounds. And more amazingly, they lost twice as much abdominal fat. (Some studies suggest that a high-protein diet helps your body control its level of cortisol, a stress hormone that causes fat to converge on the abdominal region.)

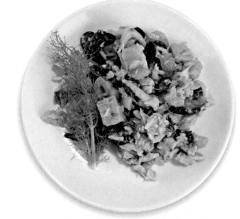

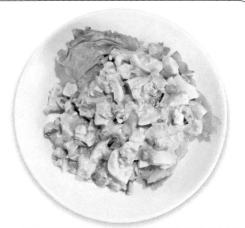

TUSCAN TUNA

2 cans tuna
½ cup diced fennel
½ cup diced celery
¼ cup chopped
olives

2 Tbsp sun-dried
tomatoes
2 Tbsp olive oil
Juice of one lemon

Add-ins like fennel and sun-dried tomato allow you to scale back the fat impact without diminishing flavor.

210 calories / 16 g fat (2 g saturated)
150 mg sodium / 2 g carbohydrates
15 g protein / 1 g fiber

FIERY EGG SALAD

8 hard-boiled eggs
1 small onion
½ cup chopped
pickle
6 Tbsp mayonnaise

Sriracha,
canned chipotle
peppers, or
favorite hot sauce
to taste

In terms of both flavor and fat, this egg salad is far superior to the week-old sludge at your local deli.

200 calories / 15 g fat (3.5 g saturated)
290 mg sodium / 2 g carbohydrates
13 g protein / 0 g fiber

Rules of the Salad

RULE #1:

DON'T DROWN.
You want just enough binder to lightly coat your ingredients and help bring them together. If you can't distinguish the individual ingredients in the salad, you've gone way too far.

RULE #2:

SEASON TO TASTE.
The difference between a good salad and a great one comes down to salt and pepper. Add each pinch by pinch, tasting as you go. A good rule of thumb is a pinch of salt and a half pinch of pepper for every cup of protein.

RULE #3:

TINKER WITH TEXTURES.
Like a regular leafy salad, protein-based salads benefit from crunch. Toasted nuts, celery, and apple are all excellent ways to bring interesting textures to the mix.

RULE #4:

FIND THE PERFECT SIDEKICK.
Don't undo the good you've done in constructing a superlative salad by setting it adrift in a massive bread boat. Instead, try piling it onto a toasted whole wheat English muffin, tossing it with a bowl of mixed baby greens, or scooping it up with Triscuits.

THE ULTIMATE SMOOTHIE SELECTOR

It's so easy it's almost science fiction: Complete human nutrition with just the push of a button. The smoothie is so efficient at delivering a human need that Philip K. Dick could have thought it up: Roll out of bed, toss fruit in a blender, hit "Liquefy." Boom! Your perfect meal is served.

Making smoothies can be a pretty freewheeling endeavor, which is certainly part of the fun, but we've established a few basic rules. Follow these and the ingredient-by-ingredient guide that follows and you'll be ready for liquid liftoff.

Perfectly Simple Supplement

1 part ground flaxseed
1 part whey protein powder

Simple? Sure, but that's the point—it's a nutritional work-horse that will take you 2 seconds to prepare. No nutrient jolts your metabolism to life quicker than protein, and the flaxseed delivers a mother lode of the famously healthy omega-3 fatty acids. Mix a big batch and store it in an airtight container in the cupboard. It's great for smoothies, but it also blends well into dozens of foods like oatmeal, cereal, yogurt, and shakes.

40 calories, 1.5 g fat
(0 g saturated), 5 mg sodium,
1 g carbohydrates,
6 g protein, 1 g fiber

per tablespoon

CHOOSE 2 OR MORE FRUITS

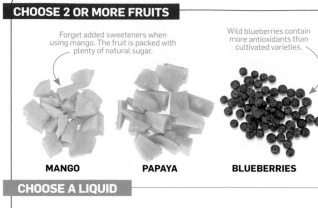

Forget added sweeteners when using mango. The fruit is packed with plenty of natural sugar.

Wild blueberries contain more antioxidants than cultivated varieties.

MANGO   **PAPAYA**   **BLUEBERRIES**

CHOOSE A LIQUID

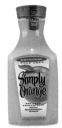

ORANGE JUICE   **POMEGRANATE JUICE**

CHOOSE THICKENERS & ENHANCERS

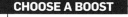

Peanut butter is nutritionally stacked, but it's also extremely dense with calories. Limit yourself to about ½ tablespoon per smoothie to keep it in the lean zone.

PEANUT BUTTER

CHOOSE A BOOST

Often sold under the name of psyllium husk (for the seeds this powder is ground from), fiber keeps you fuller longer and creates a more stable ride for your blood sugar.

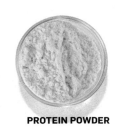
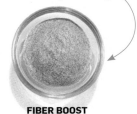

PROTEIN POWDER   **FIBER BOOST**

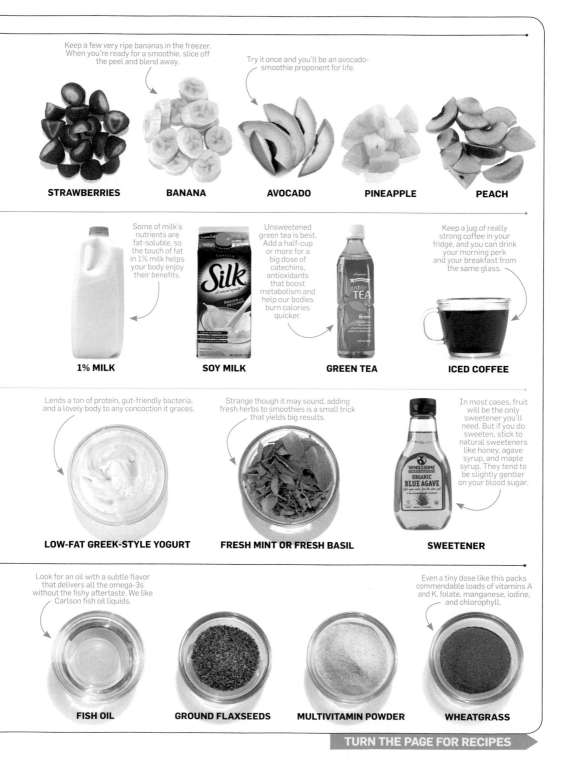

Keep a few very ripe bananas in the freezer. When you're ready for a smoothie, slice off the peel and blend away.

Try it once and you'll be an avocado-smoothie proponent for life.

STRAWBERRIES

BANANA

AVOCADO

PINEAPPLE

PEACH

Some of milk's nutrients are fat-soluble, so the touch of fat in 1% milk helps your body enjoy their benefits.

Unsweetened green tea is best. Add a half-cup or more for a big dose of catechins, antioxidants that boost metabolism and help our bodies burn calories quicker.

Keep a jug of really strong coffee in your fridge, and you can drink your morning perk and your breakfast from the same glass.

1% MILK

SOY MILK

GREEN TEA

ICED COFFEE

Lends a ton of protein, gut-friendly bacteria, and a lovely body to any concoction it graces.

Strange though it may sound, adding fresh herbs to smoothies is a small trick that yields big results.

In most cases, fruit will be the only sweetener you'll need. But if you do sweeten, stick to natural sweeteners like honey, agave syrup, and maple syrup. They tend to be slightly gentler on your blood sugar.

LOW-FAT GREEK-STYLE YOGURT

FRESH MINT OR FRESH BASIL

SWEETENER

Look for an oil with a subtle flavor that delivers all the omega-3s without the fishy aftertaste. We like Carlson fish oil liquids.

Even a tiny dose like this packs commendable loads of vitamins A and K, folate, manganese, iodine, and chlorophyll.

FISH OIL

GROUND FLAXSEEDS

MULTIVITAMIN POWDER

WHEATGRASS

TURN THE PAGE FOR RECIPES

SUPER SMOOTHIES

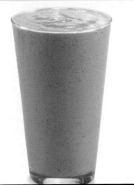

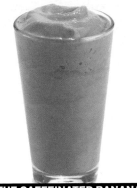

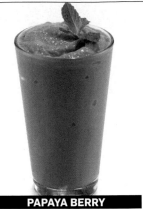

ETNT POWER SMOOTHIE

1 banana
½ cup milk
½ cup Greek-style yogurt
¼ cup orange juice
½ Tbsp peanut butter
1 Tbsp fiber powder
2 Tbsp *ETNT* Perfectly Simple
Supplement

*Place all the ingredients in
a blender and puree.*

350 calories
12 g fat (5 g saturated)
195 mg sodium
49 g carbohydrates
30 g sugars
16 g protein
7.5 g fiber

THE CAFFEINATED BANANA

1 very ripe banana
½ cup strong coffee
½ cup milk
1 Tbsp peanut butter
1 Tbsp agave syrup
1 cup ice

*With protein, healthy fat, and
caffeine, this works perfectly as
a start to your day or as a low-cal
substitute for a milk shake.*

311 calories
10 g fat (2.5 g saturated)
135 mg sodium
52 g carbohydrates
38 g sugars
10 g protein
4 g fiber

PAPAYA BERRY

¾ cup frozen papaya
¾ cup frozen strawberries
½ cup milk
½ cup orange juice
1Tbsp chopped fresh mint

*This is like a liquid multivitamin,
loaded with vitamins A and C,
plus disease-fighting carotenoids
and lycopene.*

188 calories
2 g fat (1 g saturated)
60 mg sodium
40 g carbohydrates
28 g sugars
6 g protein
5 g fiber

Rules of the Smoothie

RULE #1:

NO ICE CREAM.
A smoothie's still a
smoothie even after
you pour in juice, milk,
coffee, or tea. But if
you start scooping in
ice cream, call it what
it is—a milk shake—
and save it for dessert.

RULE #2:

**USE A STRONG
BLENDER.**
A weak blender won't
be able to crush the ice
quickly enough, which
means it melts and
ultimately dilutes your
precious creation
rather than giving it
that bracing, velvety
texture you want.

RULE #3:

RESPECT THE RATIO.
Once you learn the
basic proportion of
liquids to solids, you
can turn anything into
a pretty drinkable
smoothie. For every
3 cups of fruit, you'll
need about 1 cup of
liquid. Keep in mind
that both yogurt
and ice will thicken
your drink.

RULE #4:

**LOOK TO THE
FREEZER.**
Frozen fruits are
every bit as nutritious
as their fresh counter-
parts, and they
allow you to make
smoothies using less
ice. That makes for
more intense, purer
flavors in your blend.

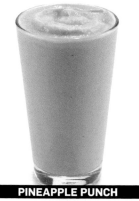

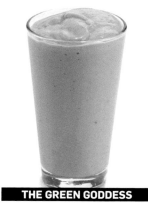

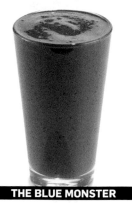

PINEAPPLE PUNCH

1 cup frozen pineapple
½ cup Greek-style yogurt
½ cup milk
½ cup orange juice

*Like a tropical island in a glass.
In fact, a shot of rum would turn this
into one heck of a healthy cocktail.*

250 calories
2 g fat (1 g saturated)
144 mg sodium
48 g carbohydrates
37 g sugars
12.5 g protein
3 g fiber

THE GREEN GODDESS

¼ avocado, peeled and pitted
1 ripe banana
1 Tbsp honey
½ cup milk
1 scoop protein powder
½ cup ice
1 tsp freshly grated ginger
(optional)

*In this untraditional but tasty
creation, fiber and protein combine
forces to vanquish any hunger.*

350 calories
12 g fat (2.5 g saturated)
180 mg sodium
59 g carbohydrates
32 g sugars
17 g protein
6 g fiber

THE BLUE MONSTER

1 cup blueberries
½ cup pomegranate or blueberry
juice
½ cup yogurt
3 or 4 cubes of ice
1 Tbsp ground flaxseed

*Between the polyphenols in the blue-
berries and the pomegranate juice
and the omega-3s in the flaxseeds,
we're talking serious brain food.*

258 calories
4 g fat (0.5 g saturated)
105 mg sodium
47 g carbohydrates
38 g sugars
10 g protein
5.5 g fiber

Should you splurge on organic fruit?

Know which produce is hardest hit by pesticides

The Environmental Working Group recently released its list of the pesticide levels of common fruits, ranked from 1 (lowest pesticide load) to 100 (highest load). The rankings, based on nearly 43,000 tests for pesticides conducted by the USDA, are surprising. Next time you're trying to decide if those organic peaches are worth the extra dollar a pound, consider these stats:

YES
(splurge on organic fruit)

PEACHES, 100
Peaches have the highest pesticide load of any fruit or vegetable.

APPLES, 89
Apples are the second most pesticide-ridden.

STRAWBERRIES, 82
We think organic strawberries taste better anyway.

PEARS, 65
One of the top 10 dirtiest fruits.

GRAPES, 43
Better to play it safe when buying grapes.

ORANGES, 42
42 is borderline; go organic when you can.

Environmental Working Group score based on pesticide load

NO
(don't need to buy organic)

BLUEBERRIES, 24
A 24 means conventional blueberries are relatively safe.

BANANAS, 16
Made the list of top 10 cleanest fruits.

PINEAPPLES, 7
Pineapples are the fourth cleanest.

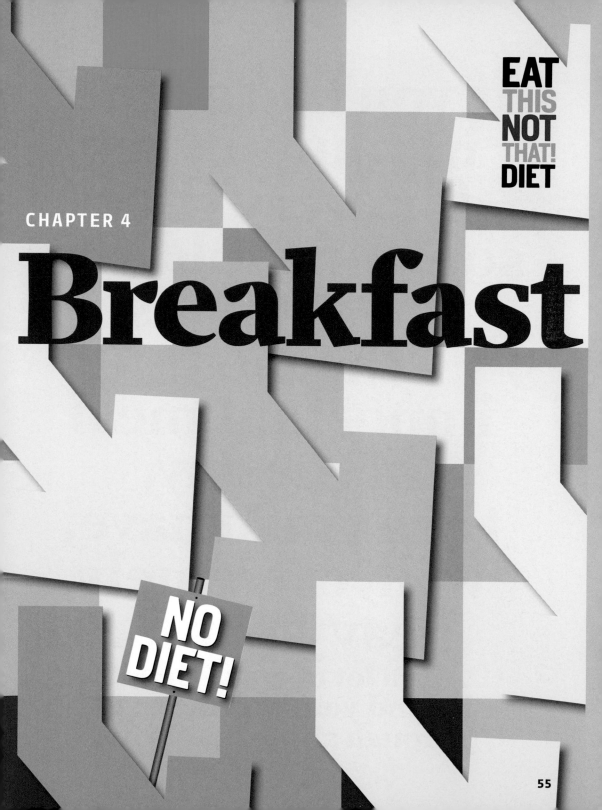

CHAPTER 4

Breakfast

NO DIET!

If you had a dime in your pocket for every time someone told you breakfast is the most important meal of the day, then you'd have, well, extremely heavy pants.

And a lot of angry people behind you, waiting to go through airport security.

But like most clichés, the one about eating breakfast is pretty right on. Studies have shown that regularly skipping breakfast increases your risk of obesity by 450 percent. And breakfast is the one meal where, calories be damned, eating more is almost always better than eating less—in an ideal world, an average American would eat between 400 and 600 calories every morning, and even someone on a low-calorie diet would devour no less than 400 calories to start the morning. (To put that in context, an Egg McMuffin has only 300 calories, so a healthy breakfast means eating more than you think!) In a 2008 study, researchers at Virginia Commonwealth University found that people who regularly ate a protein-rich, 600-calorie breakfast lost significantly more weight in 8 months than those who consumed only 300 calories and a quarter of the protein. The big-breakfast eaters lost an average of 40 pounds and had an easier time sticking with the diet, even though both groups were permitted about the same number of total daily calories.

But it's not just the number of calories. Like any good country-club snob, you want to usher in only "the right kind" of calories. So how do you know if the breakfast you're eating measures up? Don't tell the ACLU, but we've done some "nutritional profiling." Here's what the "right kind" of breakfast should look like.

→ **It's got protein.** Lots of it. Protein requires a lot of energy to digest, so eating protein first thing in the morning makes your body start burning calories fast and furiously. Look for no less than 20 grams of protein for each breakfast, and more if you can get it.

→ **It's got dairy.** Have a glass of milk, a bite of cheese. It's not only a way to reach your protein quotient, but also a source of calcium, which lowers blood pressure and heart disease risk. A study at Harvard Medical School found that people who ate three servings of low-fat dairy foods daily were 60 percent less likely to be overweight than people who consumed less.

→ **It's packed with fiber.** The more fiber your breakfast has, the longer it will take you to digest it. That means you'll have long, slow-burning energy to power you through the first half of your day. Breakfast foods like oatmeal and most cereals are relatively high in fiber, and earning fiber should be your goal. Aim for 5 to 10 grams to start your day.

→ *It's got vitamins and minerals (especially from fruits).* Is it going to hurt you to order half a grapefruit with your eggs? Breakfast is the place where whole fruits and fruit salads naturally fit. (Be careful about juices, though—even 100 percent juice is high in sugar and low in fiber.) Start off with fruit and you'll be on your way to hitting your goal of at least five servings of produce a day.

ARBY'S

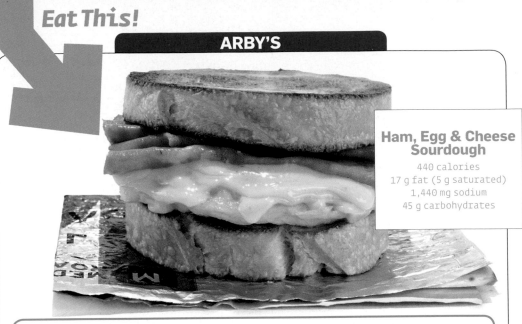

Ham, Egg & Cheese Sourdough

440 calories
17 g fat (5 g saturated)
1,440 mg sodium
45 g carbohydrates

Arby's sodium levels are uncomfortably high. In fact, only one breakfast sandwich has fewer than 1,000 milligrams. So why choose this one? Because it has the most belly-filling protein, and because the sourdough will help stabilize your blood sugar. A 2007 Italian study found that compared with those who ate regular white bread, people who ate sourdough had 25 percent lower blood sugar levels 30 minutes after mealtime.

ETNT DIET STRATEGY

FIBER BOOST!

Arby's breakfast menu is sorely lacking in the plant matter that gives us fiber, which, along with protein, is the most important nutrient of the morning hours as fiber will keep your belly feeling full as you begin to tussle with the day's demands. Compensate by munching an apple along with your sandwich or as a mid-morning snack. Each medium red delicious packs about 4.5 grams of fiber into fewer than a hundred calories.

Plus This!

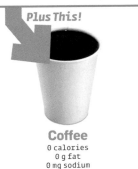

Coffee

0 calories
0 g fat
0 mg sodium
0 g carbohydrates

= Best Breakfast

440 calories
17 g fat
(5 g saturated)
1,440 mg sodium
45 g carbohydrates

----

26 g protein
2 g fiber

NUTRITION 101

COFFEE

You know that deep, complex flavor you've come to love in your morning joe? It's partially the result of the coffee bean's antioxidant concentration. According to a study from the University of Scranton, coffee is the single richest source of antioxidants in the average American's diet.

Not That!

Ham, Egg & Cheese Wrap

520 calories
24 g fat (8 g saturated)
1,900 mg sodium
45 g carbohydrates

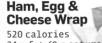

ATLANTA BREAD COMPANY

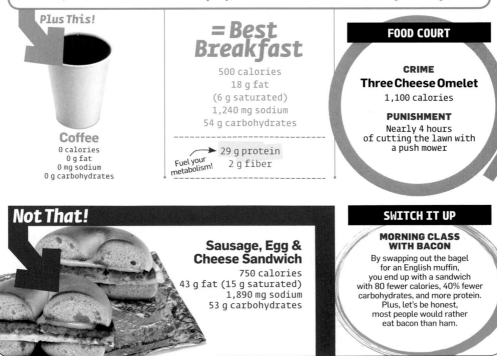

Honey Maple Ham, Egg & Cheddar Cheese Sandwich on Bagel

500 calories
18 g fat (6 g saturated)
1,240 mg sodium
54 g carbohydrates

When it comes to breakfast, you can't do much better than the classic breakfast sandwich —meat, egg, and cheese on a small bun or English muffin creates an ideal ratio of protein to carbohydrates (read: more protein, fewer carbs). Be careful about what type of meat you choose, though—sausage makes bacon look downright healthy. But whenever available, like at Atlanta Bread Company, ham is the best of the morning meat options.

Plus This!

Coffee
0 calories
0 g fat
0 mg sodium
0 g carbohydrates

= Best Breakfast

500 calories
18 g fat
(6 g saturated)
1,240 mg sodium
54 g carbohydrates

Fuel your metabolism! → 29 g protein
2 g fiber

FOOD COURT

CRIME
Three Cheese Omelet

1,100 calories

PUNISHMENT
Nearly 4 hours of cutting the lawn with a push mower

Not That!

Sausage, Egg & Cheese Sandwich

750 calories
43 g fat (15 g saturated)
1,890 mg sodium
53 g carbohydrates

SWITCH IT UP

MORNING CLASS WITH BACON
By swapping out the bagel for an English muffin, you end up with a sandwich with 80 fewer calories, 40% fewer carbohydrates, and more protein. Plus, let's be honest, most people would rather eat bacon than ham.

Eat This!

AU BON PAIN

Large Apple Cinnamon Oatmeal
370 calories
6 g fat (1 g saturated)
15 mg sodium
75 g carbohydrates

Normally we'd steer you away from a breakfast with more than 90 grams of carbohydrates, but these carbs are of the good, slow-burning variety that come from whole grains and natural sugars found within fruit. The fiber found in both oatmeal and fruit (in this case, combining for an impressive 10 grams) help slow down digestion, helping limit any dramatic spikes in blood sugar and ultimately keeping you feeling fuller, longer.

SUPER SNACK ALERT!

APPLES, BLUE CHEESE, AND CRANBERRIES
200 calories
10 g fat (4 g saturated)
27 g carbohydrates
270 mg sodium
3 g fiber

Cheese and fruit combine for a nutritionally balanced snack that's great for squashing hunger. The bonus? It's delicious.

Plus This!

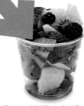

Small Fruit Cup
70 calories
0 g fat
15 mg sodium
18 g carbohydrates

= Best Breakfast
440 calories,
6 g fat (1 g saturated)
30 mg sodium
93 g carbohydrates

Cut your cholesterol!

----

12 g protein, 10 g fiber

35% DV (daily value) vitamin A, 64% DV vitamin C, 22% DV iron

----

RESTAURANT SURVIVAL GUIDE

BEWARE THE BREAD
Café-style chains like Starbucks, Panera, and Au Bon Pain are set up to encourage spur-of-the-moment purchases of baked goods, all of which hang out conveniently close to the cash register. Ignore the muffins and breads—all empty carbs and added sugars—and always opt for something hot. If it's hot, it's likely to have more protein and fewer carbs.

Not That!

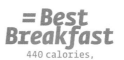

Sausage, Egg, and Cheddar on Asiago Bagel
810 calories
46 g fat (20 g saturated)
1,340 mg sodium
57 g carbohydrates

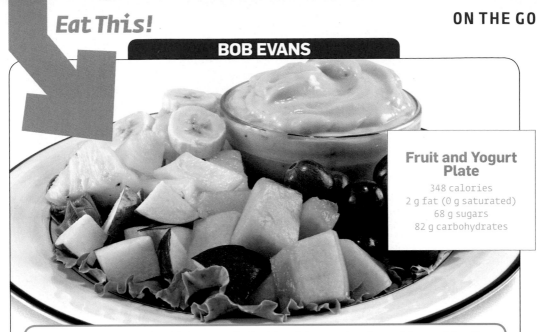

BOB EVANS

Fruit and Yogurt Plate

348 calories
2 g fat (0 g saturated)
68 g sugars
82 g carbohydrates

Yogurt is a verifiable health hero, packed with calcium and replete with gut-friendly bacteria that mimic those already living in your intestines. Add in the fruit and you've got enough natural sugars to make yourself forget all about your craving for pancakes—not to mention save you a few hundred calories of empty starch. The only thing this meal lacks is a protein punch, but you can pick that up easily with a side of scrambled or fried eggs.

Plus This!

2 Scrambled Eggs
168 calories
22 g fat (6 g saturated)
476 mg sodium
2 g carbohydrates

= Best Breakfast

516 calories
24 g fat
(6 g saturated)
549 mg sodium
84 g carbohydrates

- - - - - - - - - - - - - - - - -

20 g protein
9 g fiber

- - - - - - - - - - - - - - - - -

RESTAURANT SURVIVAL GUIDE

DRINK UP
A study presented at a meeting of the American Chemical Society found that low-calorie dieters who drank 2 cups of water—16 ounces—before each meal lost nearly 5 more pounds in 12 weeks than dieters who didn't focus on water. The reason? Water, like food, takes up space in the stomach, effectively blunting appetite.

Not That!

Stacked & Stuffed Strawberry Banana Cream Hotcakes
1,096 calories
29 g fat
(16 g saturated)
173 mg sodium
199 g carbohydrates

NUTRITION 101

PROBIOTICS

Healthy bacteria found in yogurt can help your body absorb the nutrients in food. What's more, in mice studies, British scientists found these bacteria—called probiotics—boosted the breakdown of fat molecules, preventing the rodents from gaining weight.

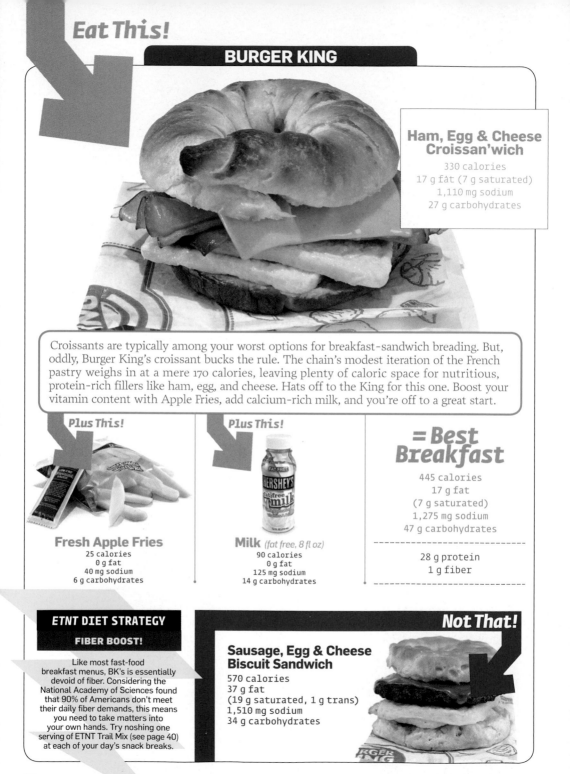

Eat This!

BURGER KING

Ham, Egg & Cheese Croissan'wich
330 calories
17 g fat (7 g saturated)
1,110 mg sodium
27 g carbohydrates

Croissants are typically among your worst options for breakfast-sandwich breading. But, oddly, Burger King's croissant bucks the rule. The chain's modest iteration of the French pastry weighs in at a mere 170 calories, leaving plenty of caloric space for nutritious, protein-rich fillers like ham, egg, and cheese. Hats off to the King for this one. Boost your vitamin content with Apple Fries, add calcium-rich milk, and you're off to a great start.

Plus This!

Fresh Apple Fries
25 calories
0 g fat
40 mg sodium
6 g carbohydrates

Plus This!

Milk *(fat free, 8 fl oz)*
90 calories
0 g fat
125 mg sodium
14 g carbohydrates

= Best Breakfast
445 calories
17 g fat
(7 g saturated)
1,275 mg sodium
47 g carbohydrates

----

28 g protein
1 g fiber

ETNT DIET STRATEGY
FIBER BOOST!

Like most fast-food breakfast menus, BK's is essentially devoid of fiber. Considering the National Academy of Sciences found that 90% of Americans don't meet their daily fiber demands, this means you need to take matters into your own hands. Try noshing one serving of ETNT Trail Mix (see page 40) at each of your day's snack breaks.

Not That!

Sausage, Egg & Cheese Biscuit Sandwich
570 calories
37 g fat
(19 g saturated, 1 g trans)
1,510 mg sodium
34 g carbohydrates

CHEESECAKE FACTORY

Shiitake Mushroom, Spinach, and Goat Cheese Scramble
570 calories
16 g saturated fat
994 mg sodium

A plain Cheesecake Factory omelette, sans toppings, packs 710 calories; most skyrocket well past 1,000. It's possible to order an omelette with more calories (2,450) than you'd find in eight McDonald's Egg McMuffins. This scramble, on the other hand, minimizes the caloric overload by cutting the eggs with a barrage of top-tier vegetables. It's long on saturated fat, but the protein and vitamin infusion are well worth 570 calories.

Plus This!

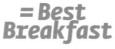

Coffee
0 calories
0 g fat
0 mg sodium
0 g carbohydrates

= Best Breakfast
570 calories
16 g saturated fat
994 mg sodium

----

*Cheesecake Factory
does not
disclose full
nutritional information.*

90◆
The number of dishes on the Factory's menu with more than 1,500 calories. That's just all the more reason to stick to the meal on this page.

Not That!

California Omelette
1,050 calories
32 g saturated fat
1,336 mg sodium

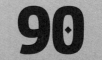

NUTRITION 101

SHIITAKE MUSHROOMS

This funky fungus is a great source of protein and contains compounds that have been found in animal studies to strengthen the immune system, ward off cancer, and improve cholesterol and blood pressure levels.

Eat This!

COSÌ

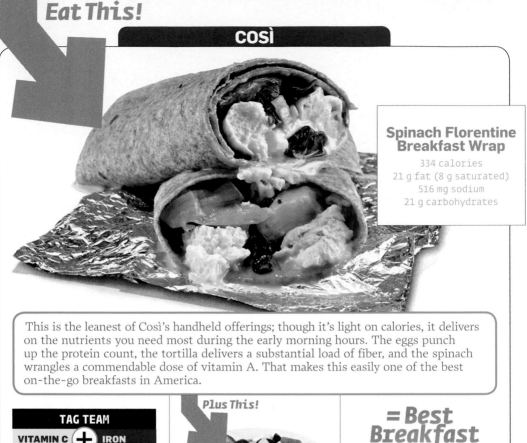

This is the leanest of Così's handheld offerings; though it's light on calories, it delivers on the nutrients you need most during the early morning hours. The eggs punch up the protein count, the tortilla delivers a substantial load of fiber, and the spinach wrangles a commendable dose of vitamin A. That makes this easily one of the best on-the-go breakfasts in America.

TAG TEAM

VITAMIN C ➕ IRON

The spinach in this wrap is loaded with iron, a mineral that's essential to your body's ability to create red blood cells. The thing is, in order for iron to pass into your bloodstream, it needs the help of vitamin C. That's where the fruit comes in—this one serving has more than your entire day's worth of vitamin C.

Plus This!

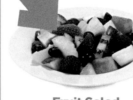

Fruit Salad
84 calories
1 g fat (0 g saturated)
21 g carbohydrates
2 g protein

= Best Breakfast
418 calories
22 g fat (8 g saturated)
534 mg sodium
42 g carbohydrates

----

26 g protein, 13 g fiber

117% DV vitamin A, 37% DV calcium, 138% DV vitamin C, 30% DV iron

Combat cancer!

80

Percentage of restaurant-served breakfasts that come from fast-food chains.

Not That!

Garden Pesto Omelette Croissant
740 calories
45 g fat
(20 g saturated)
1,491 mg sodium
56 g carbohydrates

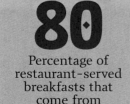

Eat This!

DENNY'S

Oatmeal
(with 8 oz milk)
290 calories
8 g fat (4 g saturated)
300 mg sodium
39 g carbohydrates

The sad truth about diners is that they rarely live up to the lean potential of the ingredients on their menus. The reason? They burden the nutritional heroes—lean meats, eggs, fruits, and whole grains—with excessive loads of fatty pork products, cheese, butter, and oils. If you want an omelet, make it at home using the recipe on page 90. Otherwise, stick to our piecemeal approach and stitch together a well-rounded start to your day.

Plus This!

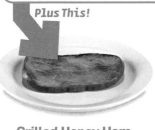

Grilled Honey Ham
120 calories
5 g fat (4 g saturated)
710 mg sodium
8 g carbohydrates

Plus This!

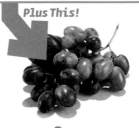

Grapes
55 calories
0 g fat
0 mg sodium
12 g carbohydrates

= Best Breakfast
465 calories
13 g fat
(8 g saturated)
1,010 mg sodium
59 g carbohydrates
----
29 g protein
8 g fiber

Not That!

Heartland Scramble
1,130 calories
63 g fat (19 g saturated)
3,180 mg sodium
110 g carbohydrates

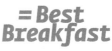

THE TRUE COST OF FREE

THE FREEBIE
ALL YOU CAN EAT
BUTTERMILK PANCAKES

THE COST
170 calories per pancake

Two stacks of three—
before butter and syrup—
socks your belly with
more than 1,000 calories.

Eat This!

DUNKIN' DONUTS

Egg White & Cheese Wake-Up Wraps (2)
300 calories
14 g fat (6 g saturated)
960 mg sodium
26 g carbohydrates

Move outside the menu's concentration of doughnuts and pastries and Dunkin' Donuts proves itself to be one of the better on-the-go breakfast joints in the country. Pair a couple of these Wake-Up Wraps with a Lite drink (or a near-zero-calorie cup of black coffee) to switch your metabolism from sleep mode to high gear. Or try the Egg, Ham, and Cheese on an English Muffin, a 360-calorie breakfast powerhouse.

1.8

Average increase, in inches, of the waistlines of people who've always skipped breakfast, according to a new study in the *American Journal of Clinical Nutrition*. Not only were breakfast skippers flabbier, but they also had worse triglycerides and LDL cholesterol levels.

Plus This!

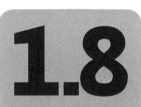

Coffee (medium)
10 calories
0 g fat
10 mg sodium
1 g carbohydrate

= Best Breakfast
310 calories
14 g fat (6 g saturated)
970 mg sodium
27 g carbohydrates

-----

16 g protein
2 g fiber

20% DV calcium

Not That!

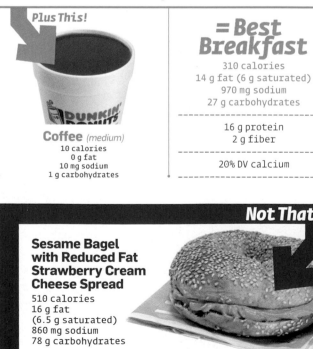

Sesame Bagel with Reduced Fat Strawberry Cream Cheese Spread
510 calories
16 g fat
(6.5 g saturated)
860 mg sodium
78 g carbohydrates

Eat This!

HARDEE'S

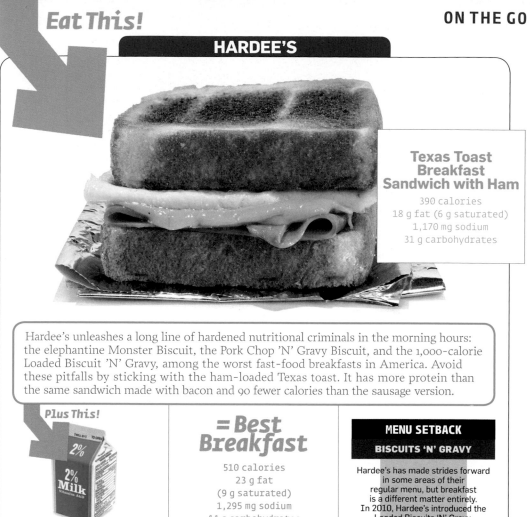

Texas Toast Breakfast Sandwich with Ham
390 calories
18 g fat (6 g saturated)
1,170 mg sodium
31 g carbohydrates

Hardee's unleashes a long line of hardened nutritional criminals in the morning hours: the elephantine Monster Biscuit, the Pork Chop 'N' Gravy Biscuit, and the 1,000-calorie Loaded Biscuit 'N' Gravy, among the worst fast-food breakfasts in America. Avoid these pitfalls by sticking with the ham-loaded Texas toast. It has more protein than the same sandwich made with bacon and 90 fewer calories than the sausage version.

Plus This!

2% Milk

Milk *(2%, 8 fl oz carton)*
120 calories
5 g fat (3 g saturated)
125 mg sodium
13 g carbohydrates

= Best Breakfast

510 calories
23 g fat
(9 g saturated)
1,295 mg sodium
44 g carbohydrates

----

32 g protein
2 g fiber

MENU SETBACK

BISCUITS 'N' GRAVY

Hardee's has made strides forward in some areas of their regular menu, but breakfast is a different matter entirely. In 2010, Hardee's introduced the Loaded Biscuits 'N' Gravy, essentially two open-faced sausage-and-egg sandwiches buried under a deluge of sausage-infused gravy. With 1,000 calories and 75 grams of fat, it's easily the chain's worst breakfast item.

Not That!

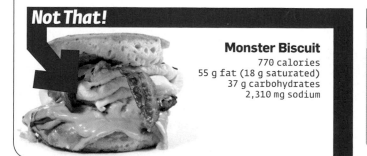

Monster Biscuit
770 calories
55 g fat (18 g saturated)
37 g carbohydrates
2,310 mg sodium

TAG TEAM

VITAMIN D 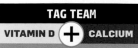 CALCIUM

In the 1930s, milk processors began fortifying their product with vitamin D in an effort to snub out the bone-decaying disease rickets. Did it work? You bet. Vitamin D helps your body absorb calcium, and calcium is essential for strong bones. Maintain a sturdy frame by keeping milk on the morning menu.

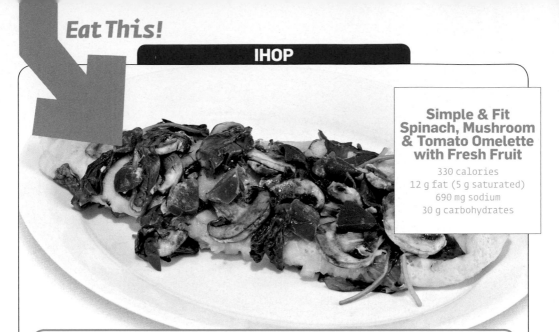

IHOP

**Simple & Fit
Spinach, Mushroom
& Tomato Omelette
with Fresh Fruit**
330 calories
12 g fat (5 g saturated)
690 mg sodium
30 g carbohydrates

Well done, IHOP—this is almost a perfect meal. In fact, it's long been a favorite of ours—probably because it used to be the only omelette on IHOP's menu that guaranteed you fewer than 1,000 calories. Luckily, they've expanded their Simple & Fit offerings to include a bit more variety, so if you're more in the mood for meat in your eggs, try the Simple & Fit Turkey Bacon Omelette with Fresh Fruit instead.

PANCAKE TOTEM POLE

ORIGINAL BUTTERMILK (3)
490 calories
18 g fat (8 g saturated)

CINNAMON APPLE (3)
510 calories
13 g fat (4.5 g saturated)

STRAWBERRY (3)
520 calories
13 g fat (4.5 g saturated)

CHOCOLATE CHIP (3)
550 calories
19 g fat (8 g saturated)

STRAWBERRY BANANA (3)
600 calories
13 g fat (4.5 g saturated)

**DOUBLE BLUEBERRY
PANCAKES (3)**
640 calories
13 g fat (4.5 g saturated)

HARVEST GRAIN 'N NUT (3)
700 calories
39 g fat (10 g saturated)

NEW YORK CHEESECAKE (3)
850 calories
34 g fat
(16 g saturated, 1.5 trans)

Plus This!

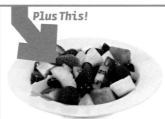

Seasonal Fruit
80 calories
0 g fat
0 mg sodium
21 g carbohydrates

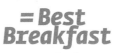

= Best
Breakfast
410 calories
12 g fat
(5 g saturated)
690 mg sodium
51 g carbohydrates

----

28 g protein
7 g fiber

Not That!

**Spinach and
Mushroom
Omelette**
(no pancakes on the side)
910 calories
71 g fat
(26 g saturated, 1 g trans)
1,580 mg sodium
23 g carbohydrates

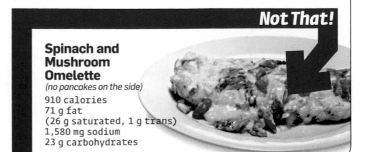

JACK IN THE BOX

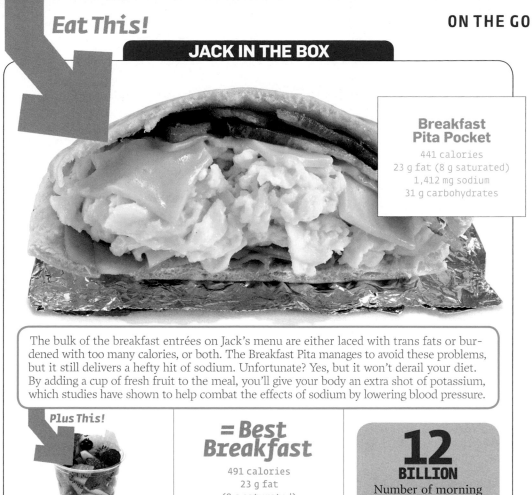

Breakfast Pita Pocket

441 calories
23 g fat (8 g saturated)
1,412 mg sodium
31 g carbohydrates

The bulk of the breakfast entrées on Jack's menu are either laced with trans fats or burdened with too many calories, or both. The Breakfast Pita manages to avoid these problems, but it still delivers a hefty hit of sodium. Unfortunate? Yes, but it won't derail your diet. By adding a cup of fresh fruit to the meal, you'll give your body an extra shot of potassium, which studies have shown to help combat the effects of sodium by lowering blood pressure.

Plus This!

Fruit Cup
50 calories
0 g fat
10 mg sodium
14 g carbohydrates

= Best Breakfast

491 calories
23 g fat
(8 g saturated)
1,422 mg sodium
45 g carbohydrates

----

29 g protein
2 g fiber

----

12 BILLION

Number of morning meals served between March 2009 and March 2010 by US restaurants, according to the research company NPD Group.

Not That!

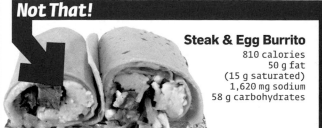

Steak & Egg Burrito

810 calories
50 g fat
(15 g saturated)
1,620 mg sodium
58 g carbohydrates

SWITCH IT UP

BACON BREAKFAST JACK
Warm croissant, eggs, melted cheese, and bacon. Doesn't sound like diet food? Well, maybe you've been on the wrong diet. With just 300 calories and 13 grams of fat, plus a good dose of protein, this isn't just a good option for those stuck at Jack in the Box, it's just a good option period.

JAMBA JUICE

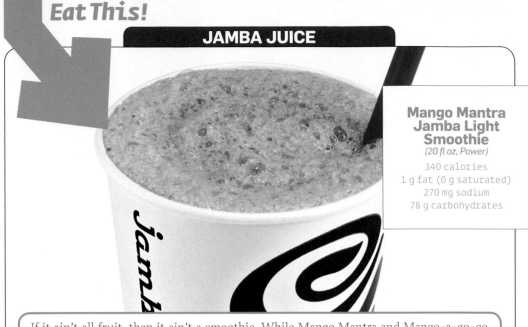

Mango Mantra Jamba Light Smoothie
(20 fl oz, Power)

340 calories
1 g fat (0 g saturated)
270 mg sodium
78 g carbohydrates

If it ain't all fruit, then it ain't a smoothie. While Mango Mantra and Mango-a-go-go may sound like two similarly healthy approaches to breakfast, the latter is built on a base of pineapple sherbert, which, in our book, makes it a milk shake. Instead, opt for a Power size (that's 32 ounces in Jamba-speak) all-fruit Mantra, and then add a whey boost. You'll end up with five times the protein and still save 160 calories.

11

Percentage of Americans who meet the recommended daily intake of fruits and vegetables.

Plus This!

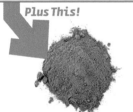

Whey Protein Boost
50 calories
0.5 g fat (0 g saturated)
25 mg sodium
1 g carbohydrates

= Best Breakfast
390 calories
1.5 g fat (0 g saturated)
295 mg sodium
79 g carbohydrates

----
20 g protein, 6 g fiber

180% DV vitamin A, 30% DV calcium,
260% DV vitamin C, 4% DV iron

NUTRITION 101
MANGOS

This tropical wonder touts too many boons to list, but its ability to nourish skin is among its most notable. Each fruit has more than 2 days' worth of vitamin C and a massive heft of beta-carotene. The former aids in the production of collagen, a skin-firming protein, and the latter helps protect your skin from premature aging.

Not That!

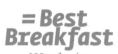

Mango-a-go-go
(20 fl oz, Power)

550 calories
2.5 g fat
(1 g saturated)
65 mg sodium
129 g carbohydrates

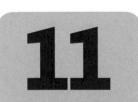

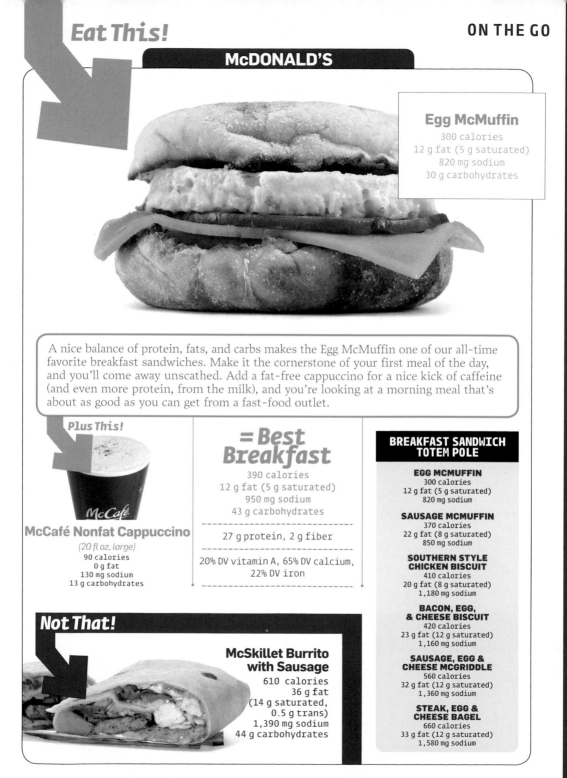

Eat This!

McDONALD'S

Egg McMuffin
300 calories
12 g fat (5 g saturated)
820 mg sodium
30 g carbohydrates

A nice balance of protein, fats, and carbs makes the Egg McMuffin one of our all-time favorite breakfast sandwiches. Make it the cornerstone of your first meal of the day, and you'll come away unscathed. Add a fat-free cappuccino for a nice kick of caffeine (and even more protein, from the milk), and you're looking at a morning meal that's about as good as you can get from a fast-food outlet.

Plus This!

McCafé Nonfat Cappuccino
(20 fl oz, large)
90 calories
0 g fat
130 mg sodium
13 g carbohydrates

= Best Breakfast
390 calories
12 g fat (5 g saturated)
950 mg sodium
43 g carbohydrates

----

27 g protein, 2 g fiber

20% DV vitamin A, 65% DV calcium, 22% DV iron

BREAKFAST SANDWICH TOTEM POLE

EGG MCMUFFIN
300 calories
12 g fat (5 g saturated)
820 mg sodium

SAUSAGE MCMUFFIN
370 calories
22 g fat (8 g saturated)
850 mg sodium

SOUTHERN STYLE CHICKEN BISCUIT
410 calories
20 g fat (8 g saturated)
1,180 mg sodium

BACON, EGG, & CHEESE BISCUIT
420 calories
23 g fat (12 g saturated)
1,160 mg sodium

SAUSAGE, EGG & CHEESE MCGRIDDLE
560 calories
32 g fat (12 g saturated)
1,360 mg sodium

STEAK, EGG & CHEESE BAGEL
660 calories
33 g fat (12 g saturated)
1,580 mg sodium

Not That!

McSkillet Burrito with Sausage
610 calories
36 g fat
(14 g saturated, 0.5 g trans)
1,390 mg sodium
44 g carbohydrates

Eat This!

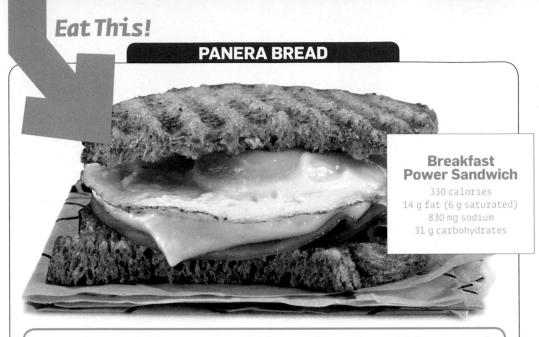

PANERA BREAD

Breakfast Power Sandwich
330 calories
14 g fat (6 g saturated)
830 mg sodium
31 g carbohydrates

What makes a sandwich a "power" sandwich? According to Panera, it's ham, egg, and cheese on whole grain bread, and we couldn't agree more. Studies show that egg-fueled breakfasts lead to fewer calories consumed throughout the day, and whole grains— all too rare on restaurant menus—have repeatedly been proven to lower the risk of cardiovascular disease. If only all sandwiches were so healthy.

RESTAURANT SURVIVAL GUIDE

STICK TO SMALL ENTRÉES

It turns out eating less won't leave you feeling deprived. In one study, Penn State researchers found that subjects ate 30 percent more food when presented with bigger portions, yet their perceived fullness didn't change. The point is it takes less food than you think to fill your stomach. Anything you eat beyond that just pushes you closer to discomfort.

Plus This!

Apple
80 calories
0 g fat
0 mg sodium
21 g carbohydrates

= Best Breakfast
410 calories
14 g fat (6 g saturated)
830 mg sodium
52 g carbohydrates
----
22 g protein, 8 g fiber

15% DV vitamin A, 20% DV calcium
15% DV iron

NUTRITION 101

QUERCETIN

Apples, specifically the skin, are replete with a compound called quercetin, which studies have shown to reduce the risk of allergies, heart attack, Alzheimer's, Parkinson's, and prostate and lung cancers. Looks like there's truth to that old saw about eating an apple every day.

Not That!

Grilled Bacon, Egg & Cheese Sandwich
510 calories
24 g fat
(10 g saturated)
1,060 mg sodium
44 g carbohydrates

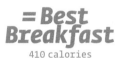

The Eat This, Not That! No-Diet Cheat Sheets

BREAKFAST SANDWICHES

		CALORIES	FAT (g)	SATURATED (g)	TRANS (g)	SODIUM (mg)	FIBER (g)	PROTEIN (g)	CARBS (g)
1.	Subway Black Forest Ham, Egg & Cheese Egg Muffin Melt (with regular egg)	180	7	2	0	650	5	15	18
2.	Dunkin' Donuts Egg White Turkey Sausage Flatbread	280	8	3	0	770	3	19	32
3.	McDonald's Egg McMuffin	300	12	5	0	820	2	18	30
4.	Jack in the Box Bacon Breakfast Jack	300	13	5	0	760	1	16	30
5.	Tim Hortons English Muffin with Bacon, Egg, and Cheese	310	14	6	0	730	1	16	32
6.	Burger King Ham, Egg & Cheese Croissan'wich	330	17	7	0	1,110	0	18	27
7.	Panera Breakfast Power Sandwich	330	14	6	0	830	4	22	31
8.	Starbucks Bacon, Gouda Cheese & Egg Frittata on Artisan Roll	350	18	7	0	840	0	17	30
9.	Au Bon Pain Turkey, Egg and Cheddar on a Skinny Bagel	380	21	9	0	830	4	30	23
10.	Hardee's Sunrise Croissaint with Ham	400	23	10	N/A	1,070	1	21	27
11.	Burger King Ham, Egg, and Cheese Biscuit	400	22	15	0.5	1,430	N/A	16	33
12.	Chick-fil-A Chicken Biscuit	440	20	8	0	1,240	3	17	47
13.	Carl's Jr. Sourdough Breakfast Sandwich	450	21	8	0	1,470	1	29	38

Eat This!

SMOOTHIE KING

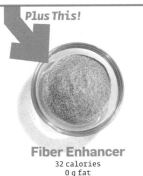

High Protein Pineapple *(20 fl oz)*

320 calories
9 g fat (1 g saturated)
336 mg sodium
29 g carbohydrates

This pineapple smoothie derives its metabolism-boosting, muscle-building chops from two forms of protein powder (whey and a protein blend), plus almonds (another good source of the muscle-strengthening material). Toss in nutrient-dense pineapple and a shot of Fiber Blend Enhancer to hit your morning's belly-filling quota, and you'll be operating at peak performance levels until the lunch hour beckons.

MENU DECODER

TURBINADO

One of the two sweeteners Smoothie King uses (the other being honey), this raw sugar is made from evaporated cane juice. Don't be fooled by the fancy name, though: It's just as bad for you as normal sugar. Order your smoothie "skinny" and they'll leave it out, eliminating 100 calories from a 20-ounce smoothie.

Plus This!

Fiber Enhancer
32 calories
0 g fat

= Best Breakfast

352 calories
9 g fat
(1 g saturated)
336 mg sodium
29 g carbohydrates

----

28 g protein
10 g fiber

SWITCH IT UP

COFFEE MOCHA

It may sound more like a dessert than a viable breakfast option, but this chocolate-laced caffeine treat is actually one of the healthiest smoothie options on the menu, low in calories and carbs and naturally high in protein. Take this smoothie to the next level by tacking on a protein boost and a fiber enhancer.

Not That!

Peanut Power Plus Strawberry *(20 fl oz)*
699 calories
22 g fat (4 g saturated)
64 mg sodium
112 g carbohydrates

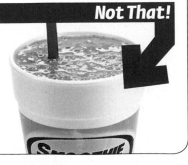

SONIC

Ham, Egg & Cheese Breakfast Burrito

440 calories
23 g fat (9 g saturated)
1,630 mg sodium
37 g carbohydrates

Tortillas are typically vessels used to house excesses of empty carbs and excess fat, making the Mexican favorite a deal-breaker for health-conscious eaters. But Sonic has reigned their breakfast burrito in, using a smaller tortilla and a healthy balance of egg, cheese, and lean ham to keep calories low and protein high. Just be sure to seek out some potassium (how about a banana?) to help balance the high sodium count.

Plus This!

Coffee (Regular)
10 calories
0 g fat
35 mg sodium
2 g carbohydrates

= Best Breakfast

450 calories
23 g fat (9 g saturated)
1,665 mg sodium
39 g carbohydrates

----

26 g protein, 2 g fiber

15% DV vitamin A,
30% DV calcium, 20% DV iron

TAG TEAM

FRUIT + FRUIT

Fruits in any form are better than most of the foods we eat, but for the strongest nutritional punch, you can't do better than fruit salad. Cornell researchers found that compared with any individual fruit, mixed fruits offered a greater antioxidant response, supporting the researchers' theory that antioxidants team together in synergistic combinations.

Not That!

CroisSONIC Breakfast Sandwich with Sausage

600 calories
46 g fat
(17.5 g saturated)
1,338 mg sodium
28 g carbohydrates

SWITCH IT UP

CROISSONIC BREAKFAST SANDWICH WITH HAM

Once again, where sausage falls short, ham steps in and saves the day. You still get to indulge in a warm croissant, rich egg, and melted cheese, but by making this one simple swap you save 170 calories and 19 grams of fat, plus you gain a few grams of protein.

Eat This!

STARBUCKS

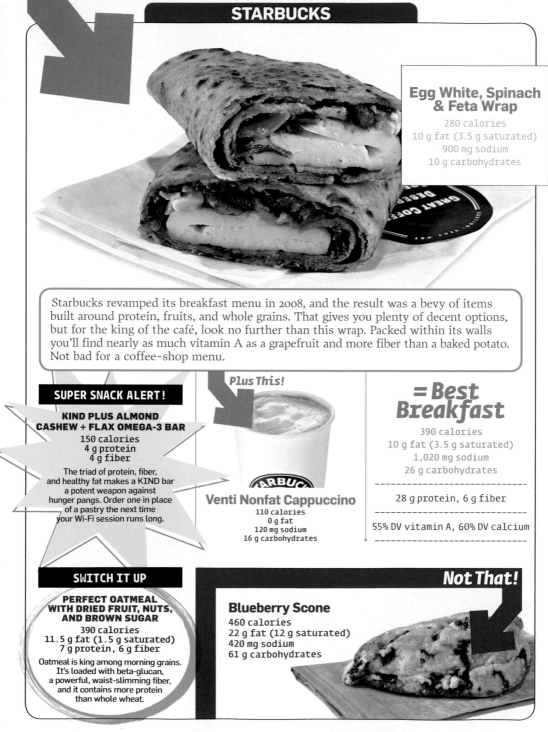

Egg White, Spinach & Feta Wrap
280 calories
10 g fat (3.5 g saturated)
900 mg sodium
10 g carbohydrates

Starbucks revamped its breakfast menu in 2008, and the result was a bevy of items built around protein, fruits, and whole grains. That gives you plenty of decent options, but for the king of the café, look no further than this wrap. Packed within its walls you'll find nearly as much vitamin A as a grapefruit and more fiber than a baked potato. Not bad for a coffee-shop menu.

SUPER SNACK ALERT!

KIND PLUS ALMOND CASHEW + FLAX OMEGA-3 BAR
150 calories
4 g protein
4 g fiber

The triad of protein, fiber, and healthy fat makes a KIND bar a potent weapon against hunger pangs. Order one in place of a pastry the next time your Wi-Fi session runs long.

Plus This!

Venti Nonfat Cappuccino
110 calories
0 g fat
120 mg sodium
16 g carbohydrates

= Best Breakfast
390 calories
10 g fat (3.5 g saturated)
1,020 mg sodium
26 g carbohydrates
----
28 g protein, 6 g fiber

55% DV vitamin A, 60% DV calcium

SWITCH IT UP

PERFECT OATMEAL WITH DRIED FRUIT, NUTS, AND BROWN SUGAR
390 calories
11.5 g fat (1.5 g saturated)
7 g protein, 6 g fiber

Oatmeal is king among morning grains. It's loaded with beta-glucan, a powerful, waist-slimming fiber, and it contains more protein than whole wheat.

Not That!

Blueberry Scone
460 calories
22 g fat (12 g saturated)
420 mg sodium
61 g carbohydrates

Eat This!

SUBWAY

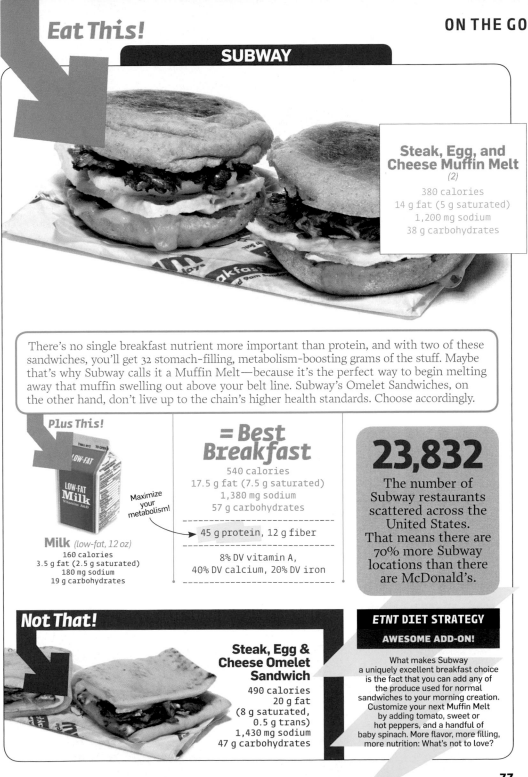

Steak, Egg, and Cheese Muffin Melt
(2)
380 calories
14 g fat (5 g saturated)
1,200 mg sodium
38 g carbohydrates

There's no single breakfast nutrient more important than protein, and with two of these sandwiches, you'll get 32 stomach-filling, metabolism-boosting grams of the stuff. Maybe that's why Subway calls it a Muffin Melt—because it's the perfect way to begin melting away that muffin swelling out above your belt line. Subway's Omelet Sandwiches, on the other hand, don't live up to the chain's higher health standards. Choose accordingly.

Plus This!

Milk *(low-fat, 12 oz)*
160 calories
3.5 g fat (2.5 g saturated)
180 mg sodium
19 g carbohydrates

Maximize your metabolism!

= Best Breakfast
540 calories
17.5 g fat (7.5 g saturated)
1,380 mg sodium
57 g carbohydrates

45 g protein, 12 g fiber

8% DV vitamin A,
40% DV calcium, 20% DV iron

23,832
The number of Subway restaurants scattered across the United States. That means there are 70% more Subway locations than there are McDonald's.

Not That!

Steak, Egg & Cheese Omelet Sandwich
490 calories
20 g fat
(8 g saturated,
0.5 g trans)
1,430 mg sodium
47 g carbohydrates

ETNT DIET STRATEGY
AWESOME ADD-ON!
What makes Subway a uniquely excellent breakfast choice is the fact that you can add any of the produce used for normal sandwiches to your morning creation. Customize your next Muffin Melt by adding tomato, sweet or hot peppers, and a handful of baby spinach. More flavor, more filling, more nutrition: What's not to love?

Eat This!

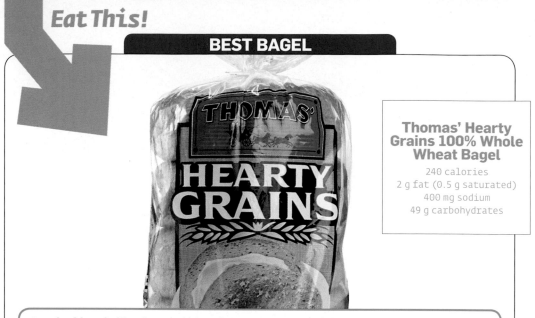

BEST BAGEL

Thomas' Hearty Grains 100% Whole Wheat Bagel
240 calories
2 g fat (0.5 g saturated)
400 mg sodium
49 g carbohydrates

Standard bagels like the one below from Sara Lee—and the oversized atrocities found at your local cafe or coffee shop—are made with refined flour, which is why the whole grain Thomas' version has more than five times the protein and six times the fiber. Skip the cream cheese in favor of creating a seriously filling breakfast sandwich, in this case, with the help of a fried egg, slices of ham, and a swipe of creamy hummus.

Plus This!

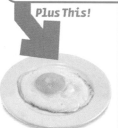

Fried egg *(large)*
70 calories
5 g fat (1.5 g saturated)
70 mg sodium
0 g carbohydrates

Plus This!

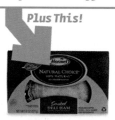

Hormel Natural Choice Smoked Deli Ham
(4 slices)
60 calories
1.5 g fat (0 g saturated)
520 mg sodium
1 g carbohydrates

Plus This!

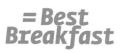

Sabra Roasted Red Pepper Hummus *(2 Tbsp)*
70 calories
6 g fat (1 g saturated)
120 mg sodium
4 g carbohydrates

= Best Breakfast

440 calories
14.5 g fat
(3 g saturated)
1,110 mg sodium
54 g carbohydrates

----

10 g protein
7 g fiber

Not That!

Sara Lee Deluxe Bagel, plain
260 calories
1 g fat (0.5 g saturated)
400 mg sodium
50 g carbohydrates

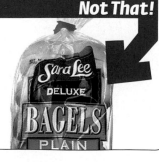

BEST CEREAL

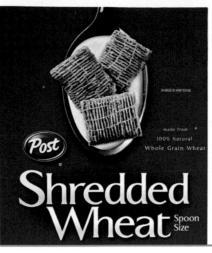

What, no cartoon characters on the box? No bold, in-your-face health claims? Nope. Post Shredded Wheat is cereal at its gimmick-free finest. Each biscuit is built entirely from one ingredient: whole wheat. That fills your bowl with fiber and protein numbers that other cereals can't match, and with just a couple of additions, you can convert this age-old grain into a powerful weapon in your battle against belly fat.

Plus This!

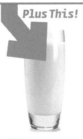

Plus This!

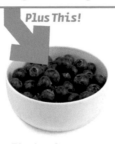

Plus This!

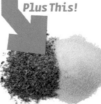

= Best Breakfast

490 calories
7 g fat
(2 g saturated)
118 mg sodium
86 g carbohydrates

Squash your hunger! 29 g protein
→ 13 g fiber

Milk *(1%, 1 cup)*
110 calories
2.5 g fat (1.5 g saturated)
108 mg sodium
13 g carbohydrates

Blueberries *(½ cup)*
40 calories
0 g fat
0 mg sodium
11 g carbohydrates

***ETNT* Perfectly Simple Supplement** *(2 Tbsp)*
(see matrix on page 50)
85 calories
3 g fat (0.5 g saturated)
10 mg sodium
2 g carbohydrates

Not That!

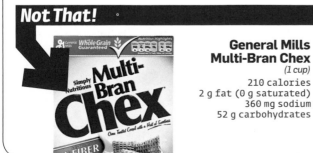

General Mills Multi-Bran Chex
(1 cup)
210 calories
2 g fat (0 g saturated)
360 mg sodium
52 g carbohydrates

STEALTH HEALTH

WHOLE GRAINS

People who incorporate whole grains into their weight-loss strategy lose more belly fat than those who stick with refined grains, according to a 2008 study from the *American Journal of Clinical Nutrition.* Nowhere is it easier to find whole grains than in the cereal aisle.

Eat This!

BEST ENGLISH MUFFIN

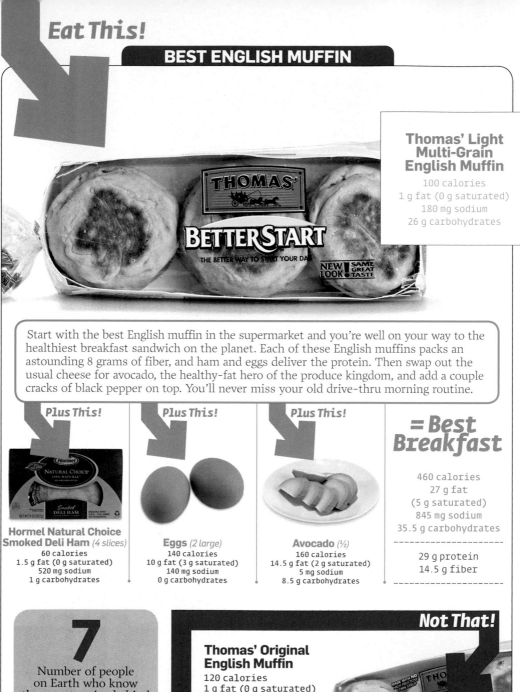

Thomas' Light Multi-Grain English Muffin
100 calories
1 g fat (0 g saturated)
180 mg sodium
26 g carbohydrates

Start with the best English muffin in the supermarket and you're well on your way to the healthiest breakfast sandwich on the planet. Each of these English muffins packs an astounding 8 grams of fiber, and ham and eggs deliver the protein. Then swap out the usual cheese for avocado, the healthy-fat hero of the produce kingdom, and add a couple cracks of black pepper on top. You'll never miss your old drive-thru morning routine.

Plus This!

Hormel Natural Choice Smoked Deli Ham *(4 slices)*
60 calories
1.5 g fat (0 g saturated)
520 mg sodium
1 g carbohydrates

Plus This!

Eggs *(2 large)*
140 calories
10 g fat (3 g saturated)
140 mg sodium
0 g carbohydrates

Plus This!

Avocado *(½)*
160 calories
14.5 g fat (2 g saturated)
5 mg sodium
8.5 g carbohydrates

= Best Breakfast

460 calories
27 g fat
(5 g saturated)
845 mg sodium
35.5 g carbohydrates

----

29 g protein
14.5 g fiber

7

Number of people on Earth who know the secret recipe behind Thomas' trademark "nooks and crannies" English muffins.

Not That!

Thomas' Original English Muffin
120 calories
1 g fat (0 g saturated)
200 mg sodium
25 g carbohydrates

BEST TOASTER PASTRY

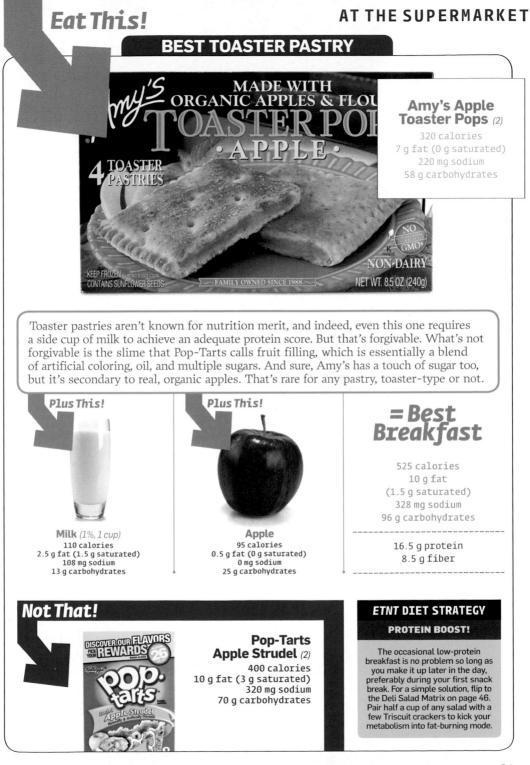

Amy's Apple Toaster Pops (2)

320 calories
7 g fat (0 g saturated)
220 mg sodium
58 g carbohydrates

Toaster pastries aren't known for nutrition merit, and indeed, even this one requires a side cup of milk to achieve an adequate protein score. But that's forgivable. What's not forgivable is the slime that Pop-Tarts calls fruit filling, which is essentially a blend of artificial coloring, oil, and multiple sugars. And sure, Amy's has a touch of sugar too, but it's secondary to real, organic apples. That's rare for any pastry, toaster-type or not.

Plus This!

Milk *(1%, 1 cup)*
110 calories
2.5 g fat (1.5 g saturated)
108 mg sodium
13 g carbohydrates

Plus This!

Apple
95 calories
0.5 g fat (0 g saturated)
0 mg sodium
25 g carbohydrates

= Best Breakfast

525 calories
10 g fat
(1.5 g saturated)
328 mg sodium
96 g carbohydrates

16.5 g protein
8.5 g fiber

Not That!

Pop-Tarts Apple Strudel (2)

400 calories
10 g fat (3 g saturated)
320 mg sodium
70 g carbohydrates

ETNT DIET STRATEGY

PROTEIN BOOST!

The occasional low-protein breakfast is no problem so long as you make it up later in the day, preferably during your first snack break. For a simple solution, flip to the Deli Salad Matrix on page 46. Pair half a cup of any salad with a few Triscuit crackers to kick your metabolism into fat-burning mode.

Eat This!

BEST PANCAKES

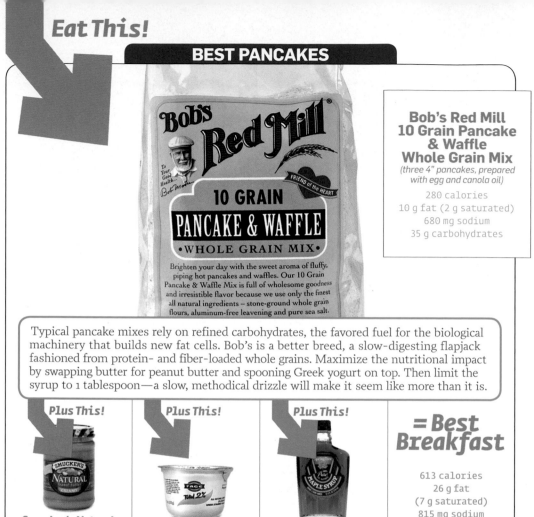

Bob's Red Mill 10 Grain Pancake & Waffle Whole Grain Mix
(three 4" pancakes, prepared with egg and canola oil)

280 calories
10 g fat (2 g saturated)
680 mg sodium
35 g carbohydrates

Typical pancake mixes rely on refined carbohydrates, the favored fuel for the biological machinery that builds new fat cells. Bob's is a better breed, a slow-digesting flapjack fashioned from protein- and fiber-loaded whole grains. Maximize the nutritional impact by swapping butter for peanut butter and spooning Greek yogurt on top. Then limit the syrup to 1 tablespoon—a slow, methodical drizzle will make it seem like more than it is.

Plus This!

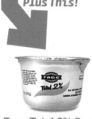

Smucker's Natural Creamy Peanut Butter
(1.5 Tbsp)
150 calories
12 g fat (2 g saturated)
70 mg sodium
4.5 g carbohydrates

Plus This!

Fage Total 2% Greek Yogurt, plain *(7 oz)*
130 calories
4 g fat (3 g saturated)
65 mg sodium
8 g carbohydrates

Plus This!

Spring Tree Pure Maple Syrup *(1 Tbsp)*
53 calories
0 g fat
0 mg sodium
13.5 g carbohydrates

= Best Breakfast

613 calories
26 g fat
(7 g saturated)
815 mg sodium
61 g carbohydrates

33.5 g protein
5.5 g fiber

Fat-burning fuel!

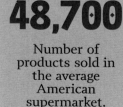

48,700

Number of products sold in the average American supermarket.

Not That!

Aunt Jemima Original Pancake Mix
(four 4" pancakes prepared with oil and egg)
250 calories
8 g fat (2 g saturated)
800 mg sodium
37 g carbohydrates

BEST WAFFLES

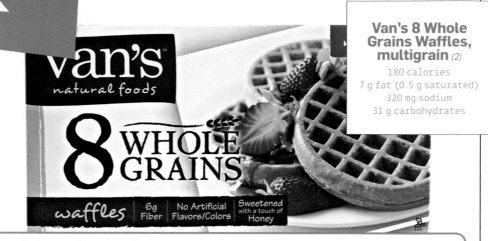

Van's 8 Whole Grains Waffles, multigrain *(2)*

180 calories
7 g fat (0.5 g saturated)
320 mg sodium
31 g carbohydrates

Sure, lighter waffles exist, but you won't find any others with Van's dedication to whole grains. This quick-prep breakfast is made with whole wheat, barley, quinoa, oats, rye, and other grains you probably don't eat enough of. That's how each serving manages to rope in 20 percent of your day's fiber needs. Bolster the protein with cheese, chicken sausage, and milk, and you've just built the foundation for a nutritionally successful day.

Plus This!

Horizon Organic Finely Shredded Cheddar Cheese *(2 Tbsp)*
55 calories
4.5 g fat (2.5 g saturated)
90 mg sodium
0 g carbohydrates

Plus This!

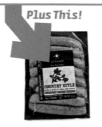

Al Fresco Country Style Chicken Sausage *(2 links)*
100 calories
6 g fat (2 g saturated)
340 mg sodium
0 g carbohydrates

Plus This!

Milk *(1%, 1 cup)*
110 calories
2.5 g fat (1.5 g saturated)
108 mg sodium
13 g carbohydrates

= Best Breakfast

445 calories
20 g fat
(6.5 g saturated)
858 mg sodium
44 g carbohydrates

26.5 g protein
6 g fiber

Not That!

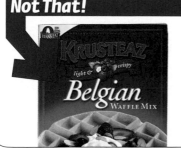

Krusteaz Belgian Waffle Mix
(½ cup prepared)
450 calories
18 g fat (3 g saturated)
899 mg sodium
58 g carbohydrates

MEAL MAKER

CHEESY CHICKEN-SAUSAGE WAFFLES

Toast the waffles and immediately top each with a tablespoon of cheese. Slice the sausage and sauté until browned, then divide among the waffles. Microwave for 20 seconds to melt the cheese. Eat them open-faced or press them together for a sausage-and-cheese breakfast sandwich on waffles.

Eat This!

BEST YOGURT

**Fage Total 2%
Greek Yogurt, plain**
(7 oz)
130 calories
4 g fat (3 g saturated)
65 mg sodium
8 g carbohydrates

You'll see Greek yogurt listed as a side dish for many of the meals in this chapter, and that's because the Greek stuff is so vastly superior to traditional varieties. Unlike American yogurt, Greek-style yogurt has had the liquids strained out, leaving it with fewer sugars and about three times as much protein. Use it to build a fruit parfait for one of the most nutritionally charged breakfasts in this entire book.

Plus This!

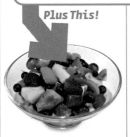

ETNT Fruit Salad *(1 cup)*
80 calories
0 g fat
0 mg sodium
20 g carbohydrates

Plus This!

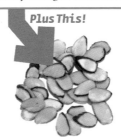

Sliced almonds *(¼ cup)*
135 calories
12 g fat (1 g saturated)
0 mg sodium
5 g carbohydrates

Plus This!

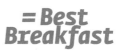

**Kashi GoLean Crisp!
Toasted Berry Crumble**
(¼ cup)
60 calories
1 g fat (0 g saturated)
42 mg sodium
12 g carbohydrates

= Best Breakfast

405 calories
17 g fat
(4 g saturated)
107 mg sodium
45 g carbohydrates

----

28 g protein
8.5 g fiber

MEAL MAKER

GREEK PARFAIT

Fill the bottom of a deep glass with a scoop of Greek yogurt, cover it with fruit salad, and then sprinkle in a few shakes of almonds and granola. (For an aromatic burst of fresh flavor, add a bit of fresh mint, too.) Repeat the process, aiming for three evenly distributed layers.

Not That!

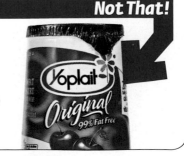

**Yoplait
99% Fat Free
Cherry Orchard**
(6 oz)
170 calories
1.5 g fat (1 g saturated)
80 mg sodium
33 g carbohydrates

BEST BREAKFAST BOWL

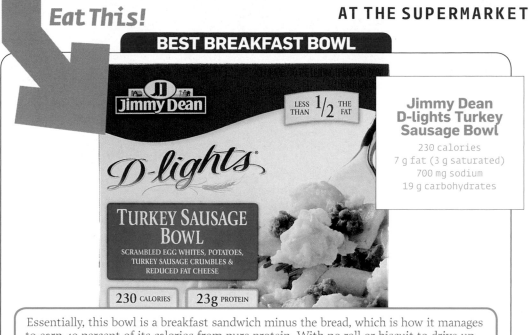

LESS THAN 1/2 THE FAT

D-lights®

TURKEY SAUSAGE BOWL
SCRAMBLED EGG WHITES, POTATOES, TURKEY SAUSAGE CRUMBLES & REDUCED FAT CHEESE

230 CALORIES   **23g** PROTEIN

Jimmy Dean D-lights Turkey Sausage Bowl
230 calories
7 g fat (3 g saturated)
700 mg sodium
19 g carbohydrates

Essentially, this bowl is a breakfast sandwich minus the bread, which is how it manages to earn 40 percent of its calories from pure protein. With no roll or biscuit to drive up the carb count, egg whites and lean turkey sausage end up contributing a disproportionate number of calories—and that's a good thing. Add a glass of milk and a full grapefruit for a complete breakfast that rivals any you could prepare from scratch.

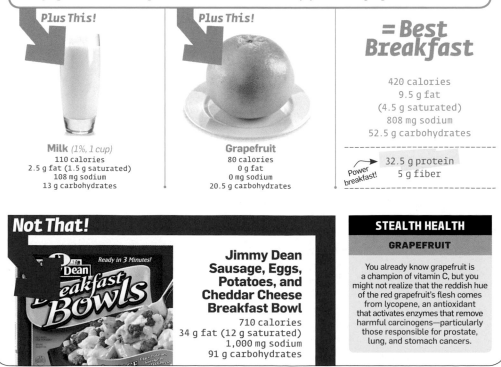

Plus This!

Milk *(1%, 1 cup)*
110 calories
2.5 g fat (1.5 g saturated)
108 mg sodium
13 g carbohydrates

Plus This!

Grapefruit
80 calories
0 g fat
0 mg sodium
20.5 g carbohydrates

= Best Breakfast

420 calories
9.5 g fat
(4.5 g saturated)
808 mg sodium
52.5 g carbohydrates

Power breakfast! → 32.5 g protein
5 g fiber

Not That!

Ready in 3 Minutes!

Jimmy Dean Sausage, Eggs, Potatoes, and Cheddar Cheese Breakfast Bowl
710 calories
34 g fat (12 g saturated)
1,000 mg sodium
91 g carbohydrates

STEALTH HEALTH

GRAPEFRUIT

You already know grapefruit is a champion of vitamin C, but you might not realize that the reddish hue of the red grapefruit's flesh comes from lycopene, an antioxidant that activates enzymes that remove harmful carcinogens—particularly those responsible for prostate, lung, and stomach cancers.

Eat This!

BEST HOT CEREAL

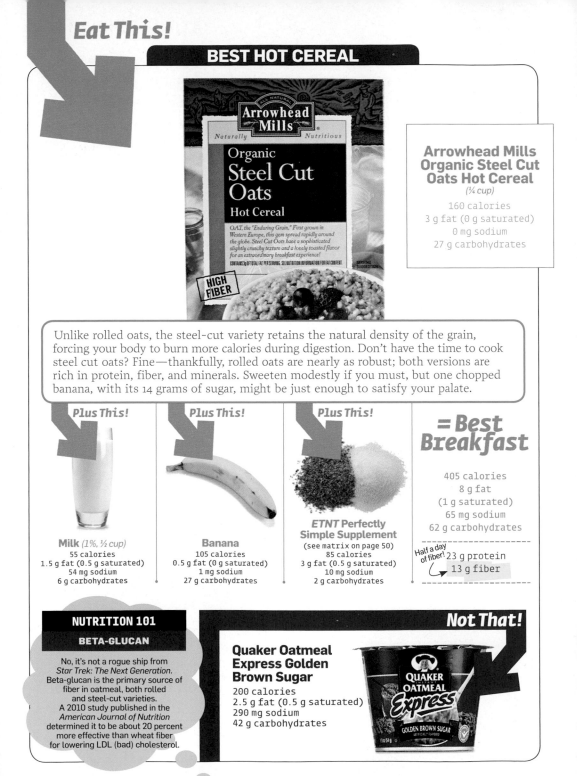

Arrowhead Mills Organic Steel Cut Oats Hot Cereal
(¼ cup)
160 calories
3 g fat (0 g saturated)
0 mg sodium
27 g carbohydrates

Unlike rolled oats, the steel-cut variety retains the natural density of the grain, forcing your body to burn more calories during digestion. Don't have the time to cook steel cut oats? Fine—thankfully, rolled oats are nearly as robust; both versions are rich in protein, fiber, and minerals. Sweeten modestly if you must, but one chopped banana, with its 14 grams of sugar, might be just enough to satisfy your palate.

Plus This!

Milk (1%, ½ cup)
55 calories
1.5 g fat (0.5 g saturated)
54 mg sodium
6 g carbohydrates

Plus This!

Banana
105 calories
0.5 g fat (0 g saturated)
1 mg sodium
27 g carbohydrates

Plus This!

ETNT Perfectly Simple Supplement
(see matrix on page 50)
85 calories
3 g fat (0.5 g saturated)
10 mg sodium
2 g carbohydrates

= Best Breakfast

405 calories
8 g fat
(1 g saturated)
65 mg sodium
62 g carbohydrates

Half a day of fiber! 23 g protein
13 g fiber

NUTRITION 101
BETA-GLUCAN

No, it's not a rogue ship from *Star Trek: The Next Generation*. Beta-glucan is the primary source of fiber in oatmeal, both rolled and steel-cut varieties.
A 2010 study published in the *American Journal of Nutrition* determined it to be about 20 percent more effective than wheat fiber for lowering LDL (bad) cholesterol.

Not That!

Quaker Oatmeal Express Golden Brown Sugar
200 calories
2.5 g fat (0.5 g saturated)
290 mg sodium
42 g carbohydrates

BEST BREAKFAST BURRITO

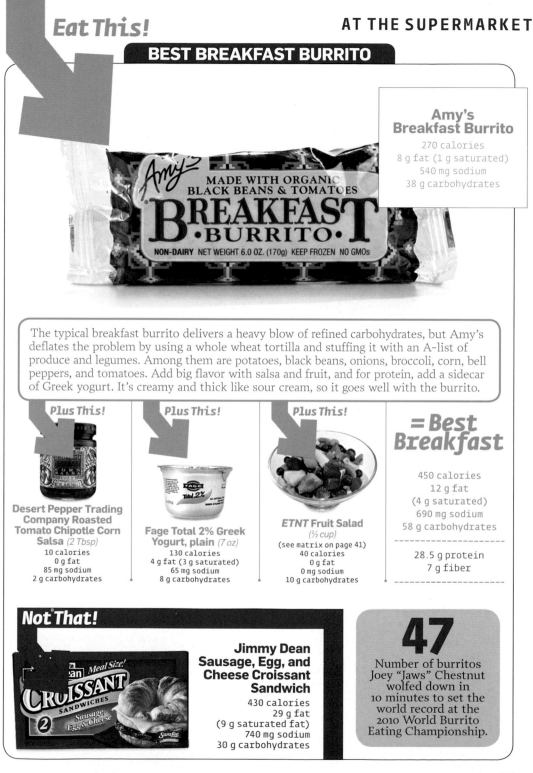

Amy's Breakfast Burrito
270 calories
8 g fat (1 g saturated)
540 mg sodium
38 g carbohydrates

The typical breakfast burrito delivers a heavy blow of refined carbohydrates, but Amy's deflates the problem by using a whole wheat tortilla and stuffing it with an A-list of produce and legumes. Among them are potatoes, black beans, onions, broccoli, corn, bell peppers, and tomatoes. Add big flavor with salsa and fruit, and for protein, add a sidecar of Greek yogurt. It's creamy and thick like sour cream, so it goes well with the burrito.

Plus This!

Desert Pepper Trading Company Roasted Tomato Chipotle Corn Salsa *(2 Tbsp)*
10 calories
0 g fat
85 mg sodium
2 g carbohydrates

Plus This!

Fage Total 2% Greek Yogurt, plain *(7 oz)*
130 calories
4 g fat (3 g saturated)
65 mg sodium
8 g carbohydrates

Plus This!

ETNT Fruit Salad
(½ cup)
(see matrix on page 41)
40 calories
0 g fat
0 mg sodium
10 g carbohydrates

= Best Breakfast
450 calories
12 g fat
(4 g saturated)
690 mg sodium
58 g carbohydrates

28.5 g protein
7 g fiber

Not That!

Jimmy Dean Sausage, Egg, and Cheese Croissant Sandwich
430 calories
29 g fat
(9 g saturated fat)
740 mg sodium
30 g carbohydrates

47
Number of burritos Joey "Jaws" Chestnut wolfed down in 10 minutes to set the world record at the 2010 World Burrito Eating Championship.

Eat This!

BEST ORGANIC BREAKFAST

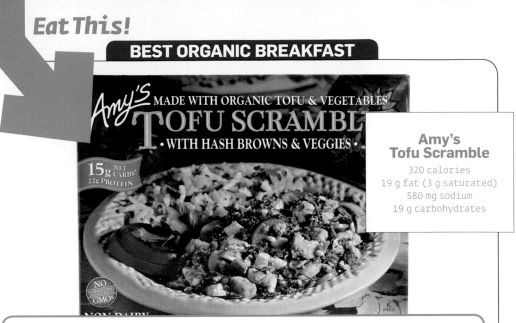

Amy's Tofu Scramble

320 calories
19 g fat (3 g saturated)
580 mg sodium
19 g carbohydrates

To those unfamiliar with tofu's soft, cheeselike curds, you'll find it to be a perfect low-calorie stand-in for scrambled eggs. Especially when sautéed, as Amy's is, in garlic and olive oil alongside a bed of spinach, zucchini, mushrooms, carrots, and tomatoes. The meal could easily stand on its own, but stack a glass of milk next to it for the extra protein you need to muscle through the morning without feeling hungry.

Plus This!

Pear
86 calories
0 g fat (0 g saturated)
1 mg sodium
23 g carbohydrates

Plus This!

Milk *(1%, 1 cup)*
110 calories
2.5 g fat (1.5 g saturated)
108 mg sodium
13 g carbohydrates

= Best Breakfast

516 calories
21.5 g fat
(4.5 g saturated)
689 mg sodium
55 g carbohydrates

----

31 g protein
9 g fiber

ETNT DIET STRATEGY

AVOID FAT-FREE MILK

Sure, fat-free milk will save you about 20 calories per glass, but much of the fat found in milk is the same heart-healthy kind found in olive oil. Plus, studies have found not just that fat will help with absorption of milk's vitamins and nutrients, but that it also helps blunt hunger.

Not That!

Jimmy Dean Bacon, Eggs, Potatoes, and Cheddar Cheese Breakfast Bowl

520 calories
34 g fat (13 g saturated)
1,490 mg sodium
22 g carbohydrates

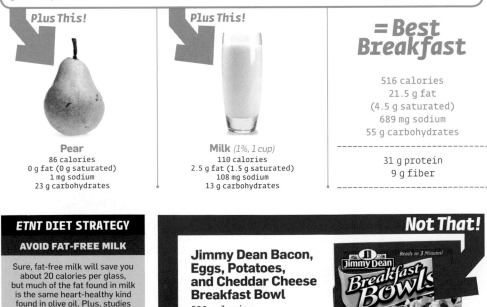

BEST BREAKFAST SANDWICH

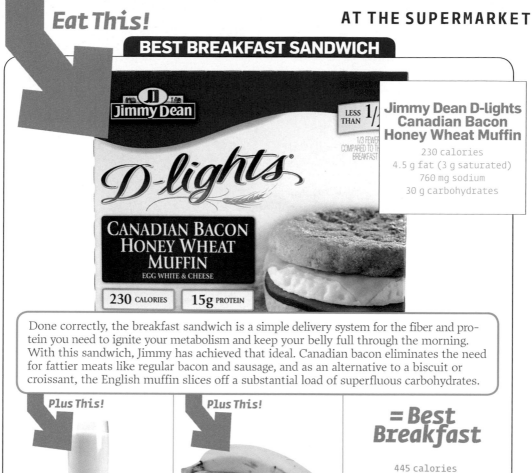

Jimmy Dean D-lights Canadian Bacon Honey Wheat Muffin

230 calories
4.5 g fat (3 g saturated)
760 mg sodium
30 g carbohydrates

Done correctly, the breakfast sandwich is a simple delivery system for the fiber and protein you need to ignite your metabolism and keep your belly full through the morning. With this sandwich, Jimmy has achieved that ideal. Canadian bacon eliminates the need for fattier meats like regular bacon and sausage, and as an alternative to a biscuit or croissant, the English muffin slices off a substantial load of superfluous carbohydrates.

Plus This!

Milk *(1%, 1 cup)*
110 calories
2.5 g fat (1.5 g saturated)
108 mg sodium
13 g carbohydrates

Plus This!

Banana
105 calories
0.5 g fat (0 g saturated)
0 mg sodium
27 g carbohydrates

= Best Breakfast

445 calories
7.5 g fat
(4.5 g saturated)
868 mg sodium
70 g carbohydrates

- - - - - - - - - - - - - - -

24.5 g protein
5 g fiber

- - - - - - - - - - - - - - -

Not That!

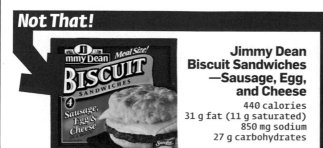

Jimmy Dean Biscuit Sandwiches —Sausage, Egg, and Cheese

440 calories
31 g fat (11 g saturated)
850 mg sodium
27 g carbohydrates

STEALTH HEALTH

BANANAS

Bananas are known for potassium, but they also claim an equally impressive, lesser-known talent. They contain enzymes that stimulate mucus that coats your stomach and effectively functions like an antacid. Work them into your daily diet and you can kiss the Tums good-bye.

Eat This!

Plus This!

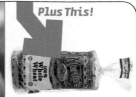

**Martin's Famous
Whole Wheat
Potato Bread**
(1 slice, toasted)
70 calories
1 g fat (0 g saturated)
125 mg sodium
14 g carbohydrates

Plus This!

**Dickinson's
Organic Strawberry
Fruit Spread**
(1 Tbsp)
45 calories
0 g fat
0 mg sodium
11 g carbohydrates
0 g protein
0 g fiber

Scrambled Eggs
with Smoked Salmon, Asparagus, and Goat Cheese
320 calories
17 g fat (6 g saturated)
540 mg sodium
3 g carbohydrates

Two eggs scrambled in a pat of butter contain approximately 200 calories. So how do so many other restaurants sling together scrambles with more than 1,000 calories? Simple: excessive fat and egregious amounts of cheese. This scramble has all the makings of hearty breakfast fare—butter, cheese, protein—but with healthy fats, fresh vegetables, and a light caloric toll. Serve it with toasted wheat bread and fresh fruit preserves.

You'll Need:

1 Tbsp butter

8 spears asparagus, woody bottoms removed, chopped into 1" pieces

Salt and ground black pepper to taste

8 eggs

2 Tbsp fat-free milk

¼ cup crumbled fresh goat cheese

4 oz smoked salmon, chopped

How to Make It:

• Heat the butter in a large nonstick skillet or sauté pan over medium heat. When the butter begins to foam, add the asparagus and cook until just tender ("crisp-tender" in kitchen par-

lance). Season with salt and pepper.

• Crack the eggs into a large bowl and whisk in the milk. Season the mixture with a few pinches of salt and pepper and add it to the pan with the asparagus. Turn the heat down to low and use a wooden spoon to constantly stir and scrape the eggs until they

begin to form soft curds. A minute before they're done, stir in the goat cheese.

• Remove the skillet from the heat when the eggs are still creamy and soft (remember, scrambled eggs are like meat—they continue to cook even after you cut the heat) and fold in the smoked salmon.

Makes 4 servings

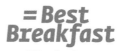

= Best
Breakfast
435 calories
18 g fat
(6 g saturated)
665 mg sodium
28 g carbohydrates
- - - - - - - - - - - - - - - - - - -
40 g protein
5 g fiber
- - - - - - - - - - - - - - - - - - -

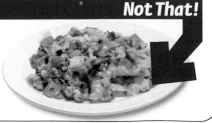

Not That!

Denny's Heartland Scramble
1,160 calories
63 g fat (19 g saturated)
2,930 mg sodium
110 g carbohydrates

Yogurt Parfait

330 calories
8 g fat (3.5 g saturated)
85 mg sodium
49 g carbohydrates

Fruit-flavored yogurts are essentially glorified ice cream, bloated with corn sweeteners and artificial colors. A better option is to buy plain, protein-rich Greek yogurt and add real fruit yourself. We do just that here, layering for visual appeal and tossing in granola for crunch. It's decadent enough to be a dessert but with exactly what you need to start your day: protein and fiber.

You'll Need:

1 cup sliced strawberries

½ cup blueberries (frozen are good, too)

2 tsp sugar

4–5 mint leaves, sliced thinly

1 container (8 oz) low-fat plain Greek-style yogurt (Fage 2% is our favorite)

¼ cup granola

How to Make It:

• Combine the fruit, sugar, and mint in a bowl and allow to sit for 3 to 4 minutes.

• Spoon half of the yogurt into a bowl or glass, top with half of the fruit and granola, then repeat with the remaining yogurt, fruit, and granola.

• Pour any accumulated juice from the fruit over the top.

SECRET WEAPON

MACERATING

Don't be put off by the cooking jargon; macerating is simply soaking or steeping something in liquid or sugar. Most fruit is plenty sweet, but by adding even the barest amount of sugar, you'll draw out the fruit's natural fructose and create a tasty syrup that works over yogurt, pancakes, or even a bowl of ice cream.

Not That!

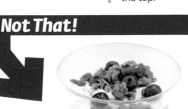

Au Bon Pain Large Vanilla Yogurt

640 calories
13 g fat (4 g saturated)
72 g sugars

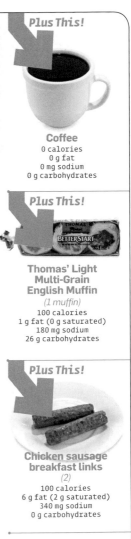

Plus This!

Coffee
0 calories
0 g fat
0 mg sodium
0 g carbohydrates

Plus This!

Thomas' Light Multi-Grain English Muffin
(1 muffin)
100 calories
1 g fat (0 g saturated)
180 mg sodium
26 g carbohydrates

Plus This!

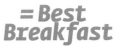

Chicken sausage breakfast links
(2)
100 calories
6 g fat (2 g saturated)
340 mg sodium
0 g carbohydrates

= Best Breakfast

530 calories
15 g fat
(5.5 g saturated)
605 mg sodium
75 g carbohydrates

----

40 g protein
15 g fiber

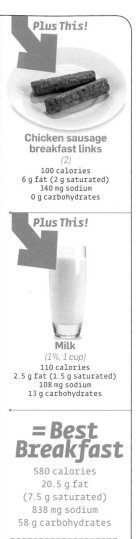

Chicken sausage breakfast links
(2)
100 calories
6 g fat (2 g saturated)
340 mg sodium
0 g carbohydrates

Plus This!

Milk
(1%, 1 cup)
110 calories
2.5 g fat (1.5 g saturated)
108 mg sodium
13 g carbohydrates

French Toast Stuffed with Strawberries
370 calories
12 g fat (4 g saturated)
390 mg sodium
45 g carbohydrates

The word "stuffed" in restaurant parlance is a sure sign of quadruple-digit caloric damage. But done correctly, stuffing can be a nutritional boon: Here, it adds a dose of low-cal protein, fiber, and all the energy-boosting vitamins of fresh strawberries. Plus, it's simple enough to pull off on a weekday morning.

= Best Breakfast
580 calories
20.5 g fat
(7.5 g saturated)
838 mg sodium
58 g carbohydrates

----

39 g protein
6 g fiber

You'll Need:

1 cup low-fat ricotta or cottage cheese

½ cup fat-free milk

2 cups sliced strawberries

2 Tbsp honey

2 Tbsp sliced almonds

1 Tbsp butter

2 eggs

¼ tsp cinnamon

1 tsp vanilla extract

8 slices whole wheat bread

Powdered sugar (optional)

Maple syrup (optional)

How to Make It:

• Place the ricotta, milk, strawberries, honey, and almonds in a mixing bowl and stir gently to combine. Set aside.

• Heat the butter in a

large cast-iron skillet or nonstick pan over medium heat. Beat the eggs with the milk, cinnamon, and vanilla in a shallow dish. Working with one slice at a time, place the bread in the egg mixture, turning it over once to thoroughly coat, then add it directly to the hot pan. Repeat until the pan is full.

• Cook each slice for 2 to 3 minutes per side, until a golden brown crust has formed.

Remove each from the pan and keep it warm in the oven until you're finished cooking. Divide the strawberry mixture to top four slices of toast, spreading it evenly to coat. Top each with another slice to make a sandwich, then slice on the diagonal to create two equal triangles. Serve with a shake of powdered sugar or a drizzle of pure maple syrup, if you prefer.

Makes 4 servings

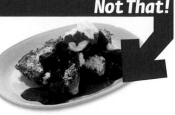

Not That!

IHOP Stuffed French Toast with Strawberry Topping and whipped cream
1,040 calories
54.5 g fat (16 g saturated)
1,160 mg sodium
155 g carbohydrates

Eat This!

Baked Egg with Mushrooms and Spinach

150 calories
9 g fat (2.5 g saturated)
560 mg sodium
8 g carbohydrates

A ramekin can be a vital weapon in the battle of the bulge. These little baking vessels allow you to combine eggs with vegetables, meat, and cheese, pop them in the oven for 10 minutes while you get ready for work, and come back to a perfectly balanced, low-calorie, and above all, delicious, breakfast.

You'll Need:

1 Tbsp olive oil

1 small onion, chopped

2 cups sliced mushrooms

4 slices Canadian bacon or deli ham, cut into thin strips

½ bag (10 oz) frozen spinach, thawed

½ can (7 oz) roasted green chilis

Salt and ground black pepper to taste

4 eggs

How to Make It:

• Preheat the oven to 375°F. Heat the oil in a large skillet over medium heat. Add the onion and cook for about 3 minutes, until translucent. Add the mushrooms and cook for about 5 minutes, until lightly browned. Stir in the bacon, spinach, and chilis and cook for a few minutes, until the spinach is heated through. If any water has accumulated in the pan, drain it into the sink. Season with salt and pepper.

• Divide the mixture among four 6-ounce oven-safe ramekins that have been lightly buttered. Carefully crack an egg into each, making sure to keep the yolks intact.

• Place the ramekins in a baking dish and bake until the whites are just set but the yolks are still runny, about 10 minutes.

Makes 4 servings

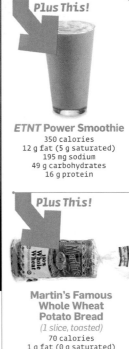

Plus This!

ETNT Power Smoothie
350 calories
12 g fat (5 g saturated)
195 mg sodium
49 g carbohydrates
16 g protein

Plus This!

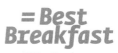

Martin's Famous Whole Wheat Potato Bread
(1 slice, toasted)
70 calories
1 g fat (0 g saturated)
125 mg sodium
14 g carbohydrates

= Best Breakfast

507 calories
22 g fat
(7.5 g saturated)
880 mg sodium
71 g carbohydrates
----
25 g protein
11.5 g fiber

Not That!

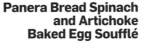

Panera Bread Spinach and Artichoke Baked Egg Soufflé
540 calories
34 g fat (19 g saturated, 0.5 g trans)
910 mg sodium
35 g carbohydrates

SECRET WEAPON

FROZEN SPINACH
The fresh stuff costs a ton, and it's mostly water. You're better off having a few boxes of this nutrient-loaded stuff in the freezer. Simply defrost and it's ready to go.

Eat This!

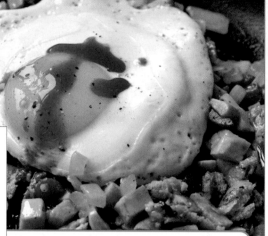

Breakfast Hash with Sweet Potatoes and Chicken Sausage

230 calories
11 g fat (4.5 g saturated)
290 mg sodium
18 g carbohydrates

Hash has long been associated with the oversalted slop that comes from a can, but when you're in control at the stovetop, it can be the base for a spectacular breakfast. Any combination of protein and vegetables qualifies as hash, but by replacing the typical beef with lean chunks of chicken sausage and the greasy spuds with crispy sweet potato nuggets and bell pepper, you end up with a whole that is far greater than the sum of its parts.

You'll Need:

2 sweet potatoes, peeled and cut into ¼" cubes

½ Tbsp olive oil

2 links uncooked chicken sausage (chicken-apple works nicely)

1 yellow onion, chopped

1 red bell pepper, chopped

⅛ tsp cayenne pepper

Salt and ground black pepper to taste

4 eggs, fried sunny-side up

Tabasco sauce

How to Make It:

• Place the potatoes in a medium saucepan and cover with water. Bring it to a boil and cook until fork-tender, about 10 minutes. Drain.

• Heat the oil in a large cast-iron or nonstick skillet over medium heat. Cut open the sausage casing and squeeze the meat directly into the pan, discarding the casing. Sauté for 4 to 5 minutes, until the meat is cooked through. Transfer it to a plate.

• Using the same pan, add the reserved sweet potatoes, the onion, and the bell pepper. Cook until the vegetables are browned, about 7 minutes. Return the sausage to the pan, season with the cayenne and salt and pepper.

• Divide the hash among four plates or bowls. Top each serving with a fried egg and Tabasco.

Makes 4 servings

Plus This!

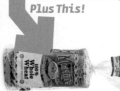

Martin's Famous Whole Wheat Potato Bread
(1 slice, toasted)
70 calories
1 g fat (0 g saturated)
125 mg sodium
14 g carbohydrates

Plus This!

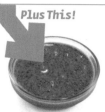

Almond Butter
(1 Tbsp)
100 calories
9 g fat (0.5 g saturated)
0 mg sodium
3 g carbohydrates
3.5 g protein

= Best Breakfast

400 calories
21 g fat
(5 g saturated)
415 mg sodium
35.5 g carbohydrates

24.5 g protein
8.5 g fiber

Not That!

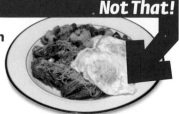

Bob Evans Pot Roast Hash

749 calories
49 g fat (16 g saturated)
1,304 mg sodium
32 g carbohydrates

Eat This!

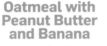

Oatmeal with Peanut Butter and Banana

320 calories
10 g fat (1 g saturated)
190 mg sodium
51 g carbohydrates

Despite its stellar reputation, oatmeal can be problematic. Plain oats are too boring to eat on a regular basis, and flavored oats carry a bevy of excess sugars and other ingredients that don't belong in your breakfast bowl. We solve both problems by using peanut butter and almonds to provide a rich base of healthy fats, and bananas for natural sweetness and a shot of potassium. This is the kind of oatmeal you could—and should—eat 5 days a week.

You'll Need:

4½ cups water
2 cups rolled oats
Pinch of salt
2 bananas, sliced
2 Tbsp peanut butter
¼ cup chopped almonds
2 Tbsp agave syrup

How to Make It:

• In a medium saucepan, bring the water to a boil. Turn the heat down to low and add the oats and salt. Cook, stirring occasionally, for about 5 minutes, until the oats are tender and have absorbed most of the liquid.

• Add the bananas, peanut butter, almonds, and agave syrup and stir to incorporate evenly. If the oatmeal is too thick, add a splash of milk.

Makes 4 servings

SECRET WEAPON

AGAVE SYRUP

Agave syrup is every bit as sweet as sugar, but becase it's made up primarily of fructose, it has a very low glycemic index. Translation: Using agave syrup instead of sugar to sweeten oatmeal or coffee or anything will have a gentler effect on your blood sugar, which in turn can help keep you trim.

Plus This!

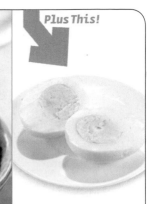

Hard-boiled egg
(1 large)
80 calories
5.5 g fat (1.5 g saturated)
60 mg sodium
0.5 g carbohydrates

Plus This!

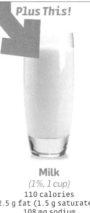

Milk
(1%, 1 cup)
110 calories
2.5 g fat (1.5 g saturated)
108 mg sodium
13 g carbohydrates

= Best Breakfast

510 calories
18 g fat
(4 g saturated)
358 mg sodium
64.5 g carbohydrates

25.5 g protein
7 g fiber

Not That!

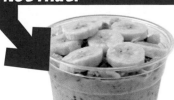

Jamba Juice Ideal Meal Chunky Strawberry

570 calories
17 g fat (2.5 g saturated)
180 mg sodium
92 g carbohydrates

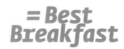

Eat This!

(see page 41)

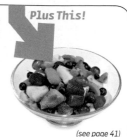

Plus This!

ETNT Fruit Salad
(½ cup)
40 calories
0 g fat
0 mg sodium
10 g carbohydrates

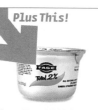

Plus This!

**Fage Total 2% Greek
Yogurt, plain**
(7 oz)
130 calories
4 g fat (3 g saturated)
65 mg sodium
8 g carbohydrates
17 g protein

= Best Breakfast

430 calories
10 g fat
(5.5 g saturated)
505 mg sodium
65 g carbohydrates

26.5 g protein
7 g fiber

Oatmeal Pancakes with Cinnamon Apples

260 calories
6 g fat (2.5 g saturated)
440 mg sodium
47 g carbohydrates

Even seemingly healthy pancakes can pack more than 1,000 calories at a restaurant, but these flapjacks boast extra fiber, protein, and plenty of delicious fresh fruit.

You'll Need:

1 ½ cups buttermilk
¾ cup instant rolled oats
¾ cup whole wheat flour
2 Tbsp milk
1 Tbsp melted butter
1½ tsp baking powder
½ tsp baking soda
Pinch + ⅛ tsp cinnamon
Pinch of nutmeg
1 Granny Smith apple, peeled, cored, and chopped
½ cup apple juice
2 Tbsp brown sugar
Butter or cooking spray
Confectioners' sugar (optional)

How to Make It:

• In a large mixing bowl, combine the buttermilk, oats, flour, milk, butter, baking powder, baking soda, pinch of cinnamon, and nutmeg. Stir to gently combine, then set aside to rest for a few minutes.

• Combine the apple, apple juice, brown sugar, and remaining ⅛ teaspoon cinnamon in a small saucepan and bring to a simmer. Cook until the apple has softened and the liquid has thickened.

• Preheat the oven to 200°F. Heat a large nonstick or cast-iron skillet over medium heat. Add a bit of butter or cooking spray to the skillet (do this before each batch you cook), pour in ¼-cup portions of batter, and use a spatula to spread each into a thin, even circle.

• Cook until small bubbles form in the top of the batter, 2 to 3 minutes, then flip and cook for another 2 minutes. Repeat with the remaining batter. Keep the pancakes warm in the oven while you finish cooking. Serve topped with the warm apples and a bit of confectioners' sugar, if you like.

Makes 4 servings

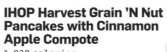

Not That!

IHOP Harvest Grain 'N Nut Pancakes with Cinnamon Apple Compote

1,030 calories
49.5 g fat (12 g saturated)
1,945 mg sodium
97 g carbohydrates

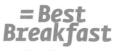

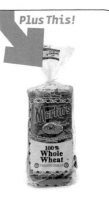

Martin's Famous Whole Wheat Potato Bread
(1 slice, toasted)
70 calories
1 g fat (0 g saturated)
125 mg sodium
14 g carbohydrates
6 g protein

Frittata with Arugula and Peppers

325 calories
21 g fat (6 g saturated)
480 mg sodium
3 g carbohydrates

A frittata is a crustless quiche that's both healthier and easier to make. Cook one at the beginning of the week, then slice off a wedge each morning for breakfast.

Plus This!

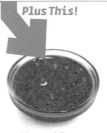

Almond Butter
(1 Tbsp)
100 calories
9 g fat (0.5 g saturated)
0 mg sodium
3 g carbohydrates
3.5 g protein

You'll Need:

½ Tbsp olive oil

¼ cup chopped bottled roasted red peppers

1 clove garlic, minced

4 cups baby arugula or baby spinach

4 thin slices prosciutto or other good ham, cut into strips

8 eggs, beaten

Salt and ground black pepper to taste

½ cup crumbled goat cheese

Other cheeses can be used with awesome

results. Try smoked Gouda, ricotta, or feta. It's your world.

How to Make It:

• Preheat the broiler. Heat the oil in a non-stick, 12" oven-safe skillet over medium-low heat. Add the roasted peppers and garlic and cook for about 1 minute, until the garlic is fragrant but not browned.

• Stir in the arugula and cook for another 2 minutes or so, until lightly wilted. Add the prosciutto, then pour

the eggs over the top. Season the eggs with a good amount of salt and pepper, then dot with the cheese.

• Cook on the stovetop for 5 to 6 minutes, until most of the egg has set. Place the pan 6 inches from the broiler's heating element and cook for about 3 minutes, until the rest of the egg has fully set and the top of the frittata has begun to brown. Cool slightly, remove from the pan, and cut into wedges.

Makes 4 servings

= Best Breakfast

495 calories
31 g fat
(6.5 g saturated)
605 mg sodium
20 g carbohydrates

39.5 g protein
6.5 g fiber

Not That!

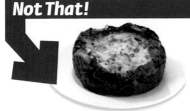

Così Quiche Lorraine
673 calories
48 g fat (26 g saturated)
1,140 mg sodium
29 g carbohydrates

Eat This!

Plus This!

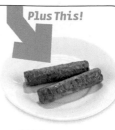

Chicken sausage breakfast links *(2)*
100 calories
6 g fat (2 g saturated)
340 mg sodium
0 g carbohydrates

Plus This!

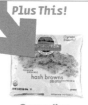

Cascadian Farm Organic Hash Browns
(1 cup)
70 calories
0 g fat
0 mg sodium
17 g carbohydrates

Breakfast Tacos with Bacon and Spinach

360 calories
17 g fat (6 g saturated)
450 mg sodium
31.5 g carbohydrates

While breakfast burritos are now commonplace in the fast food world, tacos remain rare in the a.m. hours. We hope to change that with this recipe, which is both healthier than a burrito (thanks to fiber-rich corn tortillas) and insanely delicious.

You'll Need:

4 strips bacon, chopped

½ onion, chopped

2 cups sliced mushrooms

1 ½ cups frozen spinach, thawed

6 eggs, beaten

Salt and ground black pepper to taste

8 corn tortillas

½ cup shredded Monterey Jack cheese

Salsa

How to Make It:

• Cook the bacon in a large nonstick skillet over medium heat for 5 minutes, until the fat renders out and the bacon begins to crisp. Remove with a slotted spoon and reserve on a paper towel.

• Discard from the pan all but a thin film of the bacon grease. Add the onion and mushrooms and cook for about 3 minutes, until the onion is translucent. Add the spinach and continue cooking until the spinach is heated through. (If any water from the spinach has accumulated in the pan, pour it out.)

• Add the eggs and use a wooden spoon to continuously scrape them from the bottom of the pan as they set. (The goal is to have light, fluffy eggs, and constant movement of the spoon will help you achieve that.) Season with salt and pepper.

• Heat the tortillas in a pan over medium heat. (Or, if short on time, wrap them all together in damp paper towels and microwave for 30 seconds.) Divide the cheese among the tortillas, top with the eggs, and spoon over as much salsa as you'd like.

Makes 4 servings

= Best Breakfast

530 calories
23 g fat
(8 g saturated)
790 mg sodium
48.5 g carbohydrates

37.5 g protein
8 g fiber

Not That!

Jack in the Box Sausage Croissant

570 calories
20 g protein
40 g fat
(16 g saturated, 1 g trans)
780 mg sodium
32 g carbohydrates

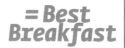

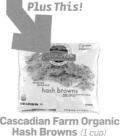

Cascadian Farm Organic Hash Browns *(1 cup)*
70 calories
0 g fat
0 mg sodium
17 g carbohydrates

Smoked Salmon Sandwich
280 calories
10 g fat (3 g saturated)
460 mg sodium
26 g carbohydrates

This is a New York classic, minus the bagel. All the great flavors that make this such a satisfying breakfast are still here—the richness of smoked salmon, the bite of onion and capers, the sweetness of tomato—but by ditching the oversized bagel in favor of whole wheat toast, you save about 200 calories and trade a ton of refined carbs for a boost of fiber. The end result is a sandwich you can feel good about eating every day of the week.

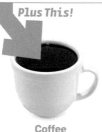

Coffee
0 calories
0 g fat
0 mg sodium
0 g carbohydrates

You'll Need:
8 slices whole wheat or 9-grain bread, toasted
¼ cup whipped cream cheese
2 Tbsp capers, rinsed and chopped
½ red onion, thinly sliced
2 cups mixed baby greens
1 large tomato, sliced

Salt and ground black pepper to taste
8 oz smoked salmon

How to Make It:
• Spread 1 tablespoon of the cream cheese on each of four slices of toast. Top each with capers, onion, greens, and a slice or two of tomato. Lightly salt the tomato, then add as much pepper as you'd like (this sandwich cries out for a lot of it). Finish by draping a few slices of smoked salmon over the tomatoes and topping each with one of the remaining slices of toasted bread.

Makes 4 sandwiches

= Best Breakfast
350 calories
10 g fat
(3 g saturated)
460 mg sodium
43 g carbohydrates

---

20 g protein
6 g fiber

SECRET WEAPON

WHIPPED CREAM CHEESE
The whipping process makes for a creamier spread, and because it's less dense, it has about a third fewer calories than regular cream cheese.

Not That!

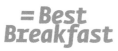

Dunkin' Donuts Multigrain Bagel with Reduced Fat Smoked Salmon Cream Cheese Spread
530 calories
19 g fat (7.5 g saturated)
820 mg sodium
71 g carbohydrates

Eat This!

(see page 41)

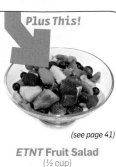

Plus This!

ETNT Fruit Salad
(½ cup)
40 calories
0 g fat
0 mg sodium
10 g carbohydrates

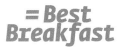

Plus This!

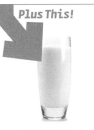

Milk (1%, 1 cup)
110 calories
2.5 g fat (1.5 g saturated)
108 mg sodium
13 g carbohydrates

Crispy Ham Omelette
with Cheese and Mushrooms

330 calories
20 g fat (9 g saturated)
570 mg sodium
3.5 g carbohydrates

Overstuffed omelettes like those at IHOP are eggs at their worst. Why not spend 5 minutes at home making a healthier, tastier version?

You'll Need:

2 Tbsp butter

½ lb mushrooms, stems removed, sliced

Salt and ground black pepper to taste

4 slices prosciutto, cut into thin strips

8 eggs

4 Tbsp milk

1 cup shredded Gruyère or other Swiss cheese

Chives or scallions, chopped (optional)

How to Make It:

• Heat 2 teaspoons of the butter in a medium skillet or sauté pan until foaming, then add the mushrooms. Cook until browned, 5 to 7 minutes. Season with salt and pepper and remove to a bowl or plate.

• Return the pan to the heat. Add the prosciutto slices and cook for a minute or two, until the pieces begin to shrink slightly and crisp up. Set the pan aside.

• Heat 1 teaspoon of the butter in a small non-stick pan over medium heat. Beat 2 of the eggs with 1 tablespoon of the milk and season with salt and pepper.

• Add the eggs to the pan and use a wooden spoon or heatproof rubber spatula to move them around, as if you were scrambling them. Do this for 30 seconds or so, until half of the eggs have set, then use your spoon to gently lift the edge of the omelette and swirl the liquid egg around so it runs underneath to the pan.

• When all but the thinnest film of egg has set, add ¼ cup of the cheese and a big spoonful of the mushrooms. Fold the omelette over and gently slide it onto a warm plate. Garnish with crispy prosciutto and chives (if using).

• Repeat to make 4 omelettes.

Makes 4 servings

= Best Breakfast

480 calories
22.5 g fat
(10.5 g saturated)
678 mg sodium
26.5 g carbohydrates

----

32 g protein
3 g fiber

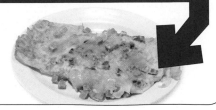

Not That!

IHOP Hearty Ham & Cheese Omelette

870 calories
60 g fat (25 g saturated)
2,270 mg sodium
18 g carbohydrates

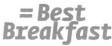

Banana
105 calories
0.5 g fat (0 g saturated)
0 mg sodium
27 g carbohydrates

Plus This!

Breakfast Burrito
415 calories
17 g fat (5 g saturated)
625 mg sodium
36 g carbohydrates

By swapping worthless white tortillas for whole wheat, trading fatty pork sausage for the lean chicken variety, and adding fiber-rich beans, we've created an ideal breakfast in burrito form.

= Best Breakfast
520 calories
17.5 g fat
(5 g saturated)
625 mg sodium
63 g carbohydrates

26.5 g protein
11 g fiber

You'll Need:

- ½ Tbsp olive oil
- 2 chicken sausage links, diced
- 1 red onion, diced
- 6 eggs, lightly beaten
- Salt and ground black pepper to taste
- Fresh cilantro, chopped
- 4 whole wheat tortillas (10")
- 1 cup black beans, rinsed, drained, and heated
- ½ cup shredded Cheddar or Monterey Jack cheese
- 1 avocado, pitted, peeled, and sliced
- Salsa
- Pickled jalapeños (optional)

How to Make It:

• Heat the oil in a large skillet or sauté pan over medium heat. Add the sausage and onion; cook for 5 minutes or until lightly browned. Turn the heat to low.

• Pour the eggs into the skillet. Cook slowly, stirring constantly with a wooden spoon until the eggs are firm but still moist. Remove from the heat, season with salt and pepper, and stir in the cilantro.

• Wrap the tortillas together in damp paper towels and heat in the microwave for 45 seconds. (Or heat them individually in a dry pan until warm and lightly toasted.) Divide the eggs, beans, cheese, and avocado among the tortillas. Roll tightly and top each burrito with salsa, more cilantro, and jalapeños (if using).

Makes 4 servings

MASTER THE TECHNIQUE

PERFECT SCRAMBLED EGGS

It's not about how fast you can scramble an egg, it's about how slow. Start by melting butter in a nonstick pan over low heat until it just begins to turn brown and nutty. Lightly beat the eggs, season with a pinch of salt and pepper, and add to the pan. Use a wooden spoon to keep the eggs in constant motion, scraping the bottom of the pan to remove the cooked egg and expose more raw egg to the hot surface. Right before they look done (while they still have a light gloss on them) cut the heat and stir in any fresh chopped herbs you have on hand.

Not That!

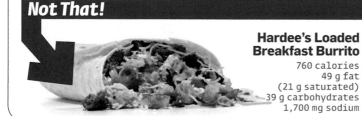

Hardee's Loaded Breakfast Burrito
760 calories
49 g fat
(21 g saturated)
39 g carbohydrates
1,700 mg sodium

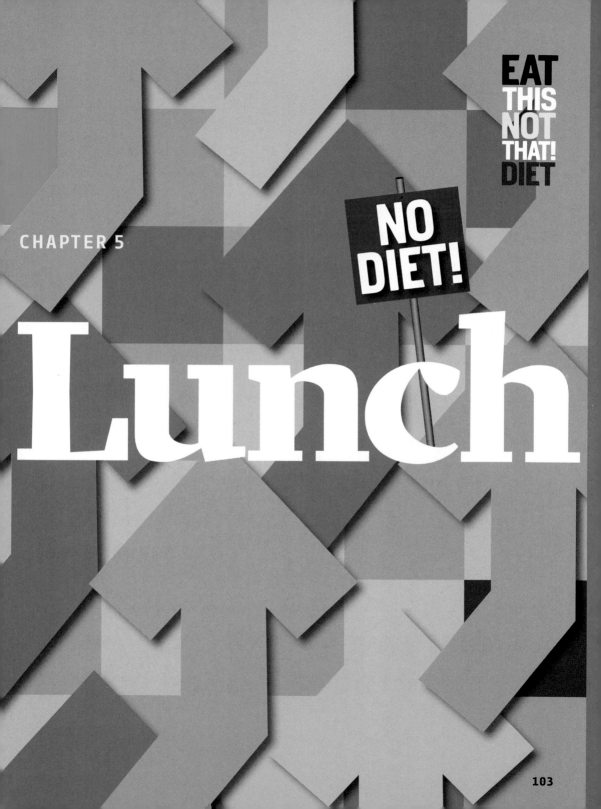

CHAPTER 5

NO
DIET!

Lunch

At most eateries in America, facing lunchtime is like being in the latest *Saw* movie: There are no good choices, and chances are, just getting out alive means that something valuable is gonna have to get lopped off.

Whether you're an office worker, a student, or a harried mom running around to doctor's appointments and school meetings, most lunchtimes consist of being held hostage to a handful of fast-food and sit-down chains. And while brown-bagging it is almost always the healthiest option, for some reason June Cleaver keeps forgetting to stop by our house and make our lunch for us each morning. What's that about?

Part of the problem is that at most restaurants, lunch is simply a slightly cheaper version of dinner. But a robust lunch should have its own nutritional standards—standards that, with a little quick thinking, are a lot easier to meet than the demands of some demented dungeon master. Especially since lunch should offer you a generous helping of calories—between 300 and 600, in fact—because you're still less than halfway through your day and you're going to need energy for later. Here's what a good lunch looks like:

➤ It's got a few more carbs than breakfast had.
This is the meal where carbs come in most handy—that's why a sandwich has bread on both sides, after all. Quick-burning energy will help you power past your 3 p.m. slump. Pasta can be a great lunchtime choice, as well, assuming you can find a bowl for under 600 calories.

➤ It's got vegetables. It's hard to fit enough vegetables into your
day, and dinner can't carry the whole load. A bowl of hearty soup can pack two or three servings of plant matter alone. Not in the mood for a slurpable lunch? Order a side salad whenever your entrée doesn't include something green. If eating out, be sure to pick restaurants that offer some form of vegetable side beyond french fries.

➤ It's got lean protein. Breakfast is the place to splurge on bacon,
fried eggs, melted cheese, and the like. At lunch, think leaner sources of protein—chicken, turkey, and fish should be toward the top of your lunchtime wish list. That will keep your body burning calories, but also begin to dial back on your fat and calorie intake for the day.

The Indisputable Laws of a Lean Lunch

Stop turning your midday meal into a Mayday meal. Avoid these common lunchtime lapses in judgment and start sculpting a leaner body today!

Mistake #1
Making it the second meal of the day

Whether by street cart, drive-thru, or all-you-can-eat buffet, the workday lunchtime is full of temptations. To resist all the creamy, chunky, chewy chow on offer, you need willpower. And how do you build up the willpower to eat less at lunch? By eating more before lunch. Indeed, a mid-morning snack is your most important defense against a fattening lunchbreak.

Here's why: Willpower—the ability to harness the brain's might to resist temptation—is fueled by glucose, another word for blood sugar. When your brain has a steady supply of blood sugar, it has the ability to make smart, well-thought-out decisions. But when it's running low on blood sugar then the next thing you know, you set out to buy a salad and come back with a salami.

So to keep your brain, and your willpower, working efficiently, pack yourself a mid-morning snack rich in fiber, protein, and healthy fats.

Mistake #2
Ordering the Deli "Salad"

On most menus, "salad" denotes some leaf-based bowl of veggies. On a deli's menu, however, it more likely means chicken, egg, or tuna suspended in a massive glut of fatty mayo. Just say no and you'll avoid monstrosities like Quizno's 1,520-calorie large Tuna Melt Classic Sub, which essentially consists of tuna salad glued to bread by mayo and a blanket of melted cheese.

Mistake #3
Hitting the Drive-Thru

This book is packed with smart strategies for making the right choices at your favorite fast-food restaurants. But still, just because you're good at running through minefields doesn't mean you should make them part of your daily routine. According to a 2005 study published in the medical journal the *Lancet*, people who eat fast food more than twice a week carry 10 more pounds of body fat than those who eat fast food less than once a week. What's more, fast-food eaters have a higher rate of insulin resistance, which puts them at risk for diabetes. The point: Whenever possible, pack your own lunch. Make it rich in protein, fiber, and healthy fats, and you'll feel full and satisfied well into the late afternoon hours.

Mistake #4
Falling for the Combo Meal

At every fast-food restaurant, as soon as you decide on an entrée, expect to face some variation of the question "Would you like to make it a combo meal?" Of course you're tempted. This is the modern-day equivalent of supersizing, wherein you get an average of 55 percent more calories for 17 percent more money. It's also the cheapest way for excess sugar, salt, and lard to get you fat in a hurry. Just say no.

Mistake #5
Hoovering It Down

Not all of us can spend our lunchtimes leisurely exercising Ye Olde Expense Account at Le Côte Snob. Sometimes, a lunch hour is a lunch hour and it takes 15 minutes to get to the nearest restaurant. But try to slow down: Dutch researchers recently found that big bites and fast chewing can lead to overeating. In the study, people who chewed large bites of food for 3 seconds consumed 52 percent more food before feeling full than those who chewed small bites for 9 seconds. The reason: Tasting food for a longer period of time (no matter how much of it you bite off) signals your brain to make you feel full sooner, say the scientists. So use the nondiet approach: You're not denying yourself food, you're just eating it more slowly. Savoring it. Allowing your body some time so you don't keep eating when you're full. Two easy ways to slow your consumption: Put your fork down while you chew, or take a sip of water between bites.

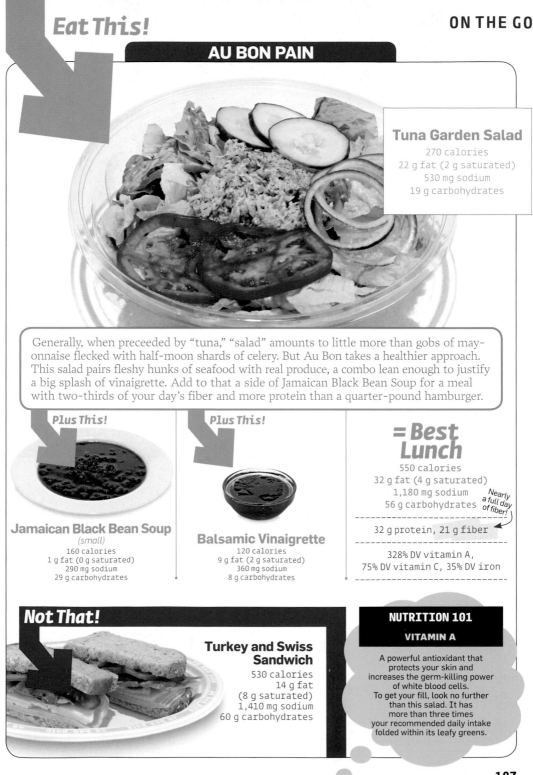

AU BON PAIN

Tuna Garden Salad
270 calories
22 g fat (2 g saturated)
530 mg sodium
19 g carbohydrates

Generally, when preceeded by "tuna," "salad" amounts to little more than gobs of mayonnaise flecked with half-moon shards of celery. But Au Bon takes a healthier approach. This salad pairs fleshy hunks of seafood with real produce, a combo lean enough to justify a big splash of vinaigrette. Add to that a side of Jamaican Black Bean Soup for a meal with two-thirds of your day's fiber and more protein than a quarter-pound hamburger.

Plus This!

Jamaican Black Bean Soup
(small)
160 calories
1 g fat (0 g saturated)
290 mg sodium
29 g carbohydrates

Plus This!

Balsamic Vinaigrette
120 calories
9 g fat (2 g saturated)
360 mg sodium
8 g carbohydrates

= Best Lunch
550 calories
32 g fat (4 g saturated)
1,180 mg sodium
56 g carbohydrates

Nearly a full day of fiber!

32 g protein, 21 g fiber

328% DV vitamin A,
75% DV vitamin C, 35% DV iron

Not That!

Turkey and Swiss Sandwich
530 calories
14 g fat
(8 g saturated)
1,410 mg sodium
60 g carbohydrates

NUTRITION 101

VITAMIN A

A powerful antioxidant that protects your skin and increases the germ-killing power of white blood cells. To get your fill, look no further than this salad. It has more than three times your recommended daily intake folded within its leafy greens.

Eat This!

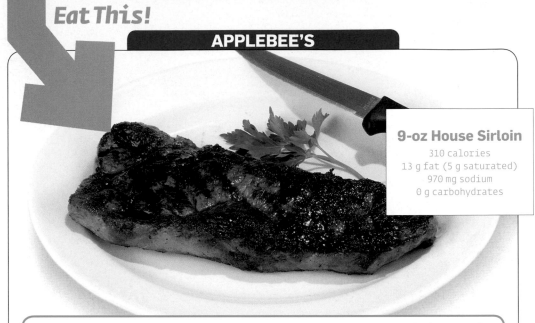

9-oz House Sirloin
310 calories
13 g fat (5 g saturated)
970 mg sodium
0 g carbohydrates

Steak for lunch? Not a problem, as long as sirloin is on the menu. It's the leanest of the commonly available steaks, and the heft of protein will guarantee you a full belly well into the dinner hour. But there's one problem: Applebee's ratchets up the calorie count by adding either a Baked Potato or Garlic Mashed Potatoes on the side. Swap out the usual spuds for Fried Red Potatoes and you'll cut the calories by more than half.

Plus This!

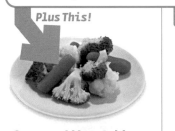

Seasonal Vegetables
45 calories
0 g fat
300 mg sodium
8 g carbohydrates

Plus This!

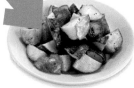

Fried Red Potatoes
150 calories
5 g fat (1 g saturated)
680 mg sodium
22 g carbohydrates

= Best Lunch
505 calories
18 g fat
(6 g saturated)
1,950 mg sodium
30 g carbohydrates

Protein powerhouse!

54 g protein
5.5 g fiber

6,750 ◆
Milligrams of sodium in Applebee's appetizer sampler. That's the equivalent of 450 Doritos Cool Ranch chips.

Not That!

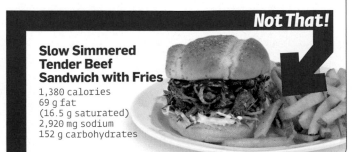

Slow Simmered Tender Beef Sandwich with Fries
1,380 calories
69 g fat
(16.5 g saturated)
2,920 mg sodium
152 g carbohydrates

ARBY'S

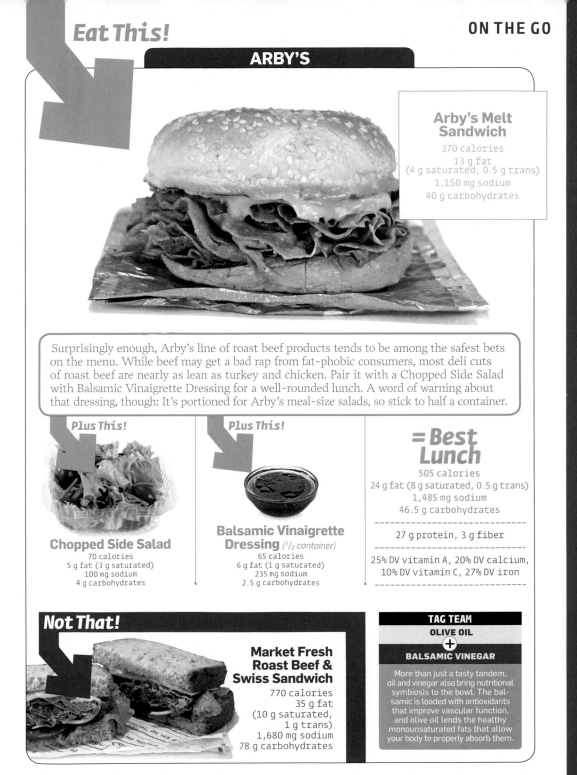

Arby's Melt Sandwich
370 calories
13 g fat
(4 g saturated, 0.5 g trans)
1,150 mg sodium
40 g carbohydrates

Surprisingly enough, Arby's line of roast beef products tends to be among the safest bets on the menu. While beef may get a bad rap from fat-phobic consumers, most deli cuts of roast beef are nearly as lean as turkey and chicken. Pair it with a Chopped Side Salad with Balsamic Vinaigrette Dressing for a well-rounded lunch. A word of warning about that dressing, though: It's portioned for Arby's meal-size salads, so stick to half a container.

Plus This!

Chopped Side Salad
70 calories
5 g fat (3 g saturated)
100 mg sodium
4 g carbohydrates

Plus This!

Balsamic Vinaigrette Dressing (½ container)
65 calories
6 g fat (1 g saturated)
235 mg sodium
2.5 g carbohydrates

= Best Lunch
505 calories
24 g fat (8 g saturated, 0.5 g trans)
1,485 mg sodium
46.5 g carbohydrates

----

27 g protein, 3 g fiber

25% DV vitamin A, 20% DV calcium,
10% DV vitamin C, 27% DV iron

Not That!

Market Fresh Roast Beef & Swiss Sandwich
770 calories
35 g fat
(10 g saturated,
1 g trans)
1,680 mg sodium
78 g carbohydrates

TAG TEAM

OLIVE OIL
+
BALSAMIC VINEGAR

More than just a tasty tandem, oil and vinegar also bring nutritional symbiosis to the bowl. The balsamic is loaded with antioxidants that improve vascular function, and olive oil lends the healthy monounsaturated fats that allow your body to properly absorb them.

Eat This!

BAJA FRESH

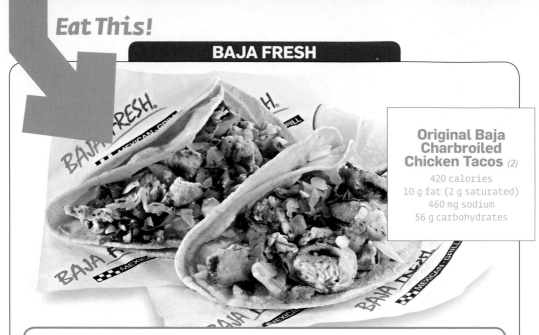

Original Baja Charbroiled Chicken Tacos *(2)*

420 calories
10 g fat (2 g saturated)
460 mg sodium
56 g carbohydrates

This swap just goes to show what sort of impact a simple change of vessel can make in a meal. By moving similar ingredients from a massive flour tortilla to two smaller corn tortillas, you'll save 460 calories, 26 grams of fat, and 1,730 milligrams of sodium. As for the Side Salad: By topping these greens with pico de gallo instead of dressing, Baja Fresh swaps out unnecessary fat for crucial doses of vitamin A.

NUTRITION 101
CILANTRO

Most people interpret cilantro's flavor as clean and citrusy, but because the plant contains aldehydes, to others it tastes soapy. That's a shame for the latter group, especially considering the 2004 study in the *Journal of Agricultural and Food Chemistry* that found that the herb displays antibacterial properties that might help decrease your risk of salmonella poisoning.

Plus This!

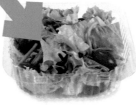

Side Salad
130 calories
6 g fat (1.5 g saturated)
430 mg sodium
16 g carbohydrates

= Best Lunch

550 calories
16 g fat
(3.5 g saturated)
890 mg sodium
72 g carbohydrates

----

29 g protein
8 g fiber

SWITCH IT UP
VEGGIE MIX

Baja's Veggie Mix, a grilled pepper, chili, and onion blend, is typically combined with cheese and sour cream and stuffed into the chain's oversized 800-calorie Grilled Veggie Burrito, but if you order it as a taco topper, you'll earn 6 grams of belly-filling fiber in a modest, 110-calorie package.

Not That!

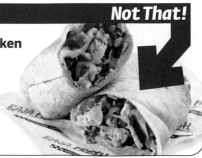

Charbroiled Chicken Baja Burrito

880 calories
36 g fat
(18 g saturated,
1 g trans)
2,190 mg sodium
84 g carbohydrates

BLIMPIE

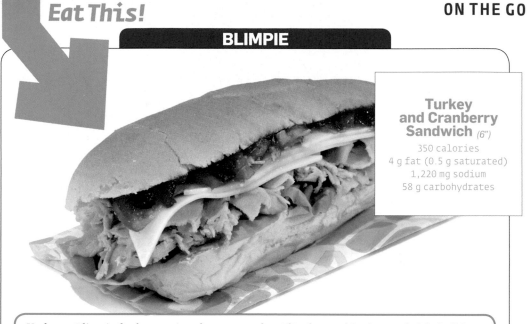

Turkey and Cranberry Sandwich *(6")*
350 calories
4 g fat (0.5 g saturated)
1,220 mg sodium
58 g carbohydrates

Kudos to Blimpie for harnessing the most underutilized spread in the sandwich-builder's arsenal. By displacing mayonnaise and other high-calorie dressings, the antioxidant-rich cranberries help make one of the leanest creations on Blimpie's menu. Try the same move at home by topping a sandwich of smoked turkey, avocado, and Swiss with a few spoonfuls of leftover cranberry sauce and you'll never go back to the fattier stuff.

Plus This!

Garden Vegetable Soup
80 calories
1 g fat (0 g saturated)
620 mg sodium
14 g carbohydrates

= Best Lunch
430 calories
5 g fat (0.5 g saturated)
1,840 mg sodium
72 g carbohydrates

---
25 g protein, 6 g fiber

47% DV vitamin A, 24% DV iron

RESTAURANT SURVIVAL GUIDE

OMIT THE OIL
There's nothing more dangerous than an apathetic sandwich maker with a bottle of oil, but unfortunately that's what you'll find behind many deli counters. At Blimpie, many sandwiches get oiled whether you ask for it or not, so if you decide to stray from the Turkey and Cranberry, be sure to specify "no oil." Otherwise, you're facing 120 calories per half ounce, and there's no telling how much of it will wind up on your lunch.

Not That!

Grilled Chicken Caesar Ciabatta
580 calories
20 g fat
(5 g saturated)
1,480 mg sodium
62 g carbohydrates

NUTRITION 101

CRANBERRIES
These tart little berries are brimming with antioxidants, and one of them, known as ellagic acid, has been shown to kill cancer cells in lab tests. One recent study found that when applied topically, ellagic acid can help prevent skin damage—including wrinkles—caused by sun exposure.

The Eat This, Not That! No-Diet Cheat Sheets

CHICKEN SANDWICHES

		CALORIES	FAT (g)	SATURATED (g)	TRANS (g)	SODIUM (mg)	FIBER (g)	PROTEIN (g)	CARBS (g)
1.	Chick-fil-A Chargrilled Chicken Sandwich	300	3.5	1	0	1,120	3	29	38
2.	Culver's Flame Roasted Chicken Sandwich	309	9	3	0	980	1	27	36
3.	Wendy's Crispy Chicken Sandwich	350	15	3	0	830	2	15	38
4.	Dairy Queen Grilled Chicken Sandwich	370	16	2.5	0	810	1	24	32
5.	Carl's Jr. Charbroiled BBQ Chicken	380	7	1.5	0	1,070	3	30	51
6.	KFC Grilled Doublicious	380	11	4	0	950	2	35	35
7.	Jamba Juice Smokehouse Chicken Flatbread	390	10	4	N/A	690	5	19	53
8.	Hardee's Charbroiled BBQ Chicken Sandwich	400	6	1	N/A	1,370	5	27	62
9.	Arby's Roasted Chicken Fillet Sandwich	400	16	3	0	870	3	24	40
10.	Starbucks Chicken Santa Fe Panini	400	11	6	0	900	11	27	47
11.	Jack in the Box Chicken Sandwich	415	21	3	0	882	2	15	41
12.	McDonald's Premium Grilled Chicken Classic Sandwich	420	10	2	0	1,190	3	32	51
13.	Burger King Tendergrill Chicken Sandwich on Ciabatta	470	18	3.5	0	1,100	2	37	40

BOB EVANS

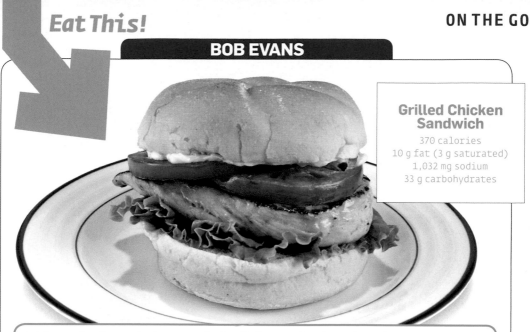

Grilled Chicken Sandwich
370 calories
10 g fat (3 g saturated)
1,032 mg sodium
33 g carbohydrates

It's becoming increasingly rare to find a chicken sandwich not buried under mountains of bacon, cheese, or ranch. To that point, Bob Evans serves three grilled chicken sandwiches that exceed 550 calories, and one of them approaches 950. Tell them to make yours simple, with a toasted bun and plenty of fresh vegetables (just like it's pictured here), and stay far away from terms like Farmstand, Smokehouse, and Club.

Plus This!

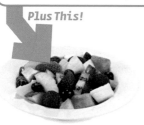

Fresh Fruit Cup
148 calories
1 g fat (0 g saturated)
8 mg sodium
38 g carbohydrates

= Best Lunch
518 calories
11 g fat
(3 g saturated)
1,040 mg sodium
71 g carbohydrates

- - - - - - - - - - - - - - - - - - - -

37 g protein
6 g fiber

- - - - - - - - - - - - - - - - - - - -

879

The average number of calories in Bob Evans beef and chicken burgers. You've been warned.

Not That!

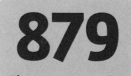

Big Farm Grilled Chicken Smokehouse Burger
941 calories
53 g fat (18 g saturated)
2,468 mg sodium
47 g carbohydrates

RESTAURANT SURVIVAL GUIDE

AVOID THE POT PIE
Seems innocuous, right?
A pie made out of vegetables?
Too bad those vegetables are
bound together with a
creamy sludge and held upright by
a buttery pastry crust.
At Bob Evans that amounts to
862 calories and more than
your entire day's intake of
saturated fat—and you can expect
similar numbers elsewhere.

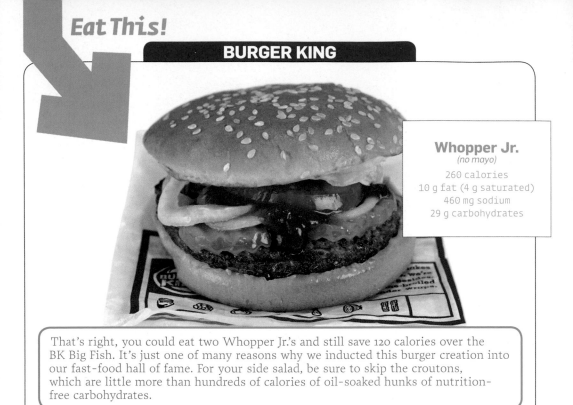

Whopper Jr.
(no mayo)

260 calories
10 g fat (4 g saturated)
460 mg sodium
29 g carbohydrates

That's right, you could eat two Whopper Jr.'s and still save 120 calories over the BK Big Fish. It's just one of many reasons why we inducted this burger creation into our fast-food hall of fame. For your side salad, be sure to skip the croutons, which are little more than hundreds of calories of oil-soaked hunks of nutrition-free carbohydrates.

14 BILLION

Number of burgers Americans eat every year.

Plus This!

Side Garden Salad with Ken's Fat Free Ranch
(no croutons)

100 calories
2 g fat (1 g saturated)
785 mg sodium
17 g carbohydrates

= Best Lunch

360 calories
12 g fat
(5 g saturated)
1,245 mg sodium
46 g carbohydrates

----

16 g protein
5 g fiber

SWITCH IT UP

TENDERGRILL CHICKEN SANDWICH ON CIABATTA

360 calories
7 g fat (1.5 g saturated)
1,010 mg sodium

Order this baby sans the heavy BK mayo application and this becomes a near-perfect sandwich, with a third more protein than a Whopper and less than half the calories.

Not That!

BK Big Fish

640 calories
32 g fat
(5 g saturated,
0.5 g trans)
1,370 mg sodium
66 g carbohydrates

CALIFORNIA PIZZA KITCHEN

Original BBQ Chicken Pizza
(3 slices)

568 calories
9.5 g saturated fat
1,284 mg sodium
68 g carbohydrates

Eating at California Pizza Kitchen is like being on Bizzaro World, where nothing is as it seems. Perfectly healthy-sounding pastas come with quadruple digit caloric price tags while lavish slices of pizza turn out to be relatively prudent picks. It's rare that you get to eat pizza and feel decent about it, so enjoy it while it lasts. (Just be sure to tack on something with real nutrients, like a glass of zero-calorie polyphenol-rich iced tea.)

Plus This!

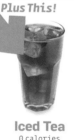

Iced Tea
0 calories
0 g fat
0 mg sodium
0 g carbohydrates

= Best Lunch

568 calories
9.5 g saturated fat
1,284 mg sodium
68 g carbohydrates

----

30 g protein
3 g fiber

SWITCH IT UP

KOREAN BBQ STEAK TACOS

454 calories
3 g saturated fat
645 mg sodium
55 g carbohydrates

You'll find this two-taco duo on the Small Cravings menu, but with 21 grams of protein and 9 grams of fiber, it has all the grit necessary to qualify as a legitimate meal.

Not That!

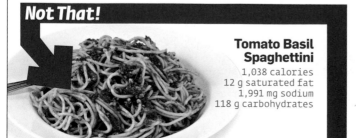

Tomato Basil Spaghettini

1,038 calories
12 g saturated fat
1,991 mg sodium
118 g carbohydrates

MENU UPGRADE

SMALL CRAVINGS MENU

We are often critical of California Pizza Kitchen's menu, but its newest addition, the Small Cravings menu, marks an impressive stride toward redemption. The nutritional safe haven for diners consists of eight small-portion dishes that all weigh in under the 500-calorie mark.

CHICK-FIL-A

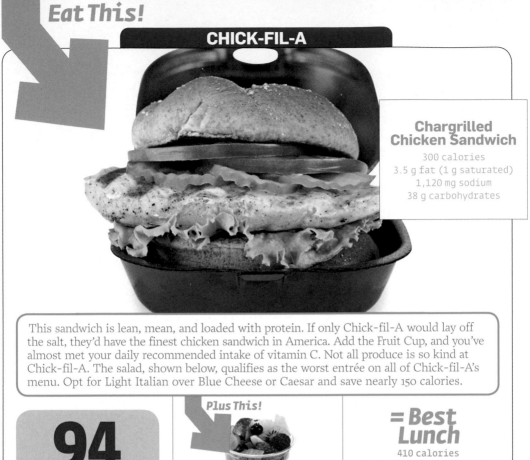

Chargrilled Chicken Sandwich

300 calories
3.5 g fat (1 g saturated)
1,120 mg sodium
38 g carbohydrates

This sandwich is lean, mean, and loaded with protein. If only Chick-fil-A would lay off the salt, they'd have the finest chicken sandwich in America. Add the Fruit Cup, and you've almost met your daily recommended intake of vitamin C. Not all produce is so kind at Chick-fil-A. The salad, shown below, qualifies as the worst entrée on all of Chick-fil-A's menu. Opt for Light Italian over Blue Cheese or Caesar and save nearly 150 calories.

94

Grams of sugar in a large Cookies & Cream Milkshake. That means sugar contributes more than half of the 700 calories in this cup.

Plus This!

Fruit Cup *(large)*
110 calories
0 g fat
5 mg sodium
27 g carbohydrates

= Best Lunch

410 calories

Boost your immune system!

3.5 g fat (1 g saturated)
1,125 mg sodium
65 g carbohydrates

30 g protein, 6 g fiber

40% DV vitamin A, 12% DV calcium, 90% DV vitamin C, 24% DV iron

SUPER SNACK ALERT!

CHICKEN NUGGETS (4 PIECE)

130 calories
6 g fat (1 g saturated)
490 mg sodium
6 g carbohydrates
14 g protein

Each nugget consists of more than 40 percent pure protein, making Chick-fil-A's the best nuggets in the industry.

Not That!

Chick-n-Strips Salad with Blue Cheese Dressing

620 calories
39 g fat (9 g saturated)
1,640 mg sodium
28 g carbohydrates

Eat This!

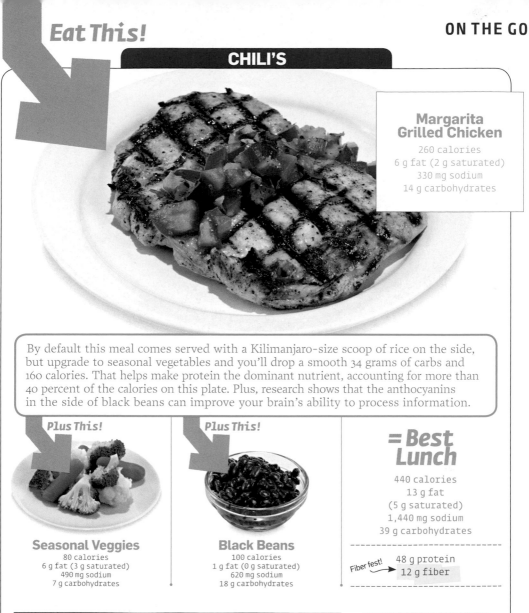

CHILI'S

Margarita Grilled Chicken

260 calories
6 g fat (2 g saturated)
330 mg sodium
14 g carbohydrates

By default this meal comes served with a Kilimanjaro-size scoop of rice on the side, but upgrade to seasonal vegetables and you'll drop a smooth 34 grams of carbs and 160 calories. That helps make protein the dominant nutrient, accounting for more than 40 percent of the calories on this plate. Plus, research shows that the anthocyanins in the side of black beans can improve your brain's ability to process information.

Plus This!

Seasonal Veggies
80 calories
6 g fat (3 g saturated)
490 mg sodium
7 g carbohydrates

Plus This!

Black Beans
100 calories
1 g fat (0 g saturated)
620 mg sodium
18 g carbohydrates

= Best Lunch

440 calories
13 g fat
(5 g saturated)
1,440 mg sodium
39 g carbohydrates

Fiber fest! ➔ 48 g protein
12 g fiber

Not That!

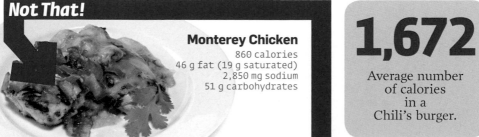

Monterey Chicken

860 calories
46 g fat (19 g saturated)
2,850 mg sodium
51 g carbohydrates

1,672

Average number
of calories
in a
Chili's burger.

Eat This!

CHIPOTLE

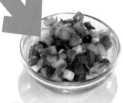

Salad
(with barbacoa, black beans, cheese, and lettuce)

400 calories
17 g fat (8 g saturated)
920 mg sodium
26 g carbohydrates

Chipotle's menu is tricky—it offers a huge range of modification options, so if you're not careful you can end up with a salad that has more calories than a burrito. That said, you can also choose your salad components wisely and end up with a really well-rounded, protein- and fiber-rich lunch. Here's a trick: Salsa provides all the flavor you need, so double up on that and skip the 260 calories in Chipotle's Chipotle-Honey Vinaigrette.

NUTRITION 101
NATURALLY RAISED BEEF

Chipotle's meat is from naturally raised cows, which means it's grass fed and lean. Compared with corn-fed cattle, the meat from cows raised on grass contains more conjugated linoleic acid—which has been shown to reduce abdominal fat and build lean muscle—and has a higher concentration of omega-3 fatty acids. Omega-3s improve your mood, boost your metabolism, sharpen your brain, and help you lose weight.

Plus This!

Tomato Salsa *(3.5 oz)*
20 calories
0 g fat
470 mg sodium
4 g carbohydrates

= Best Lunch

420 calories
17 g fat (8 g saturated)
1,390 mg sodium
30 g carbohydrates

Potent anti-viral agent!

41 g protein, 11 g fiber

108% DV vitamin A, 30% DV calcium, 38% DV vitamin C, 31% DV iron

16

Miles you would need to bike to burn off the 570 calories in a serving of Chipotle tortilla chips.

Not That!

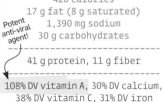

Salad
(with steak, pinto beans, cheese, corn salsa, and Chipotle-Honey Vinaigrette)

750 calories
42 g fat
(11 g saturated)
1,940 mg sodium
51 g carbohydrates

The Eat This, Not That! No-Diet Cheat Sheets

ENTRÉE SALADS WITH DRESSING	CALORIES	FAT (g)	SATURATED (g)	TRANS (g)	SODIUM (mg)	FIBER (g)	PROTEIN (g)	CARBS (g)
1. Chick-fil-A Chargrilled & Fruit Salad with Reduced Fat Berry Balsamic Vinaigrette	300	8	3.5	0	800	4	22	35
2. Così Shanghai Chicken Salad	313	13	2	0	839	4	26	26
3. Quiznos Raspberry Vinaigrette Chicken Small Chopped Salad with flatbread	330	12	3.5	0	760	2	14	37
4. Romano's Macaroni Grill Scallops & Spinach Salad	340	31	6	N/A	820	4	8	11
5. Denny's Cranberry Apple Salad with Chicken and Low Fat Balsamic Vinaigrette	355	11	2	N/A	540	3	36	29
6. California Pizza Kitchen Classic Caesar with Grilled Shrimp (Half)	372	N/A	8	N/A	823	4	27	16
7. Applebee's Steak and Potato Salad	380	12	4	0	1,860	6	35	32
8. Bob Evans Wildfire Grilled Chicken Salad	389	13	5	0	963	6	32	37
9. Panera Full Asian Sesame Chicken Salad	400	20	3.5	0	810	3	31	31
10. Au Bon Pain Mediterranean Chicken Salad with Balsamic Vinaigrette	410	25	8	0	1,590	3	23	20
11. Così Bombay Chicken Salad	481	32	5	N/A	1,094	4	25	17
12. Uno Chicago Grill Walnut Crusted Goat Cheese	500	34	12	0	420	4	20	N/A

Eat This!

DAIRY QUEEN

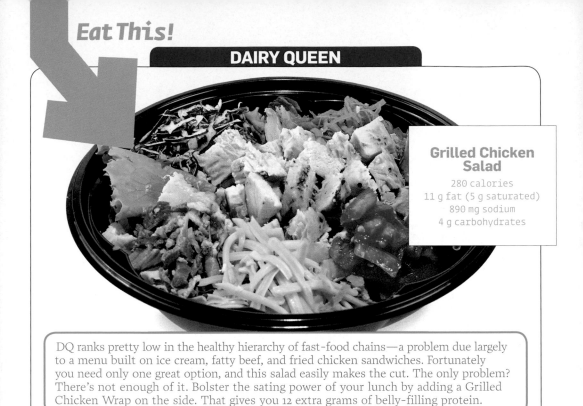

DQ ranks pretty low in the healthy hierarchy of fast-food chains—a problem due largely to a menu built on ice cream, fatty beef, and fried chicken sandwiches. Fortunately you need only one great option, and this salad easily makes the cut. The only problem? There's not enough of it. Bolster the sating power of your lunch by adding a Grilled Chicken Wrap on the side. That gives you 12 extra grams of belly-filling protein.

Plus This!

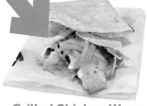

Fat-Free Italian
15 calories
0 g fat
360 mg sodium
4 g carbohydrates

Plus This!

Grilled Chicken Wrap
200 calories
13 g fat (3.5 g saturated)
450 mg sodium
9 g carbohydrates

= Best Lunch
495 calories
24 g fat (8.5 g saturated)
1,700 mg sodium
17 g carbohydrates

---

43 g protein, 5 g fiber

Boost bone strength! 140% DV vitamin A, 80% DV calcium, 26% DV iron

---

MENU UPGRADE
MINI BLIZZARD

In 2010, Dairy Queen introduced a 7-ounce version of its infamous Blizzard, which is 40 percent smaller than its previous "small." That drops a Snickers Blizzard from 670 to 390 calories—still rich, but inching closer to manageable. Split one with a friend and you've got a perfectly portioned dessert.

Not That!

Chicken Quesadilla Basket
1,200 calories
60 g fat
(27 g saturated)
2,740 mg sodium
115 g carbohydrates

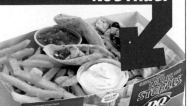

Eat This!

DENNY'S

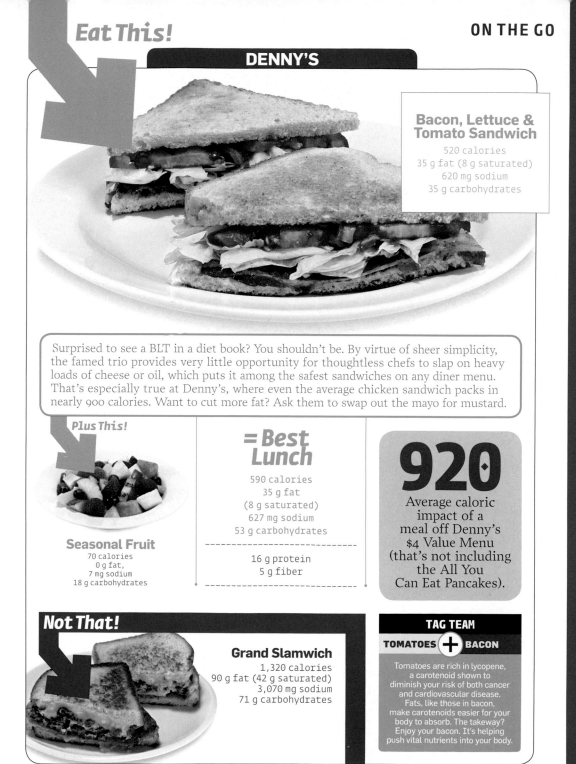

Bacon, Lettuce & Tomato Sandwich
520 calories
35 g fat (8 g saturated)
620 mg sodium
35 g carbohydrates

Surprised to see a BLT in a diet book? You shouldn't be. By virtue of sheer simplicity, the famed trio provides very little opportunity for thoughtless chefs to slap on heavy loads of cheese or oil, which puts it among the safest sandwiches on any diner menu. That's especially true at Denny's, where even the average chicken sandwich packs in nearly 900 calories. Want to cut more fat? Ask them to swap out the mayo for mustard.

Plus This!

Seasonal Fruit
70 calories
0 g fat,
7 mg sodium
18 g carbohydrates

= Best Lunch
590 calories
35 g fat
(8 g saturated)
627 mg sodium
53 g carbohydrates

----

16 g protein
5 g fiber

920◆
Average caloric impact of a meal off Denny's $4 Value Menu (that's not including the All You Can Eat Pancakes).

Not That!

Grand Slamwich
1,320 calories
90 g fat (42 g saturated)
3,070 mg sodium
71 g carbohydrates

TAG TEAM
TOMATOES ➕ BACON

Tomatoes are rich in lycopene, a carotenoid shown to diminish your risk of both cancer and cardiovascular disease. Fats, like those in bacon, make carotenoids easier for your body to absorb. The takeway? Enjoy your bacon. It's helping push vital nutrients into your body.

Eat This!

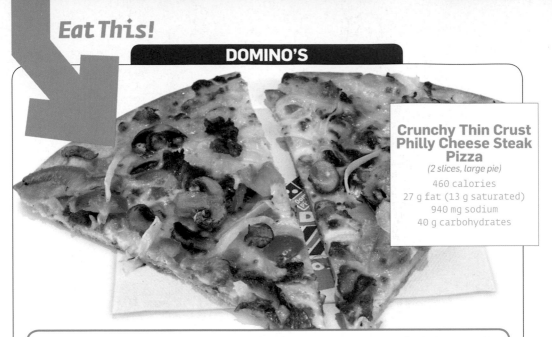

Crunchy Thin Crust Philly Cheese Steak Pizza
(2 slices, large pie)
460 calories
27 g fat (13 g saturated)
940 mg sodium
40 g carbohydrates

A broad selection of toppings and one of the leanest thin-crust pies in the industry make Domino's a surprisingly safe place to grab a meal. Order this pizza exactly like it's pictured here and you save calories in two significant ways: By avoiding fattier meats (Domino's ultra-lean Philly meat has 75 percent fewer calories than sausage) and by dodging the hand-tossed pie, which adds 120 calories to this quarter-pie serving.

MEAT TOPPING TOTEM POLE

(PER 2 MEDIUM SLICES)

HAM
23 calories
1 g fat (<1 g saturated)
255 mg sodium

PHILLY MEAT
23 calories
<1 g fat (<1 g saturated)
125 mg sodium

ANCHOVIES
28 calories
2 g fat, 828 mg sodium

CHICKEN
35 calories
1 g fat (<1 g saturated)
183 mg sodium

PEPPERONI
60 calories
5 g fat (2 g saturated)
255 mg sodium

BEEF
75 calories
6.5 g fat (3 g saturated fat)
143 mg sodium

Plus This!

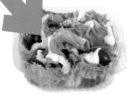

Side Garden Salad
70 calories
3.5 g fat (2.5 g saturated)
80 mg sodium
5 g carbohydrates

= Best Lunch
530 calories
30.5 g fat (15.5 g saturated)
1,020 mg sodium
45 g carbohydrates

----

26 g protein, 4 g fiber

136% DV vitamin A,
54% DV calcium

Not That!

Hand Tossed Sausage and Pepperoni Pizza
(2 slices, large pie)
670 calories
31 g fat (13 g saturated)
1,590 mg sodium
69 g carbohydrates

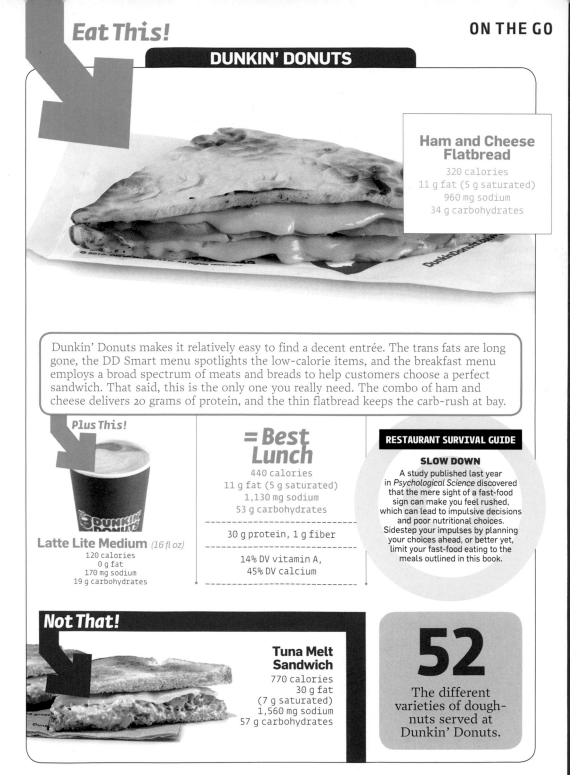

DUNKIN' DONUTS

Ham and Cheese Flatbread
320 calories
11 g fat (5 g saturated)
960 mg sodium
34 g carbohydrates

Dunkin' Donuts makes it relatively easy to find a decent entrée. The trans fats are long gone, the DD Smart menu spotlights the low-calorie items, and the breakfast menu employs a broad spectrum of meats and breads to help customers choose a perfect sandwich. That said, this is the only one you really need. The combo of ham and cheese delivers 20 grams of protein, and the thin flatbread keeps the carb-rush at bay.

Plus This!

Latte Lite Medium *(16 fl oz)*
120 calories
0 g fat
170 mg sodium
19 g carbohydrates

= Best Lunch
440 calories
11 g fat (5 g saturated)
1,130 mg sodium
53 g carbohydrates
————————————————
30 g protein, 1 g fiber
————————————————
14% DV vitamin A,
45% DV calcium

RESTAURANT SURVIVAL GUIDE

SLOW DOWN
A study published last year in *Psychological Science* discovered that the mere sight of a fast-food sign can make you feel rushed, which can lead to impulsive decisions and poor nutritional choices. Sidestep your impulses by planning your choices ahead, or better yet, limit your fast-food eating to the meals outlined in this book.

Not That!

Tuna Melt Sandwich
770 calories
30 g fat
(7 g saturated)
1,560 mg sodium
57 g carbohydrates

52
The different varieties of dough-nuts served at Dunkin' Donuts.

Eat This!

IHOP

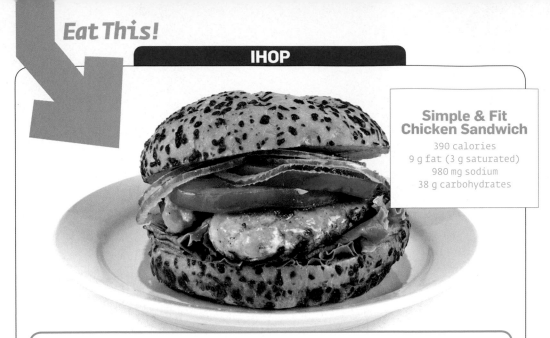

Simple & Fit Chicken Sandwich

390 calories
9 g fat (3 g saturated)
980 mg sodium
38 g carbohydrates

It's difficult to get behind any restaurant that regularly assaults its customers' arteries with a battery of butterfat and bacon grease, but with the Simple & Fit menu, IHOP is making small steps toward healthier fare. This chicken sandwich, a result of those efforts, has as much protein as a 7-ounce sirloin steak and fewer calories than a Tendergrill Garden Salad from Burger King. The pancakes, unfortunately, are still off limits.

RESTAURANT SURVIVAL GUIDE

KEEP IT SIMPLE

The rule of menu nomenclature: The longer and more embellished the name of the food, the more fat, sugar, and sodium it contains. For example, IHOP's French toast carries 640 calories, but the Strawberry Banana French Toast carries 1,060. Similarly, a Hamburger at Applebee's delivers 790 calories, while the fancier Steakhouse Burger with A.1. Sauce swells to 1,190. Stick to basic entrées you know and love and you'll come out ahead almost every time.

Plus This!

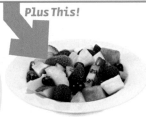

Fresh Fruit

80 calories
0 g fat
0 mg sodium
21 g carbohydrates

= Best Lunch

470 calories
9 g fat
(3 g saturated)
980 mg sodium
59 g carbohydrates

----

42 g protein
5 g fiber

MENU UPGRADE

In 2010, IHOP debuted its SIMPLE & FIT menu, which highlights more than 30 items under 600 calories. The rest of the menu is still atrocious and should be avoided at all costs, but we salute progress of any sort.

Not That!

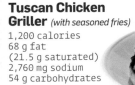

Tuscan Chicken Griller *(with seasoned fries)*

1,200 calories
68 g fat
(21.5 g saturated)
2,760 mg sodium
54 g carbohydrates

KFC

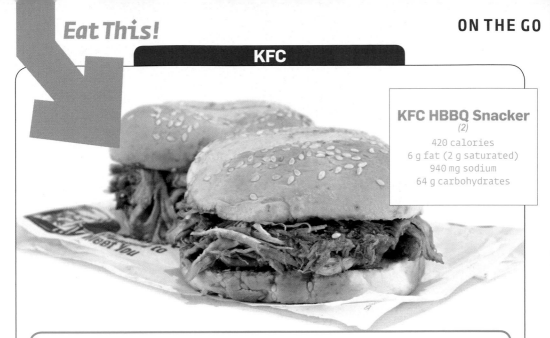

KFC HBBQ Snacker
(2)
420 calories
6 g fat (2 g saturated)
940 mg sodium
64 g carbohydrates

What's great about KFC is that it offers a variety of small dishes (like these Snacker sandwiches, and the Three Bean Salad) that you can combine to form reasonable meals. The surprising thing here is that the HBBQ Snacker, chicken slathered in hickory Honey BBQ Sauce, is the leanest of all of KFC's Snackers (surprising because "honey barbecue sauce" is usually code for "drowning in sugary syrup"). The worst? The Fish Snacker.

Plus This!

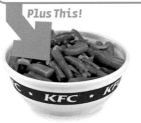

Green Beans
20 calories
0 g fat
290 mg sodium
3 g carbohydrates

= Best Lunch

440 calories
6 g fat
(2 g saturated)
1,230 mg sodium
67 g carbohydrates

----

29 g protein
7 g fiber

CHICKEN
TOTEM POLE

GRILLED DRUMSTICK
80 calories
4 g fat (1 g saturated)

ORIGINAL RECIPE DRUMSTICK
120 calories
7 g fat (1.5 g saturated)

EXTRA CRISPY DRUMSTICK
150 calories
10 g fat (2 g saturated)

HOT & SPICY DRUMSTICK
160 calories
10 g fat (2 g saturated)

HBBQ HOT WINGS (3)
240 calories
12 g fat (1.5 g saturated)

CRISPY STRIPS (3)
340 calories
11 g fat (4 g saturated)

POPCORN CHICKEN (INDIVIDUAL)
400 calories
26 g fat (6 g saturated)

Not That!

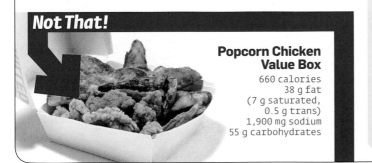

Popcorn Chicken Value Box
660 calories
38 g fat
(7 g saturated,
0.5 g trans)
1,900 mg sodium
55 g carbohydrates

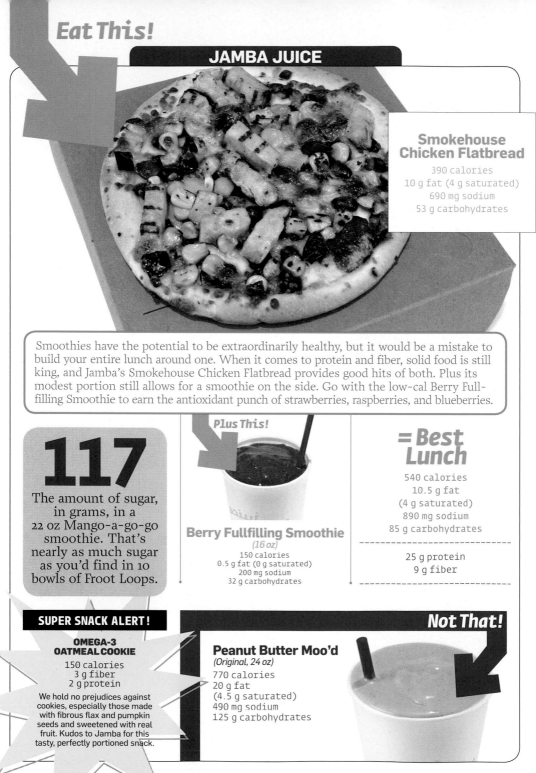

Eat This!

JAMBA JUICE

Smokehouse Chicken Flatbread
390 calories
10 g fat (4 g saturated)
690 mg sodium
53 g carbohydrates

Smoothies have the potential to be extraordinarily healthy, but it would be a mistake to build your entire lunch around one. When it comes to protein and fiber, solid food is still king, and Jamba's Smokehouse Chicken Flatbread provides good hits of both. Plus its modest portion still allows for a smoothie on the side. Go with the low-cal Berry Full-filling Smoothie to earn the antioxidant punch of strawberries, raspberries, and blueberries.

117

The amount of sugar, in grams, in a 22 oz Mango-a-go-go smoothie. That's nearly as much sugar as you'd find in 10 bowls of Froot Loops.

Plus This!

Berry Fullfilling Smoothie
(16 oz)
150 calories
0.5 g fat (0 g saturated)
200 mg sodium
32 g carbohydrates

= Best Lunch
540 calories
10.5 g fat
(4 g saturated)
890 mg sodium
85 g carbohydrates

----
25 g protein
9 g fiber

SUPER SNACK ALERT!

OMEGA-3 OATMEAL COOKIE
150 calories
3 g fiber
2 g protein

We hold no prejudices against cookies, especially those made with fibrous flax and pumpkin seeds and sweetened with real fruit. Kudos to Jamba for this tasty, perfectly portioned snack.

Not That!

Peanut Butter Moo'd
(Original, 24 oz)
770 calories
20 g fat
(4.5 g saturated)
490 mg sodium
125 g carbohydrates

The Eat This, **Not That!**
No-Diet **Cheat Sheets**

FAST-FOOD BURGERS	CALORIES	FAT (g)	SATURATED (g)	TRANS (g)	SODIUM (mg)	FIBER (g)	PROTEIN (g)	CARBS (g)
1. Wendy's Jr. Hamburger	230	8	3	0	480	1	12	26
2. In-N-Out Protein Style Hamburger w/ Onion	240	17	4	0	370	3	13	11
3. McDonald's Hamburger	250	9	3.5	0.5	520	2	12	31
4. Burger King Whopper Jr. (w/o mayo)	260	10	4	0	440	2	13	28
5. Hardee's Regular Cheeseburger	350	19	4	NA	730	1	16	32
6. Culver's Original ButterBurger	351	16	6	1	670	1	19	36
7. Wendy's Double Stack	360	18	8	1	760	1	23	27
8. A&W Hamburger	380	19	6	0.5	860	3	21	33
9. McDonald's McDouble	390	19	8	1	920	2	22	33
10. McDonald's Quarter-Pounder	410	19	7	1	730	2	24	37
11. McDonald's Big N' Tasty	460	24	8	1.5	720	3	24	37
12. Carl's Jr. Big Hamburger	470	17	8	0.5	1,010	3	24	55
13. Wendy's ¼ Pound	470	21	8	1	880	2	26	43
14. Five Guys Little Hamburger	480	26	11.5	0	380	2	23	39
15. Dairy Queen ¼ lb Grillburger	490	24	8	0.5	690	2	26	43
16. Jack in the Box Jumbo Jack	499	27	11	1	782	1	18	45

Eat This!

McDONALD'S

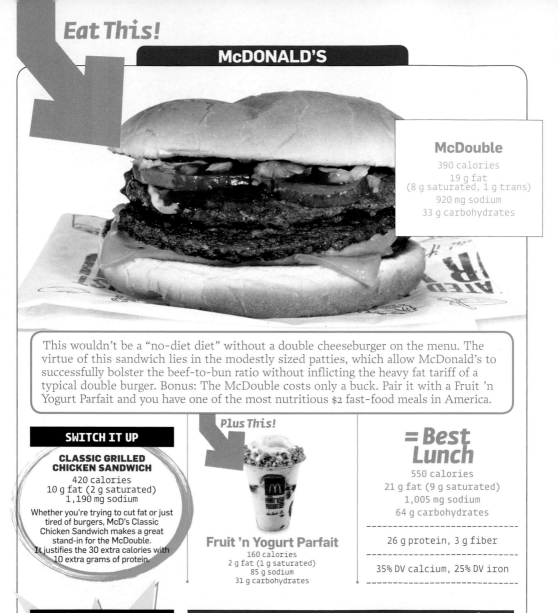

McDouble
390 calories
19 g fat
(8 g saturated, 1 g trans)
920 mg sodium
33 g carbohydrates

This wouldn't be a "no-diet diet" without a double cheeseburger on the menu. The virtue of this sandwich lies in the modestly sized patties, which allow McDonald's to successfully bolster the beef-to-bun ratio without inflicting the heavy fat tariff of a typical double burger. Bonus: The McDouble costs only a buck. Pair it with a Fruit 'n Yogurt Parfait and you have one of the most nutritious $2 fast-food meals in America.

SWITCH IT UP

CLASSIC GRILLED CHICKEN SANDWICH

420 calories
10 g fat (2 g saturated)
1,190 mg sodium

Whether you're trying to cut fat or just tired of burgers, McD's Classic Chicken Sandwich makes a great stand-in for the McDouble. It justifies the 30 extra calories with 10 extra grams of protein.

Plus This!

Fruit 'n Yogurt Parfait
160 calories
2 g fat (1 g saturated)
85 g sodium
31 g carbohydrates

= Best Lunch
550 calories
21 g fat (9 g saturated)
1,005 mg sodium
64 g carbohydrates

----

26 g protein, 3 g fiber

35% DV calcium, 25% DV iron

SUPER SNACK ALERT!

McNUGGETS
(4 Piece)
190 calories
12 g fat (2 g saturated)
400 mg sodium

These nuggets don't offer much in the fiber department, but with 2.5 grams of hunger-quashing protein apiece, you can afford a fiber-less snack.

Not That!

Angus Deluxe
750 calories
39 g fat
(16 g saturated,
2 g trans)
1,700 mg sodium
61 g carbohydrates

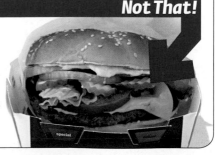

OLIVE GARDEN

Ravioli di Portobello
(lunch portion)
450 calories
19 g fat (11 g saturated)
960 mg sodium
53 g carbohydrates

When it comes to noodle numbers, stuffed pastas like ravioli and manicotti almost always trump regular piles of spaghetti and fettuccine. It seems counterintuitive, but normal noodles are heaped onto plates in indiscriminate mountains, whereas restaurants narrowly define the serving size for a plate of ravioli (say, six for lunch, eight for dinner). It's more than enough to fill you up, but not so much that it fills you out.

Plus This!

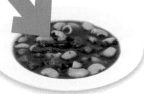

Minestrone Soup
100 calories
1 g fat (0 g saturated)
1,020 mg sodium
18 g carbohydrates

= Best Lunch
550 calories
20 g fat (11 g saturated)
1,980 mg sodium
71 g carbohydrates

- - - - - - - - - - - - - - - - - - - -

11 g fiber

- - - - - - - - - - - - - - - - - - - -

Olive Garden does not disclose protein information.

- - - - - - - - - - - - - - - - - - - -

THE TRUE COST OF FREE

THE FREEBIE
GARLIC BREADSTICKS, UNLIMITED

THE COST
150 calories each

You eat one with your salad, another while you wait, perhaps a third with your entrée without thinking about it. An additional 450 calories just once a week will add nearly 7 pounds of flab in a year.

Not That!

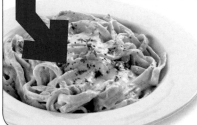

Chicken Alfredo
910 calories
52 g fat
(30 g saturated)
1,150 mg sodium
71 g carbohydrates

SWITCH IT UP

PASTA E FAGIOLI
130 calories
2.5 g fat (1 g saturated)
680 mg sodium
6 g fiber

Don't fall back on salad and breadsticks. This bean-based soup is similar to minestrone, but it harbors twice as much fiber and 33 percent less sodium.

Eat This!

Jalapeño-BBQ Salmon
320 calories
17 g fat (5 g saturated)
305 mg sodium
5 g carbohydrates

Far too many restaurants seem bent on blunting salmon's health boons by drowning it in puddles of cream and butter, but with this fillet, On the Border has taken a smarter approach. The tender fish is dressed in a light glaze and topped with pico de gallo, which, in our book, is one of the world's great condiments. The fact that it's also loaded with antioxidants—and carries almost zero calories—is just a bonus.

Plus This!

Black Beans
180 calories
3 g fat (1 g saturated)
830 mg sodium
29 g carbohydrates

Plus This!

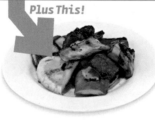

Grilled Vegetables
90 calories
1 g fat (0 g saturated)
85 mg sodium
11 g carbohydrates

= Best Lunch
590 calories
21 g fat
(6 g saturated)
1,220 mg sodium
45 g carbohydrates

96% of your DV! 54 g protein
24 g fiber

NUTRITION 101
OMEGA-3 FATTY ACIDS

Omega-3s are concentrated in fatty fish such as salmon and sardines, and they're credited with an incredibly wide range of health benefits. Among them are preventing heart disease and stroke, bolstering brain function, fighting depression, and improving skin tone.

Not That!

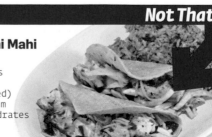

Grilled Mahi Mahi Tacos

1,130 calories
58 g fat
(13 g saturated)
2,150 mg sodium
116 g carbohydrates

OUTBACK STEAKHOUSE

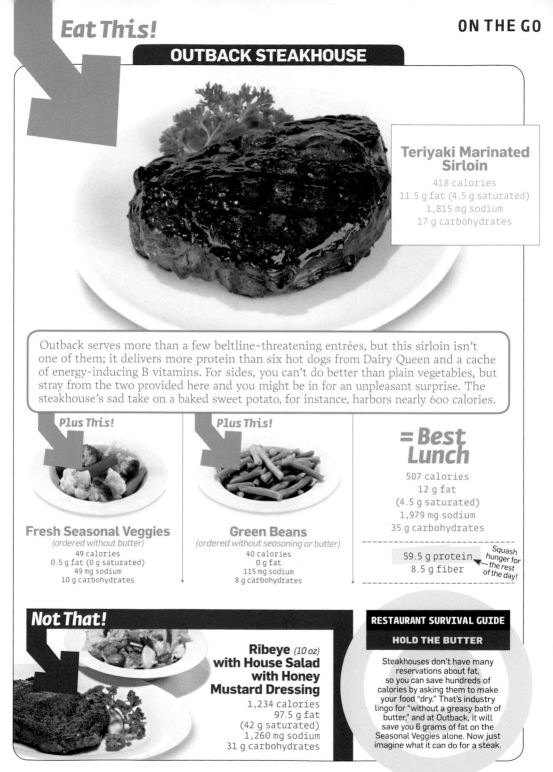

Teriyaki Marinated Sirloin

418 calories
11.5 g fat (4.5 g saturated)
1,815 mg sodium
17 g carbohydrates

Outback serves more than a few beltline-threatening entrées, but this sirloin isn't one of them; it delivers more protein than six hot dogs from Dairy Queen and a cache of energy-inducing B vitamins. For sides, you can't do better than plain vegetables, but stray from the two provided here and you might be in for an unpleasant surprise. The steakhouse's sad take on a baked sweet potato, for instance, harbors nearly 600 calories.

Plus This!

Fresh Seasonal Veggies
(ordered without butter)
49 calories
0.5 g fat (0 g saturated)
49 mg sodium
10 g carbohydrates

Plus This!

Green Beans
(ordered without seasoning or butter)
40 calories
0 g fat
115 mg sodium
8 g carbohydrates

= Best Lunch

507 calories
12 g fat
(4.5 g saturated)
1,979 mg sodium
35 g carbohydrates

- -

59.5 g protein
8.5 g fiber

Squash hunger for the rest of the day!

Not That!

Ribeye *(10 oz)* with House Salad with Honey Mustard Dressing

1,234 calories
97.5 g fat
(42 g saturated)
1,260 mg sodium
31 g carbohydrates

RESTAURANT SURVIVAL GUIDE

HOLD THE BUTTER

Steakhouses don't have many reservations about fat, so you can save hundreds of calories by asking them to make your food "dry." That's industry lingo for "without a greasy bath of butter," and at Outback, it will save you 6 grams of fat on the Seasonal Veggies alone. Now just imagine what it can do for a steak.

Eat This!

P.F. CHANG'S

Buddha's Feast Lunch Bowl

(steamed and on brown rice)

420 calories
4 g fat (0 g saturated)
160 mg sodium
78 g carbohydrates

P.F. Chang's menu is a minefield of entrées hovering around 1,000 calories and packing unthinkable loads of sodium. But follow Buddha to reach nutritional nirvana. Not only does this dish help you avoid the more nefarious items on the menu, but it also pads your belly with a stout load of fiber and flab-melting nutrients. Just be sure to order it steamed—the stir-fry treatment adds 160 additional calories.

RESTAURANT SURVIVAL GUIDE

STICK TO SMALL ENTRÉES

As it turns out, eating less food won't leave you feeling deprived. In one study, Penn State researchers found that subjects ate 30 percent more food when presented with bigger portions, yet their perceived fullness didn't change. The point is it takes less food than you think to fill your stomach. Anything you eat beyond that just adds inches to your waistline.

Plus This!

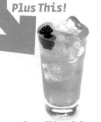

Jasmine Blackberry Tea
0 calories
0 g fat
0 mg sodium
0 g carbohydrates

= Best Lunch

420 calories
4 g fat
(0 g saturated)
160 mg sodium
78 g carbohydrates

----

20 g protein
10 g fiber

NUTRITION 101

BROWN RICE

When food processors leave rice's germ and bran layers intact, the result is brown rice. So how does it compare to the traditional white stuff? It packs an extra payload of B vitamins, an extra touch of protein, and about 6 times as much fiber.

Not That!

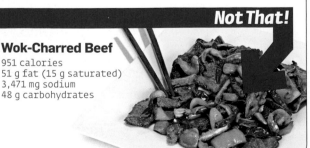

Wok-Charred Beef
951 calories
51 g fat (15 g saturated)
3,471 mg sodium
48 g carbohydrates

PANDA EXPRESS

Mushroom Chicken
220 calories
13 g fat (3 g saturated)
780 mg sodium
9 g carbohydrates

Like so many chain restaurants, Panda Express sets you up for failure by the very nature of their menu concept. Unless you order à la carte, Panda meals come with rice or noodles, each packing more than 400 calories of empty carbohydrates onto your plate. Thankfully, there's an easy fix: Nix the starch and combine two meat dishes instead. You'll have more protein, more vegetables, and more flavor for about half the calories.

Plus This!

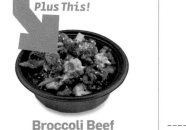

Broccoli Beef
180 calories
9 g fat (2 g saturated)
670 mg sodium
11 g carbohydrates

= Best Lunch
400 calories
22 g fat
(5 g saturated)
1,450 mg sodium
20 g carbohydrates

----

30 g protein
5 g fiber

NUTRITION 101
STARCH

You know starch can make your shirts stiffer, but it can also make what's under your shirt softer. Starches, or "simple carbohydrates," are long chains of easily digestible sugar molecules that spike your blood sugar and force your body into fat-storage mode. That's why studies find that people who cut starches, like Panda's white rice or chow mein noodles, from their diets are more successful at preventing weight gain.

Not That!

Orange Chicken with Steamed Rice
820 calories
20 g fat
(3.5 g saturated)
640 mg sodium
135 g carbohydrates

SUPER SNACK ALERT!

VEGGIE SPRING ROLLS (2)
160 calories
7 g fat (1 g saturated)
540 mg sodium
4 g fiber

Sure they're fried, but for half the calories and fat you end up with four times the amount of fiber you'd find in a typical side of fast food french fries.

Eat This!

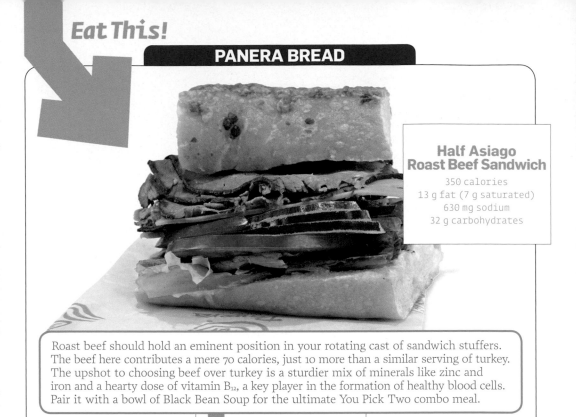

Half Asiago Roast Beef Sandwich

350 calories
13 g fat (7 g saturated)
630 mg sodium
32 g carbohydrates

Roast beef should hold an eminent position in your rotating cast of sandwich stuffers. The beef here contributes a mere 70 calories, just 10 more than a similar serving of turkey. The upshot to choosing beef over turkey is a sturdier mix of minerals like zinc and iron and a hearty dose of vitamin B$_{12}$, a key player in the formation of healthy blood cells. Pair it with a bowl of Black Bean Soup for the ultimate You Pick Two combo meal.

SOUP SELECTOR

(PER CUP)

CHICKEN NOODLE
90 calories
3 g fat (0 g saturated)
1,160 mg sodium

LOW-FAT GARDEN VEGETABLE WITH PESTO
110 calories
2 g fat (0 g saturated)
830 mg sodium

VEGETARIAN BLACK BEAN
110 calories
2.5 g fat (1 g saturated)
980 mg sodium

BROCCOLI CHEDDAR
190 calories
10 g fat (6 g saturated)
1,020 mg sodium

CREAMY TOMATO SOUP WITH CROUTONS
300 calories
18 g fat (9 g saturated)
580 mg sodium

NEW ENGLAND CLAM CHOWDER
300 calories
23 g fat (13 g saturated)
790 mg sodium

Plus This!

Low-Fat Vegetarian Black Bean Soup
110 calories
2.5 g fat (1 g saturated)
980 mg sodium
18 g carbohydrates

= Best Lunch

460 calories
15.5 g fat (8 g saturated)
1,610 mg sodium
50 g carbohydrates

----
30 g protein, 4 g fiber

20% DV vitamin A, 30% DV calcium,
50% DV vitamin C, 35% DV iron

Not That!

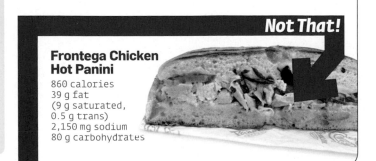

Frontega Chicken Hot Panini
860 calories
39 g fat
(9 g saturated,
0.5 g trans)
2,150 mg sodium
80 g carbohydrates

PAPA JOHN'S

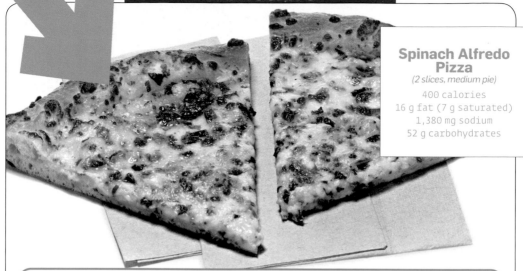

Spinach Alfredo Pizza
(2 slices, medium pie)

400 calories
16 g fat (7 g saturated)
1,380 mg sodium
52 g carbohydrates

Just call it the "business-meets-pleasure" pizza. Spinach? That's your business. And Alfredo, well, that's creamy pleasure, plain and simple. Yet, surprisingly, this pie still manages to land itself among the leanest on Papa John's specialty pizza menu, matched in calories only by the Garden Fresh Pizza. What's even better, this two-slice serving undercuts John's Favorite Pizza by a staggering 180 calories and 14 grams of fat.

Plus This!

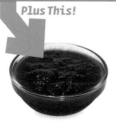

Pizza Sauce *(1 cup)*
20 calories
1 g fat (0 g saturated)
230 mg sodium
3 g carbohydrates

= Best Lunch
420 calories
17 g fat (7 g saturated)
1,610 mg sodium
55 g carbohydrates

----

16 g protein, 2 g fiber

34% DV vitamin A,
40% DV calcium, 16% DV iron

DIP SELECTOR

(PER CUP)

BUFFALO
15 calories
0.5 g fat, 1,030 mg sodium

PIZZA
20 calories
1 g fat, 230 mg sodium

CHEESE
40 calories
3.5 g fat (1 g saturated)
160 mg sodium

BBQ
45 calories
0 g fat, 240 mg sodium

HONEY MUSTARD
150 calories
15 g fat (2.5 g saturated)
120 mg sodium

GARLIC
150 calories
17 g fat (3 g saturated)
310 mg sodium

BLUE CHEESE
160 calories
16 g fat (3.5 g saturated)
250 mg sodium

Not That!

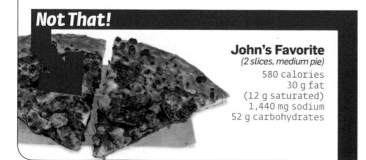

John's Favorite
(2 slices, medium pie)
580 calories
30 g fat
(12 g saturated)
1,440 mg sodium
52 g carbohydrates

Eat This!

PIZZA HUT

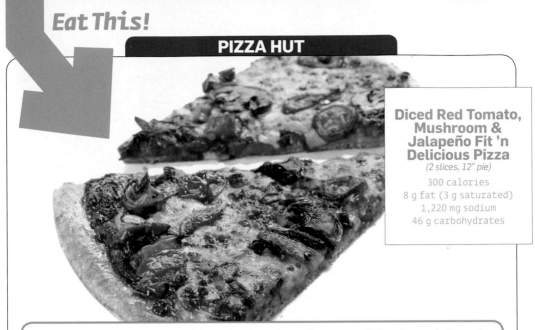

Diced Red Tomato, Mushroom & Jalapeño Fit 'n Delicious Pizza
(2 slices, 12" pie)

300 calories
8 g fat (3 g saturated)
1,220 mg sodium
46 g carbohydrates

It might not taste like a slice of Naples, but this—thin crust, light cheese, balanced topping distribution—is closer to the Italian ideal than that Supreme Pan Pizza. See, when it comes to a healthy slice of pie, crust is everything. Go thin and crispy over deep and doughy and you'll cut hundreds of calories from your plate without having to sacrifice any toppings.

BUFFALO WING
TOTEM POLE

(PER TWO PIECES)

ALL AMERICAN TRADITIONAL WINGS
80 calories
5 g fat (1.5 g saturated)
290 mg sodium

BAKED HOT WINGS
100 calories
6 g fat (2 g saturated)
430 mg sodium

HONEY BBQ TRADITIONAL WINGS
140 calories
5 g fat (1.5 g saturated)
530 mg sodium

MEDIUM BUFFALO BONE OUT WINGS
190 calories
9 g fat (1.5 g saturated)
990 mg sodium

SPICY ASIAN CRISPY BONE IN WINGS
250 calories
14 g fat (2.5 g saturated)
710 mg sodium

Plus This!

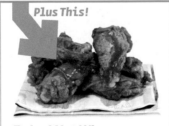

Baked Hot Wings *(2 pieces)*
100 calories
6 g fat (2 g saturated)
430 mg sodium
1 g carbohydrates

= Best Lunch

400 calories
14 g fat
(5 g saturated)
1,650 mg sodium
47 g carbohydrates

----

22 g protein
4 g fiber

Not That!

Supreme Pan Pizza
(2 slices, 12" crust)
580 calories
28 g fat (10 g saturated)
1,300 mg sodium
54 g carbohydrates

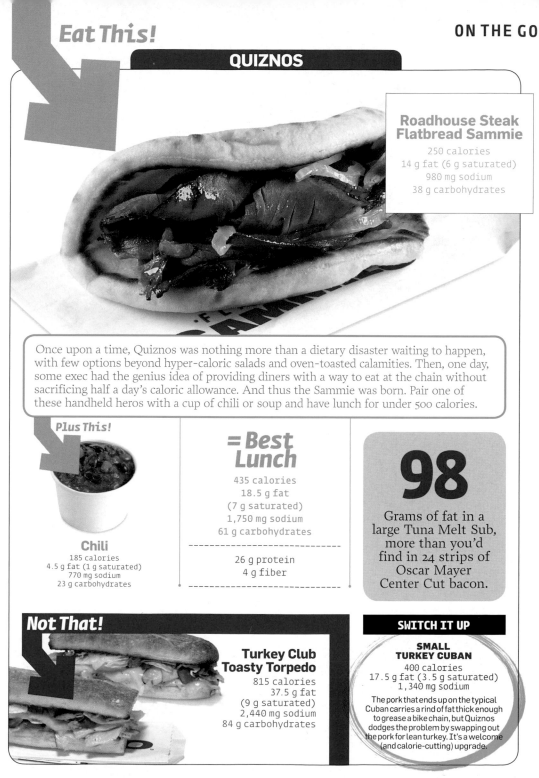

QUIZNOS

Roadhouse Steak Flatbread Sammie

250 calories
14 g fat (6 g saturated)
980 mg sodium
38 g carbohydrates

Once upon a time, Quiznos was nothing more than a dietary disaster waiting to happen, with few options beyond hyper-caloric salads and oven-toasted calamities. Then, one day, some exec had the genius idea of providing diners with a way to eat at the chain without sacrificing half a day's caloric allowance. And thus the Sammie was born. Pair one of these handheld heros with a cup of chili or soup and have lunch for under 500 calories.

Plus This!

Chili
185 calories
4.5 g fat (1 g saturated)
770 mg sodium
23 g carbohydrates

= Best Lunch

435 calories
18.5 g fat
(7 g saturated)
1,750 mg sodium
61 g carbohydrates

----

26 g protein
4 g fiber

98

Grams of fat in a large Tuna Melt Sub, more than you'd find in 24 strips of Oscar Mayer Center Cut bacon.

Not That!

Turkey Club Toasty Torpedo
815 calories
37.5 g fat
(9 g saturated)
2,440 mg sodium
84 g carbohydrates

SWITCH IT UP

SMALL TURKEY CUBAN
400 calories
17.5 g fat (3.5 g saturated)
1,340 mg sodium

The pork that ends up on the typical Cuban carries a rind of fat thick enough to grease a bike chain, but Quiznos dodges the problem by swapping out the pork for lean turkey. It's a welcome (and calorie-cutting) upgrade.

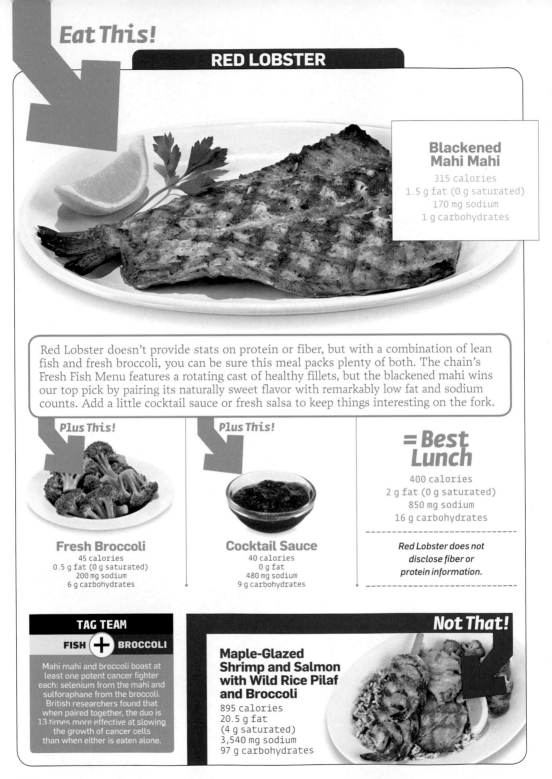

RED LOBSTER

Blackened Mahi Mahi
315 calories
1.5 g fat (0 g saturated)
170 mg sodium
1 g carbohydrates

Red Lobster doesn't provide stats on protein or fiber, but with a combination of lean fish and fresh broccoli, you can be sure this meal packs plenty of both. The chain's Fresh Fish Menu features a rotating cast of healthy fillets, but the blackened mahi wins our top pick by pairing its naturally sweet flavor with remarkably low fat and sodium counts. Add a little cocktail sauce or fresh salsa to keep things interesting on the fork.

Plus This!

Fresh Broccoli
45 calories
0.5 g fat (0 g saturated)
200 mg sodium
6 g carbohydrates

Plus This!

Cocktail Sauce
40 calories
0 g fat
480 mg sodium
9 g carbohydrates

= Best Lunch
400 calories
2 g fat (0 g saturated)
850 mg sodium
16 g carbohydrates

Red Lobster does not disclose fiber or protein information.

TAG TEAM
FISH + BROCCOLI

Mahi mahi and broccoli boast at least one potent cancer fighter each: selenium from the mahi and sulforaphane from the broccoli. British researchers found that when paired together, the duo is 13 times more effective at slowing the growth of cancer cells than when either is eaten alone.

Not That!

Maple-Glazed Shrimp and Salmon with Wild Rice Pilaf and Broccoli
895 calories
20.5 g fat
(4 g saturated)
3,540 mg sodium
97 g carbohydrates

ROMANO'S MACARONI GRILL

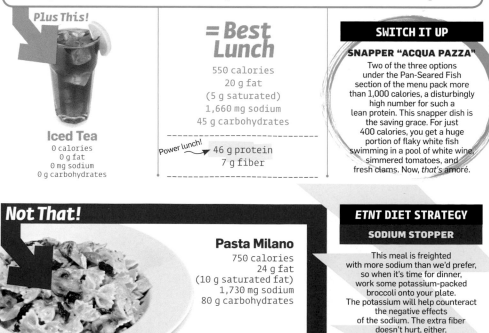

Pollo Caprese
550 calories
20 g fat (5 g saturated)
1,660 mg sodium
45 g carbohydrates

Americans love a good tale of redemption, and few are more dramatic than Macaroni Grill's. Once among the worst restaurants in America, the Italian chain underwent a sweeping overhaul of their offerings in 2009 and now claim one of the healthiest menus you'll find outside of your own kitchen. Dishes like the Pollo Caprese, with a perfect balance of carbs, fat, and protein, are now the rule, not the exception.

Plus This!

Iced Tea
0 calories
0 g fat
0 mg sodium
0 g carbohydrates

= Best Lunch
550 calories
20 g fat
(5 g saturated)
1,660 mg sodium
45 g carbohydrates

Power lunch! → 46 g protein
7 g fiber

SWITCH IT UP

SNAPPER "ACQUA PAZZA"
Two of the three options under the Pan-Seared Fish section of the menu pack more than 1,000 calories, a disturbingly high number for such a lean protein. This snapper dish is the saving grace. For just 400 calories, you get a huge portion of flaky white fish swimming in a pool of white wine, simmered tomatoes, and fresh clams. Now, *that's* amoré.

Not That!

Pasta Milano
750 calories
24 g fat
(10 g saturated fat)
1,730 mg sodium
80 g carbohydrates

ETNT DIET STRATEGY

SODIUM STOPPER

This meal is freighted with more sodium than we'd prefer, so when it's time for dinner, work some potassium-packed broccoli onto your plate. The potassium will help counteract the negative effects of the sodium. The extra fiber doesn't hurt, either.

The Eat This, Not That! No-Diet Cheat Sheets

FRIES	CALORIES	FAT (g)	SATURATED (g)	TRANS (g)	SODIUM (mg)	FIBER (g)	PROTEIN (g)	CARBS (g)
1. **KFC Potato Wedges**	260	13	2.5	0	740	3	4	33
2. **Dairy Queen Regular Fries**	310	13	2	0	640	3	4	43
3. **Sonic Medium French Fries**	330	13	2.5	0	440	4	4	48
4. **McDonald's Medium French Fries**	380	19	2.5	0	270	5	4	48
5. **Culver's Crinkle Cut Regular Fries**	385	17	3	0	56	4	5	53
6. **In-N-Out Burger French Fries**	395	18	5	0	245	2	7	54
7. **Wendy's Medium Natural-Cut French Fries**	420	20	3.5	0	500	6	5	54
8. **Jack in the Box Medium Fries**	443	20	2	0	809	4	5	60
9. **Chick-fil-A Waffle Medium Potato Fries**	380	21	4	0	190	4	4	45
10. **Red Robin Steak Fries**	434	18	N/A	N/A	774	4	6	60
11. **Burger King Medium Fries**	440	22	4.5	0	670	5	5	56
12. **Carl's Jr. Medium Natural-Cut Fries**	430	21	4	0	870	5	5	56

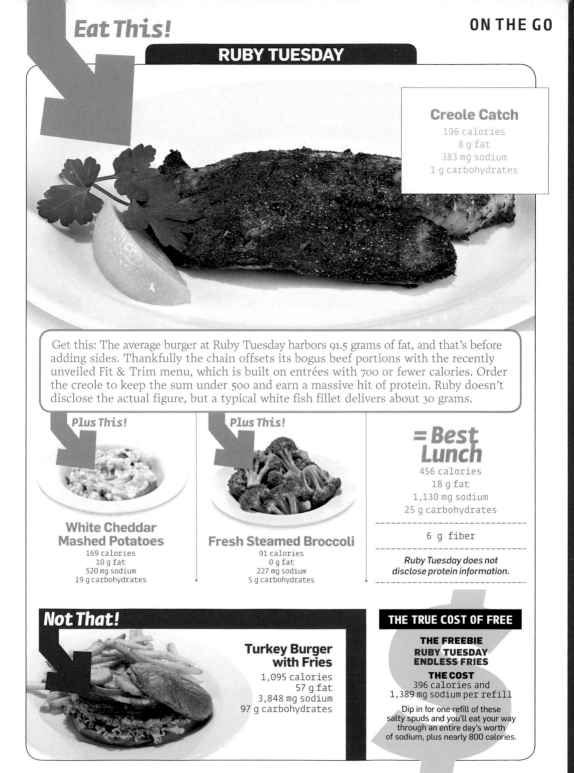

Eat This!

RUBY TUESDAY

Creole Catch
196 calories
8 g fat
383 mg sodium
1 g carbohydrates

Get this: The average burger at Ruby Tuesday harbors 91.5 grams of fat, and that's before adding sides. Thankfully the chain offsets its bogus beef portions with the recently unveiled Fit & Trim menu, which is built on entrées with 700 or fewer calories. Order the creole to keep the sum under 500 and earn a massive hit of protein. Ruby doesn't disclose the actual figure, but a typical white fish fillet delivers about 30 grams.

Plus This!

White Cheddar Mashed Potatoes
169 calories
10 g fat
520 mg sodium
19 g carbohydrates

Plus This!

Fresh Steamed Broccoli
91 calories
0 g fat
227 mg sodium
5 g carbohydrates

= Best Lunch
456 calories
18 g fat
1,130 mg sodium
25 g carbohydrates

----

6 g fiber

Ruby Tuesday does not disclose protein information.

Not That!

Turkey Burger with Fries
1,095 calories
57 g fat
3,848 mg sodium
97 g carbohydrates

THE TRUE COST OF FREE

THE FREEBIE
RUBY TUESDAY ENDLESS FRIES

THE COST
396 calories and
1,389 mg sodium per refill

Dip in for one refill of these salty spuds and you'll eat your way through an entire day's worth of sodium, plus nearly 800 calories.

Eat This!

STARBUCKS

Roma Tomato & Mozzarella Sandwich

380 calories
18 g fat (7 g saturated)
580 mg sodium
40 g carbohydrates

The new free Wi-Fi at Starbucks means you may be sticking around the store more, so you'll need solid sustenance beyond the pastries the coffee shop is better known for. This well-balanced vegetarian sandwich delivers a good shot of protein for just 380 calories. Pair it with a Grande Nonfat Cappuccino (as opposed to a latte—cappuccinos have fewer calories because they contain less milk).

SWITCH IT UP

CHICKEN SANTA FE PANINI

A toasted sandwich laced with green chili sour cream and melted pepper jack cheese may sound decadent, but this crispy grab-and-go lunch contains just 400 calories and 11 grams of fat. In general, as long as you steer clear of ones with the word "salad" in the title, Starbucks' sandwiches are a solid lunch option.

Plus This!

Grande Nonfat Cappuccino

80 calories
0 g fat
90 mg sodium
12 g carbohydrates

= Best Lunch

460 calories
18 g fat (7 g saturated)
670 mg sodium
52 g carbohydrates

----
24 g protein, 2 g fiber

33% DV vitamin A, 45% DV calcium, 15% DV iron

CALORIE-CUTTING LINGO

Hold the whip: Cuts the cream and saves you anywhere from 50 to 110 calories
Nonfat: Uses fat-free milk instead of whole or 2%
Sugar-free syrup: Use instead of regular syrup and save up to 150 calories a drink
Skinny: Your drink will be made with sugar-free syrup and fat-free milk

Not That!

Egg Salad Sandwich with Grande Tazo Iced Chai Tea Latte

730 calories
26 g fat
(7 g saturated)
945 mg sodium
98 g carbohydrates

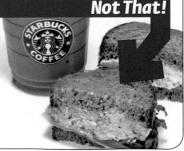

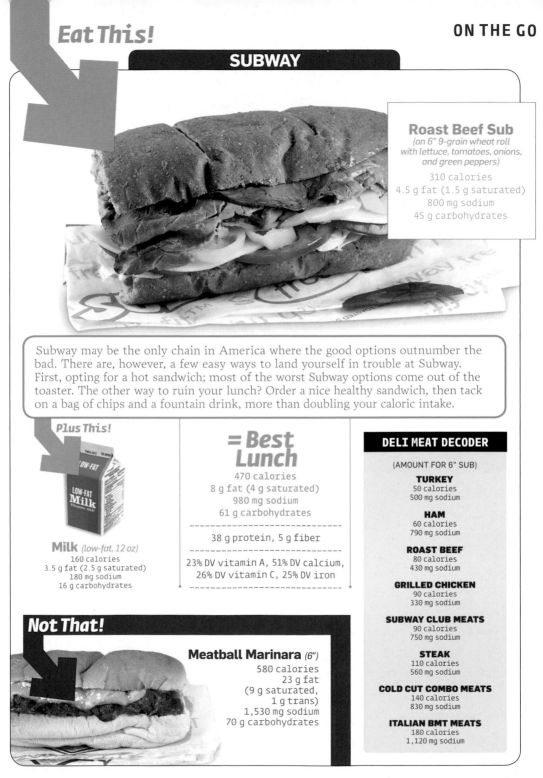

SUBWAY

Roast Beef Sub
(on 6" 9-grain wheat roll with lettuce, tomatoes, onions, and green peppers)
310 calories
4.5 g fat (1.5 g saturated)
800 mg sodium
45 g carbohydrates

Subway may be the only chain in America where the good options outnumber the bad. There are, however, a few easy ways to land yourself in trouble at Subway. First, opting for a hot sandwich; most of the worst Subway options come out of the toaster. The other way to ruin your lunch? Order a nice healthy sandwich, then tack on a bag of chips and a fountain drink, more than doubling your caloric intake.

Plus This!

Milk *(low-fat, 12 oz)*
160 calories
3.5 g fat (2.5 g saturated)
180 mg sodium
16 g carbohydrates

= Best Lunch
470 calories
8 g fat (4 g saturated)
980 mg sodium
61 g carbohydrates
----
38 g protein, 5 g fiber

23% DV vitamin A, 51% DV calcium,
26% DV vitamin C, 25% DV iron

DELI MEAT DECODER

(AMOUNT FOR 6" SUB)

TURKEY
50 calories
500 mg sodium

HAM
60 calories
790 mg sodium

ROAST BEEF
80 calories
430 mg sodium

GRILLED CHICKEN
90 calories
330 mg sodium

SUBWAY CLUB MEATS
90 calories
750 mg sodium

STEAK
110 calories
560 mg sodium

COLD CUT COMBO MEATS
140 calories
830 mg sodium

ITALIAN BMT MEATS
180 calories
1,120 mg sodium

Not That!

Meatball Marinara *(6")*
580 calories
23 g fat
(9 g saturated,
1 g trans)
1,530 mg sodium
70 g carbohydrates

Eat This!

T.G.I. FRIDAY'S

Cobb Salad
590 calories
15 g saturated fat
1,480 mg sodium
19 g carbohydrates

A salad is a salad, right? Not quite. Would you ever guess that you could eat one of them —and two Big Macs—and still consume 200 fewer calories than if you chose the other? And it's not like the Cobb skimps on the good stuff—avocado, bacon, chicken, and blue cheese will all work to squash your hunger. Proposterously enough, the Cobb and Strawberry Fields are the only Friday's salads with fewer than 1,000 calories.

SALAD DRESSING
TOTEM POLE

(PER SERVING)

GINGER-LIME SPLASH
130 calories
2 g saturated fat
280 mg sodium

LOW FAT BALSAMIC VINAIGRETTE
130 calories
0.5 g saturated fat
440 mg sodium

HOUSE VINAIGRETTE
300 calories
5 g saturated fat
1,230 mg sodium

AVOCADO CHIPOTLE RANCH
420 calories
6 g saturated fat (0.5 g trans)
700 mg sodium

BALSAMIC VINAIGRETTE
460 calories
7 g saturated fat (0.5 g trans)
580 mg sodium

HONEY MUSTARD
470 calories
7 g saturated fat
690 mg sodium

Plus This!

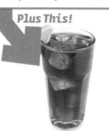

Iced Tea
0 calories
0 g fat
0 mg sodium
0 g carbohydrates

= Best Lunch
590 calories
15 g saturated fat
1,480 mg sodium
19 g carbohydrates

T.G.I. Friday's does not disclose full nutritional information.

Not That!

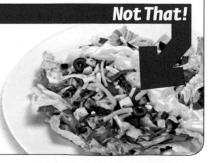

Santa Fe Chopped Salad
1,830 calories
29 g saturated fat (2 g trans)
3,450 mg sodium
97 g carbohydrates

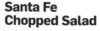

TACO BELL

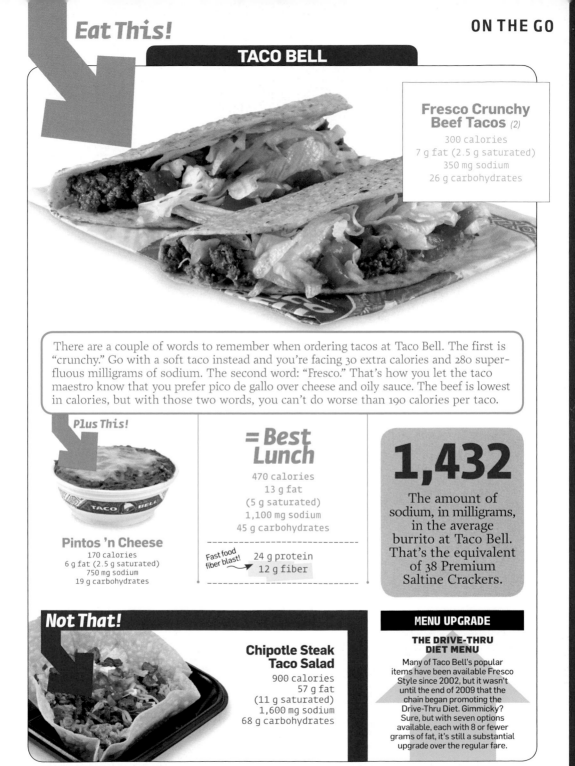

Fresco Crunchy Beef Tacos *(2)*
300 calories
7 g fat (2.5 g saturated)
350 mg sodium
26 g carbohydrates

There are a couple of words to remember when ordering tacos at Taco Bell. The first is "crunchy." Go with a soft taco instead and you're facing 30 extra calories and 280 superfluous milligrams of sodium. The second word: "Fresco." That's how you let the taco maestro know that you prefer pico de gallo over cheese and oily sauce. The beef is lowest in calories, but with those two words, you can't do worse than 190 calories per taco.

Plus This!

Pintos 'n Cheese
170 calories
6 g fat (2.5 g saturated)
750 mg sodium
19 g carbohydrates

= Best Lunch
470 calories
13 g fat
(5 g saturated)
1,100 mg sodium
45 g carbohydrates

Fast food fiber blast!
24 g protein
12 g fiber

1,432

The amount of sodium, in milligrams, in the average burrito at Taco Bell. That's the equivalent of 38 Premium Saltine Crackers.

Not That!

Chipotle Steak Taco Salad
900 calories
57 g fat
(11 g saturated)
1,600 mg sodium
68 g carbohydrates

MENU UPGRADE

THE DRIVE-THRU DIET MENU

Many of Taco Bell's popular items have been available Fresco Style since 2002, but it wasn't until the end of 2009 that the chain began promoting the Drive-Thru Diet. Gimmicky? Sure, but with seven options available, each with 8 or fewer grams of fat, it's still a substantial upgrade over the regular fare.

Eat This!

UNO CHICAGO GRILL

Roasted Eggplant, Spinach & Feta Thin Crust Pizza
(½ pizza on Five Grain Crust)

435 calories
16.5 g fat (5.5 g saturated)
840 mg sodium
55 g carbohydrates

Uno spares no breath in boasting about its deep dish pizza, but we have evidence suggesting the chain shouldn't be so proud. So let us submit to you this fact: Not one of the individual-size deep dish pies, not even the pastorally named "Farmer's Market Pie," has fewer than 1,560 calories. That doesn't mean you can't still eat pizza; just make it a thin-crust and split it with a friend. Then pair it with a side salad for a complete lunch.

Plus This!

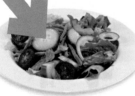

Plus This!

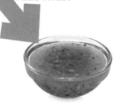

= Best Lunch

555 calories
21.5 g fat (6.5 g saturated)
1,135 mg sodium
70 g carbohydrates

15.5 g protein, 9 g fiber

45% DV vitamin A,
30% DV calcium

House Side Salad
90 calories
5 g fat (1 g saturated)
95 mg sodium
10 g carbohydrates

Fat Free Vinaigrette
30 calories
0 g fat
200 mg sodium
5 g carbohydrates

MENU UPGRADE

WHOLE GRAIN PENNE

In 2009, Uno introduced whole grain penne as an alternative to the standard noodles in all of its pasta dishes, an upgrade that earns you an extra 4 grams of fiber per plate. Seems simple enough, yet most restaurants have yet to provide a whole grain option. Kudos to Uno for jumping ahead of the curve.

Not That!

Chicago Classic Deep Dish Pizza
(½ individual size)

1,155 calories
82.5 g fat
(27 g saturated)
2,460 mg sodium
60 g carbohydrates

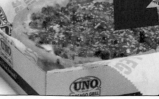

WENDY'S

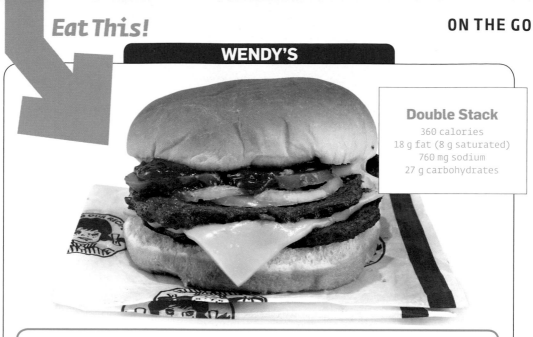

Double Stack
360 calories
18 g fat (8 g saturated)
760 mg sodium
27 g carbohydrates

Scoring a decent meal at Wendy's is just about as easy as scoring a bad one, and that's an impressive feat for a burger joint. Modestly sized burgers help, but it's the whole-some selection of sides that really sets Wendy's apart. Take the chili; it delivers 6 grams of hunger-killing fiber, a nutrient that's particularly difficult to find at less-evolved fast-food chains. Plus it just might make this America's most filling drive-thru lunch.

Plus This!

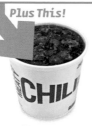

Chili *(small)*
220 calories
7 g fat (3 g saturated)
870 mg sodium
22 g carbohydrates

= Best Lunch
580 calories
25 g fat (11 g saturated)
1,630 mg sodium
49 g carbohydrates

----

41 g protein, 7 g fiber

18% DV calcium,
35% DV iron

NUTRITION 101
BEANS

A study published in the *Journal of the American College of Nutrition* found that compared with those who don't eat beans, those who eat ¾ cup per day have lower blood pressures and smaller waist sizes. This is likely related to two factors, one being that beans are among the most antioxidant-rich foods on the planet, and the other that they boast laudable loads of flab-melting fiber.

Not That!

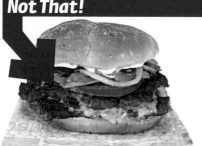

Double with Everything and Cheese
750 calories
42 g fat
(18 g saturated)
1,370 mg sodium
44 g carbohydrates

SWITCH IT UP

ULTIMATE CHICKEN GRILL
370 calories
7 g fat (1.5 g saturated)
1,150 mg sodium

This sandwich makes a great alternative to the coveted burgers on Wendy's menu. We don't much care for the extra hit of sodium, but we firmly salute the 11 extra grams of protein.

BEST CHILI

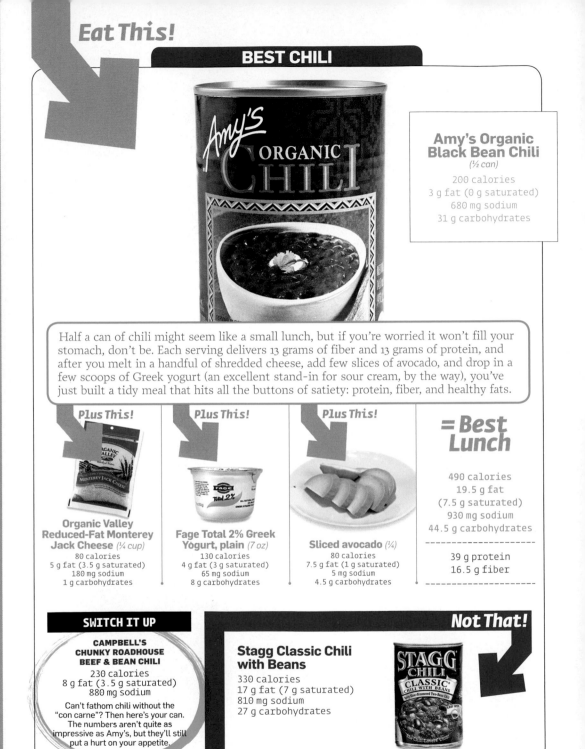

Amy's Organic Black Bean Chili
(½ can)

200 calories
3 g fat (0 g saturated)
680 mg sodium
31 g carbohydrates

Half a can of chili might seem like a small lunch, but if you're worried it won't fill your stomach, don't be. Each serving delivers 13 grams of fiber and 13 grams of protein, and after you melt in a handful of shredded cheese, add few slices of avocado, and drop in a few scoops of Greek yogurt (an excellent stand-in for sour cream, by the way), you've just built a tidy meal that hits all the buttons of satiety: protein, fiber, and healthy fats.

Plus This!

Organic Valley Reduced-Fat Monterey Jack Cheese *(¼ cup)*
80 calories
5 g fat (3.5 g saturated)
180 mg sodium
1 g carbohydrates

Plus This!

Fage Total 2% Greek Yogurt, plain *(7 oz)*
130 calories
4 g fat (3 g saturated)
65 mg sodium
8 g carbohydrates

Plus This!

Sliced avocado *(¼)*
80 calories
7.5 g fat (1 g saturated)
5 mg sodium
4.5 g carbohydrates

= Best Lunch

490 calories
19.5 g fat
(7.5 g saturated)
930 mg sodium
44.5 g carbohydrates

----

39 g protein
16.5 g fiber

SWITCH IT UP

CAMPBELL'S CHUNKY ROADHOUSE BEEF & BEAN CHILI
230 calories
8 g fat (3.5 g saturated)
880 mg sodium

Can't fathom chili without the "con carne"? Then here's your can. The numbers aren't quite as impressive as Amy's, but they'll still put a hurt on your appetite.

Not That!

Stagg Classic Chili with Beans
330 calories
17 g fat (7 g saturated)
810 mg sodium
27 g carbohydrates

BEST SOUP

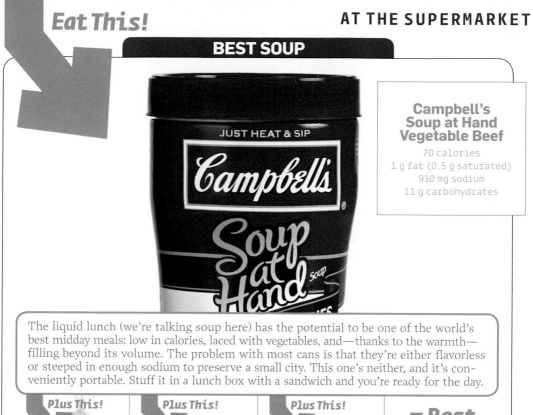

JUST HEAT & SIP

Campbell's Soup at Hand Vegetable Beef

70 calories
1 g fat (0.5 g saturated)
930 mg sodium
11 g carbohydrates

The liquid lunch (we're talking soup here) has the potential to be one of the world's best midday meals: low in calories, laced with vegetables, and—thanks to the warmth—filling beyond its volume. The problem with most cans is that they're either flavorless or steeped in enough sodium to preserve a small city. This one's neither, and it's conveniently portable. Stuff it in a lunch box with a sandwich and you're ready for the day.

Plus This!

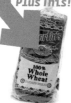

Martin's Famous Whole Wheat Potato Bread
(2 slices)
140 calories
2 g fat (0 g saturated)
250 mg sodium
28 g carbohydrates

Plus This!

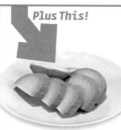

Sliced avocado *(½)*
160 calories
14.5 g fat (2 g saturated)
5 mg sodium
8.5 g carbohydrates

Plus This!

Curried Chicken Salad
(½ cup)
160 calories
8 g fat (1 g saturated)
160 mg sodium
10 g carbohydrates

=Best Lunch

530 calories
25.5 g fat
(3.5 g saturated)
1,345 mg sodium
57.5 g carbohydrates

- - - - - - - - - - - - - -

22 g protein
12.5 g fiber   *50% of your DV!*

- - - - - - - - - - - - - -

Not That!

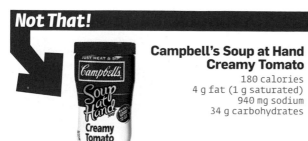

JUST HEAT & SIP

Campbell's Soup at Hand Creamy Tomato

180 calories
4 g fat (1 g saturated)
940 mg sodium
34 g carbohydrates

MEAL MAKER

SOUP AND SANDWICH

A hot cup of soup can be deceptively filling, but a sandwich on the side can provide the protein and fiber you need to make that fullness last. Build a lean rendition of a deli sandwich by stuffing slices of toasted wheat bread with our Curried Chicken Salad (see page 48) and thick slices of avocado.

Eat This!

BEST HOT DOG

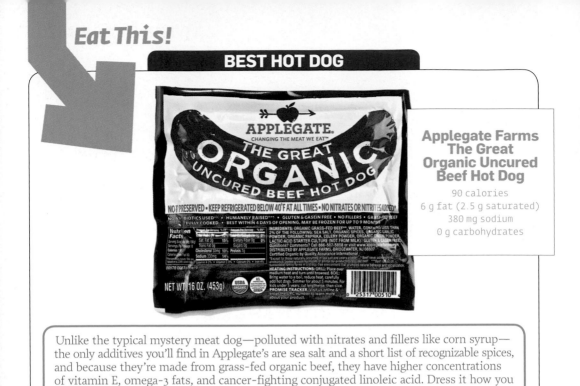

Applegate Farms The Great Organic Uncured Beef Hot Dog

90 calories
6 g fat (2.5 g saturated)
380 mg sodium
0 g carbohydrates

Unlike the typical mystery meat dog—polluted with nitrates and fillers like corn syrup—the only additives you'll find in Applegate's are sea salt and a short list of recognizable spices, and because they're made from grass-fed organic beef, they have higher concentrations of vitamin E, omega-3 fats, and cancer-fighting conjugated linoleic acid. Dress it how you like it and pair with a crisp apple and a side of egg salad for a hugely satisfying lunch.

Plus This!

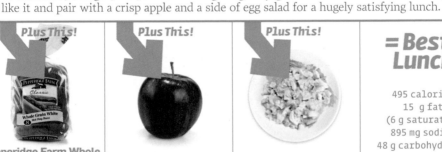

Pepperidge Farm Whole Grain White Hot Dog Bun
110 calories
1 g fat (0 g saturated)
220 mg sodium
21 g carbohydrates

Plus This!

Apple
95 calories
0.5 g fat (0 g saturated)
0 mg sodium
25 g carbohydrates

Plus This!

Fiery Egg Salad
200 calories
15 g fat (3.5 g saturated)
290 mg sodium
2 g carbohydrates

= Best Lunch

495 calories
15 g fat
(6 g saturated)
895 mg sodium
48 g carbohydrates

----

24 g protein
7 g fiber

----

150 MILLION

Number of hot dogs Americans eat every year on the 4th of July, according to the National Hot Dog and Sausage Council.

Not That!

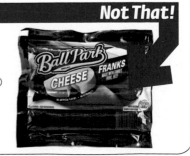

Ball Park Cheese Frank

190 calories
16 g fat (7 g saturated)
550 mg sodium
5 g carbohydrates

BEST TUNA

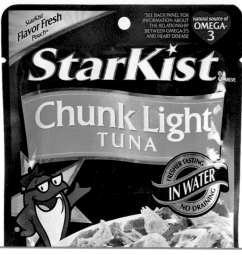

Starkist Chunk Light Tuna in Water
(2.6-oz pouch)
80 calories
0.5 g fat (0 g saturated)
300 mg sodium
1 g carbohydrates

Outside of the 4 or 5 fat calories in this bag, you're looking at what essentially amounts to pure protein, the ideal sustenance in a lunchtime sandwich, or, paired with sweet relish and whole wheat crackers, a hunger-squelching midday snack. But one word of advice: If you stray from the pouch pictured here, remember one thing: Chunk light tuna has one-third as much neurotoxic methylmercury as albacore.

Plus This!

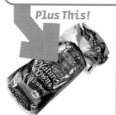

Nature's Own Double Fiber Wheat Bread *(2 slices)*
100 calories
1 g fat (0 g saturated)
270 mg sodium
26 g carbohydrates

Plus This!

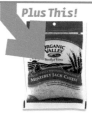

Organic Valley Monterey Jack Reduced Fat Cheese
(¼ cup)
80 calories
5 g fat (3.5 g saturated)
180 mg sodium
1 g carbohydrates

Plus This!

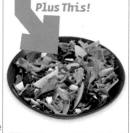

ETNT Simple Side Salad
170 calories
14 g fat (2 g saturated)
95 mg sodium
10 g carbohydrates

= Best Lunch

430 calories
20.5 g fat
(5.5 g saturated)
845 mg sodium
38 g carbohydrates

Stay full for hours!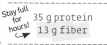
35 g protein
13 g fiber

Not That!

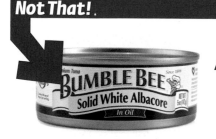

Bumble Bee Solid White Albacore in Oil
(1 can, drained)
160 calories
6 g fat
(1 g saturated)
280 mg sodium

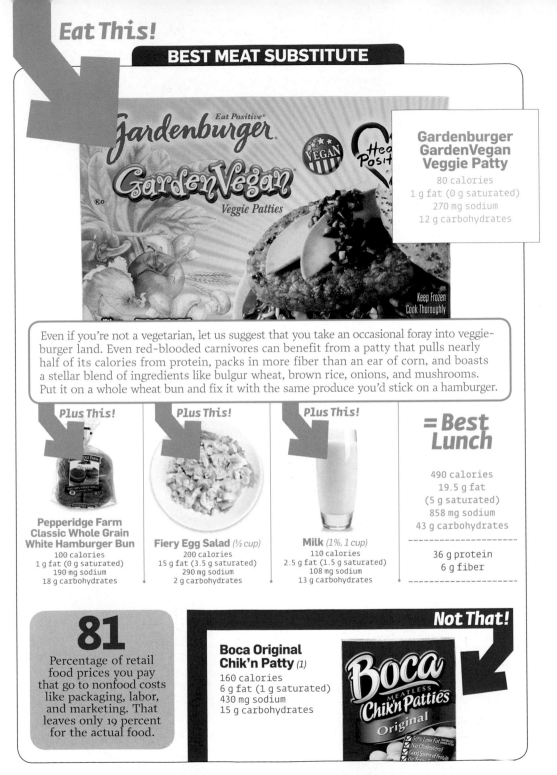

BEST MEAT SUBSTITUTE

**Gardenburger
GardenVegan
Veggie Patty**
80 calories
1 g fat (0 g saturated)
270 mg sodium
12 g carbohydrates

Even if you're not a vegetarian, let us suggest that you take an occasional foray into veggie-burger land. Even red-blooded carnivores can benefit from a patty that pulls nearly half of its calories from protein, packs in more fiber than an ear of corn, and boasts a stellar blend of ingredients like bulgur wheat, brown rice, onions, and mushrooms. Put it on a whole wheat bun and fix it with the same produce you'd stick on a hamburger.

Plus This!

**Pepperidge Farm
Classic Whole Grain
White Hamburger Bun**
100 calories
1 g fat (0 g saturated)
190 mg sodium
18 g carbohydrates

Plus This!

Fiery Egg Salad *(½ cup)*
200 calories
15 g fat (3.5 g saturated)
290 mg sodium
2 g carbohydrates

Plus This!

Milk *(1%, 1 cup)*
110 calories
2.5 g fat (1.5 g saturated)
108 mg sodium
13 g carbohydrates

**= Best
Lunch**

490 calories
19.5 g fat
(5 g saturated)
858 mg sodium
43 g carbohydrates
----
36 g protein
6 g fiber

81

Percentage of retail food prices you pay that go to nonfood costs like packaging, labor, and marketing. That leaves only 19 percent for the actual food.

Not That!

**Boca Original
Chik'n Patty** *(1)*
160 calories
6 g fat (1 g saturated)
430 mg sodium
15 g carbohydrates

BEST FROZEN CHICKEN ENTRÉE

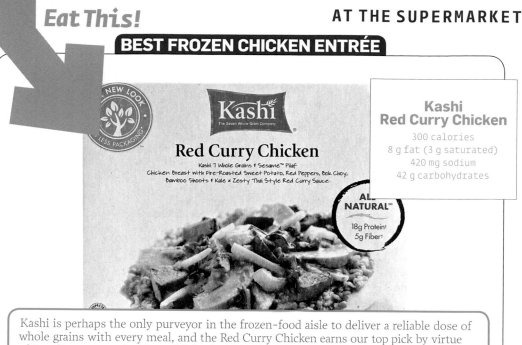

Kashi
The Seven Whole Grain Company®

Red Curry Chicken

Kashi 7 Whole Grains + Sesame™ Pilaf
Chicken Breast with Fire-Roasted Sweet Potato, Red Peppers, Bok Choy,
Bamboo Shoots + Kale + Zesty Thai Style Red Curry Sauce

ALL NATURAL®

18g Protein
5g Fiber

Kashi
Red Curry Chicken

300 calories
8 g fat (3 g saturated)
420 mg sodium
42 g carbohydrates

Kashi is perhaps the only purveyor in the frozen-food aisle to deliver a reliable dose of whole grains with every meal, and the Red Curry Chicken earns our top pick by virtue of its reliance on antioxidant-rich herbs and spices that don't typically see much action in American kitchens. It's a small meal though, so take the opportunity to work in a side dish that adds protein and healthy fat. Walnuts swirled into Greek yogurt do just that.

Plus This!

Fage Total 2% Greek Yogurt,
plain *(7 oz)*
130 calories
4 g fat (3 g saturated)
65 mg sodium
8 g carbohydrates

Plus This!

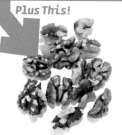

Chopped walnuts *(2 Tbsp)*
95 calories
9.5 g fat (1 g saturated)
0 mg sodium
2 g carbohydrates

= Best
Lunch

525 calories
21.5 g fat
(7 g saturated)
485 mg sodium
52 g carbohydrates

----

36 g protein
7 g fiber

Not That!

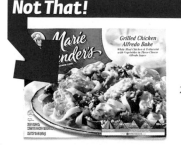

Marie Callender's
Grilled Chicken
Alfredo Bake

500 calories
26 g fat (14 g saturated)
1,230 mg sodium
34 g carbohydrates

STEALTH HEALTH

CURRY

Ginger, coriander, and turmeric are common in curry, and Kashi includes all three. Ginger is known to reduce inflammation, coriander helps regulate blood sugar, and turmeric delivers antioxidants that might help slow the progression of both Alzheimer's disease and multiple sclerosis.

Eat This!

BEST FROZEN BEEF ENTRÉE

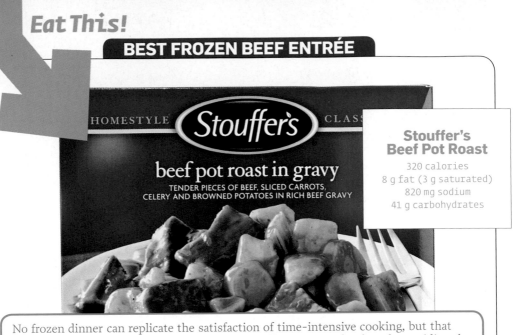

HOMESTYLE **Stouffer's** CLASSIC

beef pot roast in gravy

TENDER PIECES OF BEEF, SLICED CARROTS,
CELERY AND BROWNED POTATOES IN RICH BEEF GRAVY

**Stouffer's
Beef Pot Roast**

320 calories
8 g fat (3 g saturated)
820 mg sodium
41 g carbohydrates

No frozen dinner can replicate the satisfaction of time-intensive cooking, but that doesn't mean it can't be equally as healthy. Stouffer's proves that here by avoiding the nutritional follies of other frozen-food purveyors. Instead of creamy sauces and cheap, starchy noodles, this meal is built on the shoulders of roasted carrots, potatoes, and celery—the same ingredients you'd likely toss into your own slow cooker at home.

Plus This!

Milk *(1%, 1 cup)*
110 calories
2.5 g fat (1.5 g saturated)
108 mg sodium
13 g carbohydrates

Plus This!

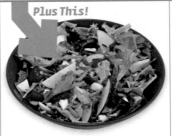

ETNT Simple Side Salad
170 calories
14 g fat (2 g saturated)
95 mg sodium
10 g carbohydrates

= Best Lunch

600 calories
24.5 g fat
(6.5 g saturated)
1,023 mg sodium
64 g carbohydrates

----

23 g protein
10 g fiber

Not That!

**Marie Callender's
Beef Pot Pie** *(½ pie)*

510 calories
29 g fat (11 g saturated)
780 mg sodium
48 g carbohydrates

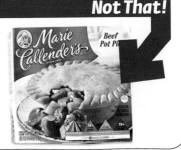

BEST FROZEN BURRITO

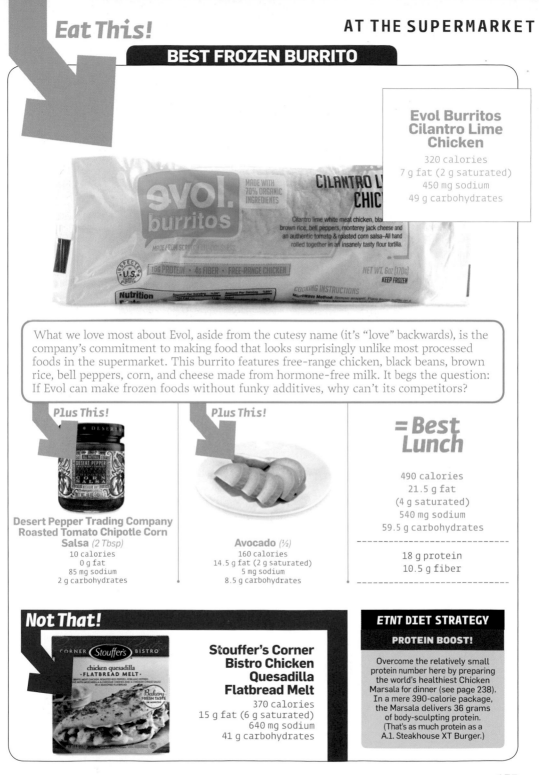

Evol Burritos Cilantro Lime Chicken

320 calories
7 g fat (2 g saturated)
450 mg sodium
49 g carbohydrates

MADE WITH 70% ORGANIC INGREDIENTS

CILANTRO L[ ]
CHIC[ ]

Cilantro lime white meat chicken, bla[ ]
brown rice, bell peppers, monterey jack cheese and
an authentic tomato & roasted corn salsa–All hand
rolled together in an insanely tasty flour tortilla.

NET WT. 6oz (170g)
KEEP FROZEN

19g PROTEIN • 4g FIBER • FREE-RANGE CHICKEN

COOKING INSTRUCTIONS

What we love most about Evol, aside from the cutesy name (it's "love" backwards), is the company's commitment to making food that looks surprisingly unlike most processed foods in the supermarket. This burrito features free-range chicken, black beans, brown rice, bell peppers, corn, and cheese made from hormone-free milk. It begs the question: If Evol can make frozen foods without funky additives, why can't its competitors?

Plus This!

Desert Pepper Trading Company Roasted Tomato Chipotle Corn Salsa *(2 Tbsp)*
10 calories
0 g fat
85 mg sodium
2 g carbohydrates

Plus This!

Avocado *(½)*
160 calories
14.5 g fat (2 g saturated)
5 mg sodium
8.5 g carbohydrates

= Best Lunch

490 calories
21.5 g fat
(4 g saturated)
540 mg sodium
59.5 g carbohydrates

- - - - - - - - - - - - - -

18 g protein
10.5 g fiber

- - - - - - - - - - - - - -

Not That!

Stouffer's Corner Bistro Chicken Quesadilla Flatbread Melt
370 calories
15 g fat (6 g saturated)
640 mg sodium
41 g carbohydrates

Eat This!

BEST FROZEN PASTA

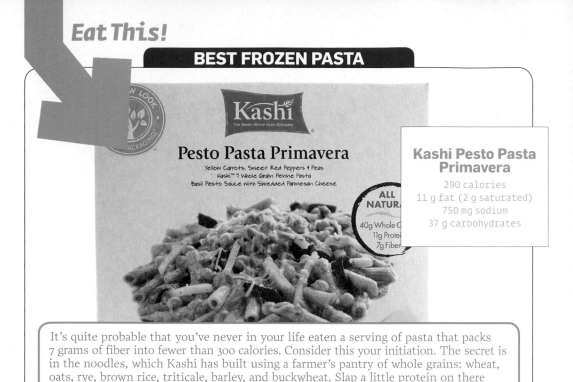

Kashi
The Seven Whole Grain Company

Pesto Pasta Primavera
Yellow Carrots, Sweet Red Peppers † Peas
Kashi™ 7 Whole Grain Penne Pasta
Basil Pesto Sauce with Shredded Parmesan Cheese

ALL NATURA...

40g Whole G...
11g Protei...
7g Fiber...

Kashi Pesto Pasta Primavera

290 calories
11 g fat (2 g saturated)
750 mg sodium
37 g carbohydrates

It's quite probable that you've never in your life eaten a serving of pasta that packs 7 grams of fiber into fewer than 300 calories. Consider this your initiation. The secret is in the noodles, which Kashi has built using a farmer's pantry of whole grains: wheat, oats, rye, brown rice, triticale, barley, and buckwheat. Slap a little protein on there and you've got a complete meal. Canned or leftover rotisserie chicken both work great.

Plus This!

Swanson White Premium Chunk Chicken Breast in Water *(½ can)*
125 calories
2.5 g fat (1.5 g saturated)
405 mg sodium
2.5 g carbohydrates

Plus This!

Milk *(1%, 1 cup)*
110 calories
2.5 g fat (1.5 g saturated)
108 mg sodium
13 g carbohydrates

= Best Lunch

525 calories
16 g fat
(5 g saturated)
1,263 mg sodium
52.5 g carbohydrates

Boost your metabolism! → 44 g protein
7 g fiber

MEAL MAKER

PROTEIN-PACKED PASTA

There's a trick to stirring chicken into frozen pasta. Microwave the tray according package directions, but pull it out a minute before it's finished. By that time the pasta will have thawed, so you can stir in the chicken, pop it back in the microwave, and enjoy fully cooked chicken pesto pasta primavera.

Not That!

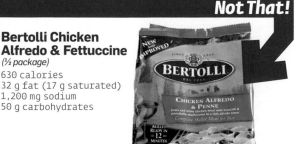

Bertolli Chicken Alfredo & Fettuccine
(½ package)
630 calories
32 g fat (17 g saturated)
1,200 mg sodium
50 g carbohydrates

BEST FROZEN VEGETARIAN ENTRÉE

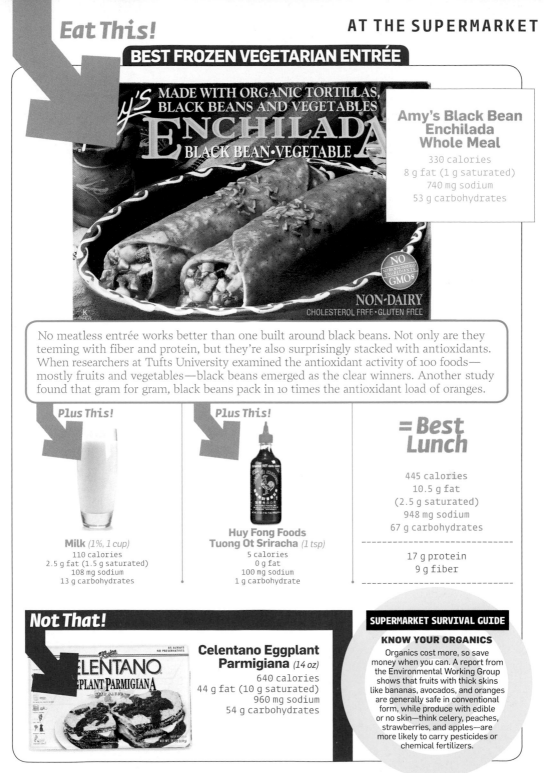

MADE WITH ORGANIC TORTILLAS, BLACK BEANS AND VEGETABLES

ENCHILADA
BLACK BEAN · VEGETABLE

NON-DAIRY
CHOLESTEROL FREE · GLUTEN FREE

NO GMOs

Amy's Black Bean Enchilada Whole Meal

330 calories
8 g fat (1 g saturated)
740 mg sodium
53 g carbohydrates

No meatless entrée works better than one built around black beans. Not only are they teeming with fiber and protein, but they're also surprisingly stacked with antioxidants. When researchers at Tufts University examined the antioxidant activity of 100 foods—mostly fruits and vegetables—black beans emerged as the clear winners. Another study found that gram for gram, black beans pack in 10 times the antioxidant load of oranges.

Plus This!

Milk *(1%, 1 cup)*
110 calories
2.5 g fat (1.5 g saturated)
108 mg sodium
13 g carbohydrates

Plus This!

Huy Fong Foods Tuong Ot Sriracha *(1 tsp)*
5 calories
0 g fat
100 mg sodium
1 g carbohydrate

= Best Lunch

445 calories
10.5 g fat
(2.5 g saturated)
948 mg sodium
67 g carbohydrates

----

17 g protein
9 g fiber

Not That!

AS ALWAYS NO PRESERVATIVES

CELENTANO
EGGPLANT PARMIGIANA

Celentano Eggplant Parmigiana *(14 oz)*

640 calories
44 g fat (10 g saturated)
960 mg sodium
54 g carbohydrates

Eat This!

(see page 45)

**ETNT Simple
Side Salad**
170 calories
14 g fat (2 g saturated)
95 mg sodium
10 g carbohydrates

Plus This!

Baked Potato Soup
220 calories
9 g fat (4 g saturated)
650 mg sodium
17 g carbohydrates

Most versions of this hearty soup pack upwards of 400 calories per bowl, but we cut the calories in half and, with a bit of bacon and cheese, still keep things exciting.

= Best Lunch
390 calories
23 g fat
(6 g saturated)
745 mg sodium
27 g carbohydrates

---

20 g protein
3 g fiber

888

The amount of potassium, in milligrams, in one medium russet potato. That's more than twice the potassium of a medium banana.

You'll Need:

3 strips bacon, sliced

4 scallions, whites and greens separated, chopped

2 cloves garlic, minced

1 Tbsp flour

8 cups low-sodium chicken stock (or a mix of stock and water)

2 medium russet potatoes, baked (leftover potatoes work great)

½ cup half-and-half

Salt and ground black pepper to taste

Shredded Cheddar cheese

Tabasco sauce to taste

How to Make It:

• Heat a large soup pot over medium heat. Add the bacon and cook for about 5 minutes, until crispy. Remove with a slotted spoon

and reserve.

• Discard all but a thin film of the bacon fat. Add the scallion whites and garlic to the pot and cook for a minute or two, until fragrant and the scallions are translucent. Add the flour and stir to coat the ingredients. Pour in the stock, whisking to prevent any lumps from forming.

• Remove and discard the peel from one of the potatoes, chop the potato meat, and add it to the pot. Use a potato masher to smash the

potato into the broth. (For a smoother, more uniform soup, you can puree the soup in a blender.) Cube the other potato, leaving the peel on, and add it to the soup, along with the half-and-half. Season with salt and pepper. Turn the heat all the way down and simmer for 5 to 10 minutes.

• When ready to serve, ladle into bowls and garnish with the bacon, scallion greens, a bit of cheese, and a few shakes of Tabasco.

Makes 4 servings

Not That!

Applebee's Baked Potato Soup (bowl)
420 calories
30 g fat (14 g saturated)
1,230 mg sodium
27 g carbohydrates

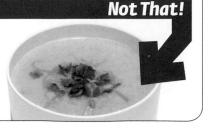

Sausage Sandwich with Peppers

370 calories
20 g fat (9 g saturated)
650 mg sodium
23.5 g carbohydrates

Pork sausage can contain up to 30 percent fat, meaning a single link can pack 400 calories. Switching to a lean chicken or turkey sausage will bring that number to fewer than 150 calories, and a tangle of sautéed onions and peppers, a bit of melted cheese, and a slick of spicy mustard will ensure that you won't miss the pig.

You'll Need:

1 Tbsp olive oil

1 red bell pepper, sliced

1 yellow bell pepper, sliced

1 yellow onion, sliced

Salt and ground black pepper to taste

½ Tbsp red wine vinegar

4 links uncooked chicken or turkey sausage

4 hot dog buns (preferably potato buns)

4 slices provolone

Spicy mustard to taste

How to Make It:

• Preheat a grill or grill pan.

• Heat the oil in a large skillet. Add the red and yellow peppers and the onion and cook, stirring occasionally, for about 10 minutes, until lightly blistered and soft. Remove from the heat, season with salt and pepper, and add the vinegar. Reserve.

• Grill the sausages until lightly charred and cooked all the way through, about 12 minutes. Heat the rolls on the grill until warm and toasted, if you like.

• Lay a slice of cheese in each roll, drizzle with mustard, then top with a sausage. Divide the peppers and onions among the four sandwiches.

Makes 4 servings

Plus This!

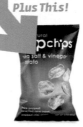

Pop Chips All Natural Sea Salt & Vinegar
(1 oz)
120 calories
4 g fat (0 g saturated)
250 mg sodium
20 g carbohydrates

= Best Lunch

490 calories
24 g fat
(9 g saturated)
900 mg sodium
43.5 g carbohydrates

28.5 g protein
6 g fiber

SECRET WEAPON

AL FRESCO CHICKEN SAUSAGES

One of our favorite products in the supermarket, Al Fresco chicken sausages are the perfect lean, flavor-packed substitute for the fattier pork and beef sausages that end up in most American refrigerators. Offered fresh or fully cooked in a dozen different varities, with just 130 calories and 7 grams per link, these are perfect for boosting a pasta, folding into a breakfast scramble, or, as seen here, eating straight off the grill with a thatch of blistered vegetables.

Not That!

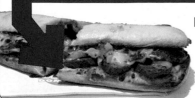

Domino's Italian Sausage and Peppers Sandwich

860 calories
45 g fat (21 g saturated, 1 g trans)
2,260 mg sodium
74 g carbohydrates

Eat This!

Chicken Fajita Burrito

355 calories
13 g fat (6 g saturated)
740 mg sodium
42 g carbohydrates

Burritos have gone off the deep end. The combination of rice, sour cream, cheese, and guacamole lifts calorie and sodium counts into the thousands. This burrito is American in spirit—hearty and generously filled—but without the excesses found at Chipotle, Baja Fresh, and the country's other burrito barons.

You'll Need:

½ Tbsp canola oil

1 large onion, sliced

1 red bell pepper, sliced

1 poblano or green bell pepper, sliced

Salt and ground black pepper to taste

½ can (14–16 oz) black beans, drained and rinsed

¼ tsp cumin

Juice of 1 lime

Hot sauce

4 (10") whole wheat tortillas

1 cup low-fat shredded Jack cheese

2 cups shredded chicken (about ½ store-bought rotisserie chicken)

Salsa (salsa verde is especially good here)

How to Make It:

• Heat the oil in a large skillet over high heat. Add the onion and red and poblano peppers and cook until browned, about 7 to 8 minutes. Season with salt and black pepper.

• Combine the beans with the cumin in a saucepan and warm. Add the lime and a few shakes of hot sauce.

• Preheat a griddle, cast-iron skillet, or large nonstick pan over medium heat. Microwave the tortillas for 20 seconds, just enough so they're pliable. Building one burrito at a time, sprinkle on some cheese, then top with some beans, onion-pepper mixture, chicken, and salsa. Roll into a tight package. Place the burritos directly on the skillet, cooking for a minute on each side until lightly toasted.

Makes 4 servings

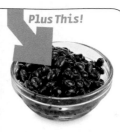

Plus This!

Black beans
(½ cup)
115 calories
0.5 g fat (0 g saturated)
205 mg sodium
20.5 g carbohydrates

= Best Lunch

470 calories
13.5 g fat
(6 g saturated)
945 mg sodium
62.5 g carbohydrates

Stay full all afternoon! → 33 g protein 16.5 g fiber

MASTER THE TECHNIQUE

BURRITO BUILDING

Most restaurant burritos are rice-heavy carbo bombs, but your home creations should focus on three elements: meat (grilled chicken, steak, or pork), beans (black or pinto, kicked up with spices), and salsa (and lots of it). Be sure to toast the tortilla before eating; it makes all the difference.

Not That!

Chipotle Grilled Chicken Burrito
with Cilantro-Lime Rice, black beans, Fajita Vegetables, cheese, sour cream, and Tomato Salsa
990 calories
38.5 g fat (17.5 g saturated)
2,290 mg sodium
101 g carbohydrates

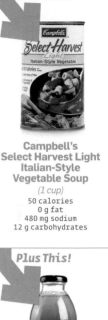

**Campbell's
Select Harvest Light
Italian-Style
Vegetable Soup**
(1 cup)
50 calories
0 g fat
480 mg sodium
12 g carbohydrates

Greek Salad
360 calories
22 g fat (7 g saturated)
580 mg sodium
21 g carbohydrates

When it comes to good eating, the Greeks have it right. Healthy fats, lots of vegetables, lean protein—all are cornerstones of their diet, the fabled Mediterranean diet, and all are captured in this simple and satisfying chopped salad. Incidentally, ask a Greek and he or she will tell you: It's not a diet, it's a lifestyle. Amen to that.

**Honest Tea
Green Tea**
(16 oz)
34 calories
0 g fat
0 mg sodium
10 mg carbohydrates

You'll Need:

2 cups shredded or chopped cooked chicken

1 large cucumber, peeled, seeded, and chopped

1 red bell pepper, chopped

4 Roma tomatoes, chopped

1 red onion, chopped

½ (14–16 oz) can chickpeas, drained

¾ cup crumbled feta cheese

2 Tbsp red wine vinegar

1 tsp dried oregano

Salt and ground black pepper to taste

¼ cup olive oil

How to Make It:

• Combine the chicken, cucumber, bell pepper, tomatoes, onion, chickpeas, and cheese in a large salad bowl. In a separate bowl, combine the vinegar and oregano with a few generous pinches of salt and black pepper. Slowly drizzle in the olive oil, whisking to combine. Toss the dressing with the salad. You can serve it right away, but it's best to let it sit in the fridge for 30 minutes or so to give all the ingredients a chance to get friendly.

Makes 4 servings

= Best Lunch

444 calories
22 g fat
(7 g saturated)
1,060 mg sodium
43 g carbohydrates

----

19 g protein
5 g fiber

Not That!

Così Greek Salad
517 calories
47 g fat (10 g saturated)
1,480 mg sodium
19 g carbohydrates

Eat This!

Grilled Vegetable Wrap

240 calories
13 g fat (3.5 g saturated)
450 mg sodium
30.5 g carbohydrates

Despite their healthy reputation, wraps from delis and cafes are among the worst lunch options out there. Slash calories and cost by building your own at home.

You'll Need:

12 asparagus spears, woody ends removed

2 portobello mushroom caps

1 red bell pepper, halved, seeds and stem removed

1 Tbsp olive oil

Salt and ground black pepper to taste

2 Tbsp olive oil mayonnaise

1 Tbsp balsamic vinegar

1 clove garlic, minced

4 large spinach or whole wheat tortillas or wraps

2 cups arugula, baby spinach, or mixed baby greens

¾ cup crumbled goat or feta cheese

How to Make It:

• Preheat a grill. Combine the asparagus, mushrooms, bell pepper, olive oil, and a few pinches of salt and black pepper in a large bowl and toss to coat evenly. Place the vegetables on the hottest part of the grill and cook, turning occasionally, until lightly charred and tender. The asparagus should take the least amount of time (about 5 minutes) and the pepper halves the most (about 10). Alternatively, you can roast the vegetables in a 450°F oven for 10 to 12 minutes. Slice the mushroom caps and pepper into thin strips. If possible, peel off the charred skin of the pepper and then slice.

• Add the mayonnaise, vinegar, and garlic to a small bowl and stir to combine. Heat the tortillas on the grill or wrap them together in damp paper towels and heat in the microwave for 30 seconds. Spread the mayo down the middle of each tortilla, then top with the greens and cheese. Divide the grilled vegetables among the tortillas, then roll up tightly and slice each wrap in half.

Makes 4 servings

Plus This!

(see page 49)

Fiery Egg Salad
200 calories
15 g fat (3.5 g saturated)
290 mg sodium
2 g carbohydrates

= Best Lunch

440 calories
28 g fat
(7 g saturated)
740 mg sodium
32.5 g carbohydrates

21.5 g protein
4.5 g fiber

MEAL MULTIPLIER

Starting with a whole wheat tortilla and a wrap can make an excellent lunch vessel. Try one of these other stellar combinations:

• Smoked turkey, Swiss, tomato, guacamole
• Grilled chicken, fresh mozzarella, roasted peppers, pesto
• Any Ultimate Deli Salad (see page 46)

Not That!

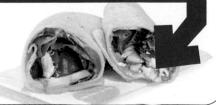

Au Bon Pain Mediterranean Wrap

610 calories
29 g fat (7 g saturated)
1,770 mg sodium
73 g carbohydrates

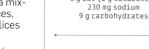

Baby carrots
(about 9 carrots)
30 calories
0 g fat
66 mg sodium
7 g carbohydrates

Plus This!

Hummus
(¼ cup)
100 calories
6 g fat (1 g saturated)
230 mg sodium
9 g carbohydrates

Italian Tuna Melt
340 calories
13 g fat (2 g saturated)
980 mg sodium
30.5 g carbohydrates

Ahh, the tuna melt: Has the potential of any sandwich been squandered more consistently than this fishy fiasco? The recipe used by most establishments tells all: 2 parts mayo to 1 part tuna. We replace the bulk of the mayo with a stronger supporting cast: pesto, lemon juice, olives, and onions. That means you can taste something other than fat when you're eating it and feel something other than fat when you're through.

You'll Need:

2 cans (5 oz each) tuna, drained

1 small red onion, diced

¼ cup chopped green olives

2 Tbsp olive oil mayonnaise

2 Tbsp jarred pesto

1 Tbsp capers, rinsed and chopped

Juice of 1 lemon

8 slices whole wheat bread

2 oz fresh mozzarella cheese, sliced (or low-fat shredded mozzarella)

1 large tomato, sliced

About 1 tsp olive oil

How to Make It:

• In a mixing bowl, combine the tuna, onion, olives, mayo, pesto, capers, and lemon juice and stir to combine. Layer the bottom halves of four slices of bread with mozzarella, then top with the tuna mixture, tomato slices, and remaining slices of bread.

• Preheat a cast-iron or nonstick pan over medium heat. Coat both sides of the sandwiches with a thin layer of olive oil and cook for 2 to 3 minutes per side, until the bread is toasted and the cheese is melted.

Makes 4 servings

= Best Lunch

470 calories
19 g fat
(3 g saturated)
1,276 mg sodium
46.5 g carbohydrates

25.5 g protein
7 g fiber

SECRET INGREDIENT

PREMIUM TUNA

Wild Planet tuna packs more omega-3s and less mercury than the leading brands. Pick up cans at wildplanetfoods.com.

Not That!

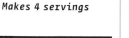

Quiznos Regular Tuna Melt Sub
1,070 calories
73 g fat (15 g saturated)
1,400 mg sodium
62 g carbohydrates

Eat This!

Gazpacho
120 calories
7 g fat (1 g saturated)
650 mg sodium
14 g carbohydrates

Eat gazpacho every day and you'll live to see 100. At least, that's what the Spaniards say, and they should know, given they live as long as almost anyone on the planet. Make big batches in the summer, when tomatoes rule, and ladle your lunch all week long.

You'll Need:

2 cups chopped tomatoes

1 red or green bell pepper, chopped

1 medium red onion, diced

1 cup diced English cucumbers

1½ cups Low Sodium V8 or other tomato juice

Juice of 1 lemon

2 Tbsp olive oil + additional for garnish

1 Tbsp white or red wine vinegar

2 cloves garlic, chopped

1 tsp salt

How to Make It:

• Combine the tomatoes, pepper, onion, and cucumber in a large mixing bowl and mix well. Transfer one-fourth of the mixture to a small bowl, cover, and refrigerate. Add the tomato juice, lemon juice, 2 tablespoons of the olive oil, vinegar, garlic, and salt to the vegetables in the large bowl and mix to combine. If you have the time, it's best at this point to allow the ingredients to mingle in the fridge for an hour or two—or even overnight.

• Working in batches if necessary, add the tomato juice mixture to a blender and puree, stopping just short of creating a smooth soup (a bit of texture is nice). If you didn't refrigerate before, place the gazpacho in the fridge for 20 to 30 minutes to chill.

• When ready to serve, divide the gazpacho among 4 to 6 bowls. Chop the reserved vegetables on a cutting board until you have a rough salsa. Garnish each bowl with a bit of the vegetable salsa and a drizzle of olive oil.

Makes 4 to 6 servings

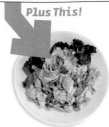

Plus This!

(see page 48)

Curried Chicken Salad
(½ cup)
160 calories
8 g fat (1 g saturated)
160 mg sodium
10 g carbohydrates

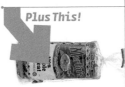

Plus This!

Martin's Famous Whole Wheat Potato Bread
(2 slices, toasted)
140 calories
2 g fat (0 g saturated)
250 mg sodium
28 g carbohydrates

= Best Lunch
420 calories
17 g fat
(2 g saturated)
1,153 mg sodium
56 g carbohydrates

----
25 g protein
12 g fiber

Not That!

Au Bon Pain Old Fashioned Tomato Soup (large)
270 calories
10 g fat (4 g saturated)
1,540 mg sodium
37 g carbohydrates

164

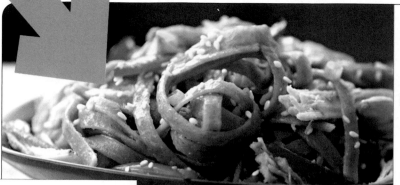

Plus This!

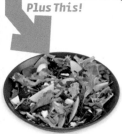

(see page 45)

ETNT Simple Side Salad
170 calories
14 g fat (2 g saturated)
95 mg sodium
10 g carbohydrates

Sesame Noodles with Chicken and Peanuts

340 calories
11 g fat (2 g saturated)
400 mg sodium

Think of this as a salad, with the noodles standing in for lettuce. Add protein and as many vegetables as you like, and toss it all with a light but powerful dressing.

= Best Lunch

510 calories
25 g fat
(4 g saturated)
495 mg sodium
46.5 g carbohydrates

33.5 g protein
10 g fiber

You'll Need:

6 oz whole wheat fettuccine

2 tsp toasted sesame oil + additional for noodles

Juice of 1 lime

2 Tbsp warm water

1½ Tbsp chunky peanut butter

1½ Tbsp low-sodium soy sauce

2 tsp chili sauce, such as sriracha

2 cups shredded chicken

1 red or yellow bell pepper, sliced

2 cups sugar snap peas

1 cup cooked and shelled edamame (optional)

Chopped peanuts, sesame seeds, or chopped scallions (optional)

How to Make It:

• Bring a large pot of salted water to a boil and cook the pasta according to the package instructions. Drain the pasta and toss it in a large bowl with a bit of sesame oil and rice wine vinegar to keep the noodles from sticking.

• Combine the 2 teaspoons of sesame oil, lime juice, water, peanut butter, soy sauce, and chili sauce in a microwaveable mixing bowl. Microwave for 45 seconds, then stir to create a uniform sauce.

• Add the sauce to the noodles and toss to mix. Stir in the chicken, bell pepper, sugar snaps, and edamame, if using. Top with peanuts, sesame seeds, or scallions if you like.

Makes 4 servings

SECRET WEAPON

RONZINI SMART TASTE PASTA

Sure, whole wheat pasta has more protein and three times the fiber of the regular white stuff, but that doesn't do you much good if it tastes like a mouthful of sand. Our taste tests have always found Ronzini's whole wheat pastas to be the most delicious in the supermarket, but their Smart Taste line is the best product yet. It has all the taste and texture of normal white pasta, but it's been enriched with 6 grams of fiber per serving, plus as much calcium as you'd find in an 8-ounce glass of milk.

Not That!

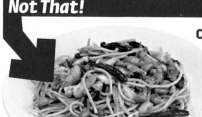

California Pizza Kitchen Kung Pao Spaghetti with Chicken

1,160 calories
8 g saturated fat
1,737 mg sodium
117 g carbohydrates

Eat This!

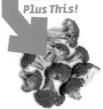

Plus This!

Steamed chopped broccoli
(1 cup)
30 calories
0 g fat
30 mg sodium
6 g carbohydrates

Plus This!

Milk
(1%, 1 cup)
110 calories
2.5 g fat (1.5 g saturated)
108 mg sodium
13 g carbohydrates

Mushroom Melt

370 calories
16 g fat (4 g saturated)
540 mg sodium
41.5 g carbohydrates

Veggie burgers may seem like nutritional safe havens, but the numbers don't lie: meatless restaurant burgers offer little refuge from the onslaught of calories, fat, and sodium found in beef burgers. This meaty, melty portobello burger is the real deal, healthy enough to eat on a daily basis (it's even great cold at your desk), delicious enough to seduce even the staunchest carnivores.

You'll Need:

2 Tbsp mayonnaise

Juice of ½ lemon

¼ cup finely chopped jarred roasted red peppers

1 clove garlic, minced

4 large portobello caps, stems removed

1 Tbsp olive oil

1 Tbsp balsamic vinegar

1 tsp dried Italian seasoning

Salt and ground black pepper to taste

½ cup shredded mozzarella

4 slices red onion

4 potato rolls or whole grain buns

A few handfuls of mixed greens, arugula, or other lettuce

How to Make It:

• Heat a grill or grill pan. Combine the mayonnaise, lemon juice, red peppers, and garlic. (For a uniformly red mayo, puree in a food processor.)

• Combine the olive oil, vinegar, Italian seasoning, salt, and black pepper in a small bowl, then rub the mushrooms with the mixture. Grill, top side down, for 2 to 3 minutes, flip, and immediately add equal portions of the cheese to the mushrooms. Cook for another 2 to 3 minutes, until the cheese is melted and the mushrooms are fully cooked. While the mushrooms cook, grill the onions until browned and toast the buns.

• Fill each bun with greens, grilled onions, a mushroom, and the red pepper mayo.

Makes 4 servings

= Best Lunch

510 calories
18.5 g fat
(5.5 g saturated)
678 mg sodium
60.5 g carbohydrates

---

24 g protein
5.5 g fiber

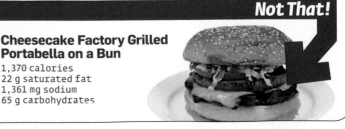

Not That!

Cheesecake Factory Grilled Portabella on a Bun

1,370 calories
22 g saturated fat
1,361 mg sodium
65 g carbohydrates

Eat This!

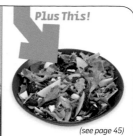

(see page 45)

ETNT Simple Side Salad
170 calories
14 g fat (2 g saturated)
95 mg sodium
10 g carbohydrates

Shrimp Roll
300 calories
9 g fat (1.5 g saturated)
470 mg sodium
24 g carbohydrates

Dead simple and insanely delicious, lobster rolls are one of America's greatest food inventions. Problem is, lobster meat is pricey and restaurants still drown it an abundance of mayo and melted butter. We sub in ultralean shrimp—one of nature's best sources of immune-boosting, blood sugar—stabilizing zinc— for the lobster and go easy on the ingredients, letting the shrimp simply speak for themselves. The result: an amazing sandwich for half the calories and a fraction of the price.

= Best Lunch
470 calories
23 g fat
(3.5 g saturated)
565 mg sodium
34 g carbohydrates

----

30 g protein
4 g fiber

You'll Need:

1 lb cooked shrimp

2 stalks celery, diced

½ small red onion, minced

2 Tbsp minced fresh chives + additional for garnish

2 Tbsp mayonnaise

Juice of 1 lemon

1 tsp hot sauce (we like sriracha)

Salt to taste

4 hot dog buns (Classic Top-Sliced Hot Dog Buns from Pepperidge Farm are best)

How to Make It:

• Heat a cast-iron skillet or sauté pan over medium heat. Add the hot dog buns and toast the outsides until they are nicely browned.

• Mix the shrimp, celery, onion, chives, mayo, lemon juice, hot sauce, and salt together in a bowl, stirring carefully to mix.

• Divide the shrimp mixture among the rolls. Garnish with more minced chives, if using.

Makes 4 servings

SECRET WEAPON

OLIVE OIL MAYONNAISE

You'll see it referenced a lot in this book, and for good reason. Not only do olive oil-based mayonnaises have about half the calories and fat of regular mayo, but since the olive oil replaces cheap soybean oil, you end up with more cholesterol-improving monounsaturated fats. Though it might sound like a fancy European condiment, both Kraft and Hellmann's make versions that are sold in supermarkets throughout the country. Use it for any sandwiches, spreads, or dips that call for mayonnaise. Saving 50 calories a swipe will add up to pounds saved over the course of a year.

Not That!

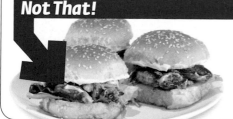

Uno Chicago Grill Lobster Sliders
640 calories
26 g fat (5 g saturated)
1,260 mg sodium
58 g carbohydrates

Eat This!

Butternut Squash Soup

150 calories
3.5 g fat (1 g saturated)
490 mg sodium
27 g carbohydrates

When it comes to vegetable soups, butternut is unbeatable. It's not just addictively delicious, but also packed with vitamin A, fiber, and omega-3s.

You'll Need:

1 large butternut squash

Olive oil

Pinch of grated nutmeg + additional to taste

Salt and ground black pepper to taste

2 strips bacon

1 small onion, diced

1 Tbsp minced or grated fresh ginger

1 green apple, peeled, cored, and chopped

4 cups low-sodium chicken broth

Chopped chives and light sour cream (optional)

How to Make It:

• Preheat the oven to 375°F. Slice the squash in half lengthwise and scoop out the seeds. Rub with oil and season with nutmeg, salt, and pepper. Place on a baking sheet and roast until the flesh is very soft, about 35 minutes.

Set aside to cool.

• Heat a large pot over medium heat. Add the bacon and cook until crispy, 5 to 7 minutes. Transfer to a plate and reserve. Add the onion and ginger to the pot and cook until the onion is translucent, about 3 minutes. Add the apple and cook until soft, another 3 minutes or so.

• When the squash is cool enough to handle, scoop out the flesh and add it to a blender or large food processor. Add the contents of

the pot and pour in enough broth to cover. (Be careful not to overfill; work in batches if necessary.) Process until very smooth and return to the pot. Stir in the remaining broth and bring to a simmer. Season with salt, black pepper, and a touch more nutmeg. Garnish with bacon and chives, and sour cream (if using).

Makes 4 servings

(see page 49)

Plus This!

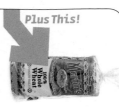

Martin's Famous Whole Wheat Potato Bread

(1 slice, toasted)
70 calories
1 g fat (0 g saturated)
125 mg sodium
14 g carbohydrates

Plus This!

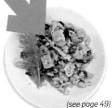

Tuscan Tuna

210 calories
16 g fat (2 g saturated)
150 mg sodium
2 g carbohydrates

= Best Lunch

430 calories
20.5 g fat
(3 g saturated)
765 mg sodium
43 g carbohydrates

26 g protein
10 g fiber

Belly-filling goodness!

Not That!

Panera Bread Creamy Tomato Soup with Croutons

370 calories
23 g fat
(12 g saturated, 1 g trans)
740 mg sodium
39 g carbohydrates

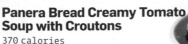

Chinese Chicken Salad

380 calories
21 g fat (3.5 g saturated)
720 mg sodium
23 g carbohydrates

Chinese chicken salad is one of the world's ultimate fusion foods. Whatever its disparate origins, it's undeniably one of the most popular—and ubiquitous—salads in America, sharing space on menus in four-star restaurants and Wendy's alike. Too bad most versions are nutritional disasters, bogged down by too much dressing and too many fried noodles. This lighter version is true to the salad's original inspiration but with about a third of the calories.

Plus This!

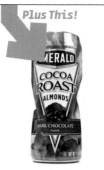

Emerald Cocoa Roast Almonds
150 calories
13 g fat (1 g saturated)
0 mg sodium
6 g carbohydrates

= Best Lunch
530 calories
34 g fat
(4.5 g saturated)
720 mg sodium
29 g carbohydrates

Power-up lunch! 42 g protein
6.5 g fiber

SECRET WEAPON

ASIAN VINAIGRETTE

1 Tbsp Dijon
½ Tbsp soy sauce
2 Tbsp rice wine vinegar
½ Tbsp sesame seed oil (toasted is best)
¼ cup peanut oil
1 tsp sugar

Most vinaigrettes are blended by slowly whisking the oil into the vinegar, but there's an easier way. Combine all ingredients in a mason jar or other sealable container and shake like crazy for 10 seconds. Then use what you need and store the rest in the container. It keeps in the refrigerator for up to a week.

You'll Need:

1 head napa cabbage
½ head red cabbage
½ Tbsp sugar
2 cups chopped or shredded cooked chicken (freshly grilled or from a store-bought rotisserie chicken)
⅓ cup Asian Vinaigrette (see recipe, right)
1 cup fresh cilantro leaves

1 cup canned mandarin oranges, drained
¼ cup sliced almonds, toasted
Salt and black pepper to taste

How to Make It:

• Slice the cabbages in half lengthwise and remove the cores. Slice the cabbage into thin strips. Toss with the sugar in a large bowl.

• If the chicken is cold, toss with a few tablespoons of vinaigrette and heat in a microwave at 50 percent power. Add to the cabbage, along with the cilantro, oranges, almonds, and the remaining vinaigrette. Toss to combine. Season with salt and pepper.

Makes 4 servings

Not That!

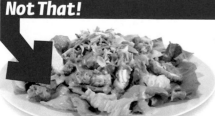

Applebee's Oriental Chicken Salad

1,430 calories
16 g saturated fat
93 g carbohydrates

Eat This!

(see page 45)

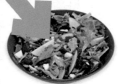

**ETNT Simple
Side Salad**
170 calories
14 g fat (2 g saturated)
95 mg sodium
10 g carbohydrates

Plus This!

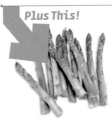

**Asparagus
spears**
(4)
40 calories
0 g fat (0 g saturated)
25 mg sodium
7 g carbohydrates

Chicken Tacos
with Salsa Verde
345 calories
12 g fat (4.5 g saturated)
800 mg sodium
18 g carbohydrates

Tossed with a good dose of bright, mildly spicy salsa verde, rotisserie chicken is the perfect filling for tacos, burritos, and even enchiladas. Indeed, there might not be a better use of a supermarket rotisserie chicken. Even freshly grilled chicken breasts won't yield better results since it's hard to top the juiciness of a spit-roasted bird.

You'll Need:

8 corn tortillas

3 cups shredded rotisserie chicken (about three-fourths of a store-bought chicken)

1½ cups bottled salsa verde

½ cup crumbled Cotija or feta cheese

1 medium onion, minced

1 cup chopped fresh cilantro

2 limes, quartered

How to Make It:

• Heat the tortillas in a large skillet or sauté pan until lightly toasted. If you're heating these up at work or on the run, wrap them in a few damp paper towels and microwave for 30 sec-

onds. (Whatever you do, don't try to eat corn tortillas cold. Trust us.)

• Combine the chicken with the salsa in a large mixing bowl, then divide evenly among the tortillas. Top with crumbled cheese, onion, and cilantro. Serve with lime wedges.

Makes 4 servings

SECRET WEAPON

STORE-BOUGHT ROTISSERIE CHICKEN

We're not afraid to admit that we rely on these succulent birds for many a meal during stressful weeks. For about $7, you get a whole chicken ready to be torn into tacos, shredded into salads and sandwiches, or eaten as is, with a side of roasted vegetables.

= Best Lunch

555 calories
28 g fat
(6.5 g saturated)
920 mg sodium
35 g carbohydrates

----

31 g protein
7 g fiber

Not That!

Chili's Crispy Chicken Tacos

1,650 calories
76 g fat (21 g saturated)
4,080 mg sodium
182 g carbohydrates

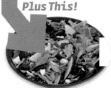

(see page 45)

Plus This!

**ETNT Simple
Side Salad**
170 calories
14 g fat (2 g saturated)
95 mg sodium
10 g carbohydrates

Minestrone
with Pesto
200 calories
5 g fat (1.5 g saturated)
490 mg sodium
41 g carbohydrates

Nearly 9 out of 10 Americans don't consume enough fruits and vegetables on
a daily basis. This hodgepodge soup
will go a long way toward making sure
you're not one of them. Keep a jar of pesto in your fridge and
crown soup—even canned soups—with a spoonful before eating.

You'll Need:

1 Tbsp olive oil

1 onion, chopped

2 cloves garlic, minced

8 oz Yukon gold or red
potatoes, cubed

2 carrots, peeled and
chopped

1 zucchini, chopped

8 oz green beans, ends
trimmed, halved

Salt and ground black
pepper to taste

1 can (14 oz) diced
tomatoes

8 cups low-sodium
chicken stock
(or water, or both)

½ tsp dried thyme

½ (14–16 oz) can white
beans, drained

Pesto

Parmesan for grating

How to Make It:

• Heat the olive oil in a
large pot over medium
heat. Add the onion
and garlic and cook until
the onion is translucent,
about 3 minutes. Stir
in the potatoes, carrots,
zucchini, and green
beans. Season with a bit
of salt and cook, stir-
ring, for 3 to 4 minutes
to release the vegeta-
bles' aromas. Add the
tomatoes, stock, and
thyme and turn the heat
down to low. Season
with salt (if needed) and
pepper to taste. Simmer
for at least 15 minutes,
and up to 45.

• Before serving, stir
in the white beans and
heat through. Serve
with a dollop of pesto
and a bit of grated
Parmesan.

Makes 4 servings

= Best
Lunch
370 calories
19 g fat
(3.5 g saturated)
585 mg sodium
51 g carbohydrates

---

21 g protein
10 g fiber

MEAL MULTIPLIER

SOUP IMPROV
Soups aren't rocket
science; most don't even
require recipes. The
formula for pureed soups
is especially simple. Just
sauté 1 chopped onion
and 2 minced garlic
cloves until translucent,
and then add any of the
following ingredients
along with 4 cups chicken
broth (the base of most
soups). Puree in a blender.

2 cans (14 oz) white
beans; add 2 Tbsp
chopped fresh rose-
mary after blending

1 can (28 oz) whole
peeled tomatoes
and ½ cup half-and-
half; add 1 cup
chopped fresh basil
after blending

2 lb sautéed mush-
rooms and ½ cup
half-and-half

2 cans (14 oz) black
beans, juice of 2 limes,
¼ tsp each cumin and
cayenne pepper

Not That!

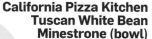

**California Pizza Kitchen
Tuscan White Bean
Minestrone (bowl)**
262 calories
3 g saturated fat
672 mg sodium
35 g carbohydrates

Eat This!

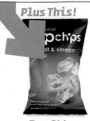

Turkey Sandwich
with guacamole and bacon

430 calories
13 g fat (4 g saturated)
1,070 mg sodium
24 g carbohydrates

As great as guacamole is with chips, it's even better slathered on a sandwich. Swapping in the avocado all-star for mayo not only shaves 70 to 100 calories from your sandwich but also replaces low-quality fats with healthy monounsaturated ones. Quiznos's creation fails because it doesn't rely solely on the guac but rather piles it on top of a slick of ranch dressing. Avoid this blunder by turning guacamole into your spread of choice for turkey, chicken, and grilled steak sandwiches.

= **Best Lunch**

550 calories
17 g fat
(4 g saturated)
1,320 mg sodium
44 g carbohydrates

---

36 g protein
3 g fiber

MASTER THE TECHNIQUE

PICKLED JALAPEÑOS

These spicy sweet chili rings make everything they touch better. Combine thinly sliced jalapeños with equal parts water and white or apple cider vinegar, plus a few pinches of salt and sugar. Let pickle at least 20 minutes. They'll keep for 2 weeks in your fridge.

You'll Need:

1 baguette

12 oz sliced turkey

4 slices Swiss cheese

1 large tomato, sliced

½ red onion, thinly sliced

Pickled Jalapeños

4 strips bacon, cooked until crisp and patted dry

¼ cup guacamole

How to Make It:

• Preheat the broiler. Carefully slice the baguette in half horizontally and place on a large baking sheet. Layer the turkey and cheese on the bottom half of the bread.

• Place the sheet in the oven 6" below the broiler. Broil for 2 to 3 minutes, until the cheese has just melted and both halves of the bread are hot, but not too brown and crunchy.

• Remove from the oven and then layer the tomato, onion, jalapeños, and bacon on top of the turkey. Spread the top half of the baguette with the guacamole. Slice the baguette into 4 individual sandwiches and serve.

Makes 4 servings

Not That!

Quiznos Regular California Club

790 calories
38 g fat (10.5 g saturated)
2,490 mg sodium
69 g carbohydrates

Plus This!

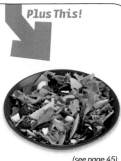

(see page 45)

ETNT Simple
Side Salad
170 calories
14 g fat (2 g saturated)
95 mg sodium
10 g carbohydrates

Chili-Mango Chicken

240 calories
8 g fat (1 g saturated)
410 mg sodium
23 g carbohydrates

Good news for lovers of sweet and heat: Studies show that flavor extremes can have a powerful effect on satiety. So not only is this super simple stir-fry packed full of flavor, it will also keep your appetite at bay well into the evening hours.

Plus This!

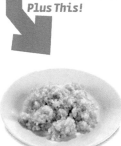

Quinoa
(½ cup cooked)
110 calories
2 g fat (0 g saturated)
10 mg sodium
20 g carbohydrates

You'll Need:

1 lb boneless, skinless chicken thighs, chopped into ½" pieces
1 Tbsp cornstarch
1 Tbsp low-sodium soy sauce
½ Tbsp sesame oil
½ Tbsp peanut or canola oil
1 red onion, chopped
1 Tbsp grated or minced fresh ginger
2 cups sugar snap peas
1 mango, peeled, pitted, and chopped
1 Tbsp chili garlic sauce
Black pepper to taste

How to Make It:

• Combine the chicken, cornstarch, soy sauce, and sesame oil in a mixing bowl and let sit for 10 minutes.

• Heat the peanut oil in a wok or large skillet over high heat. Add the onion and ginger and cook for 1 to 2 minutes, until the onion is translucent. Add the sugar snaps and stir-fry for 1 minute, using a metal spatula to keep the vegetables in near constant motion. Add the chicken and its marinade and stir-fry for about 2 minutes, until the meat begins to brown on the outside. Add the mango, chili sauce, and black pepper and stir-fry for 1 minute longer, until the chicken is cooked through and the mango has softened almost to a saucelike consistency. Serve over brown rice.

Makes 4 servings

= Best Lunch

520 calories
24 g fat
(3 g saturated)
515 mg sodium
53 g carbohydrates

----

30 g protein
7.5 g fiber

Not That!

Applebee's Crispy Orange Chicken

1,550 calories
58 g fat
(11 g saturated, 1 g trans)
3,520 mg sodium
204 g carbohydrates

Eat This!

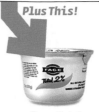

Curry with Cauliflower and Butternut Squash

260 calories
8 g fat (4.5 g saturated)
510 mg sodium
41 g carbohydrates

Such is the food world we live in that even a simple vegetable stir-fry at a restaurant packs nearly 1,000 calories and a day's worth of sodium. This Indian-style curry takes no more than 25 minutes to prepare, yet it will taste like it's been simmering away all day. The balance of the creamy coconut milk, the sweet cubes of squash, and the subtle heat of the curry could make even the most dedicated meat eater forget he was eating only vegetables.

Plus This!

Brown rice
(½ cup cooked)
110 calories
1 g fat (0 g saturated)
0 mg sodium
23 g carbohydrates

You'll Need:

½ Tbsp canola oil

1 medium onion, diced

½ Tbsp minced fresh ginger

2 cups cubed butternut squash

1 head cauliflower, cut into florets

1 can (14–16 oz) chickpeas, drained

1 jalapeño pepper, minced, wear gloves when handling

1 Tbsp yellow curry powder

1 can (14 oz) diced tomatoes

1 can (14 oz) light coconut milk

Juice of 1 lime

Salt and ground black pepper to taste

Chopped cilantro

How to Make It:

• Heat the oil in a large sauté pan or pot over medium heat. Add the onion and ginger and cook for about 2 minutes, until the onion is soft and translucent. Add the squash, cauliflower, chickpeas, jalapeño pepper, and curry powder. Cook for 2 minutes, until the curry powder is fragrant and coats the vegetables evenly. Stir in the tomatoes and coconut milk and turn the heat down to low. Simmer for 15 to 20 minutes, until the vegetables are tender. Add the lime juice and season with salt and black pepper. Serve garnished with the chopped cilantro.

Makes 4 servings

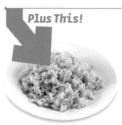

= Best Lunch

500 calories
13 g fat
(7.5 g saturated)
575 mg sodium
72 g carbohydrates

28.5 g protein
11 g fiber

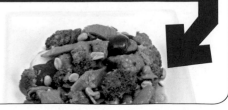

(see page 48)

Riviera Salmon
(½ cup)
197 calories
16 g fat (3.5 g saturated)
410 mg sodium
1 g carbohydrates

Caprese Sandwich
300 calories
17 g fat (4.5 g saturated)
410 mg sodium
32 g carbohydrates

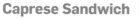

The pairing of creamy fresh mozzarella, juicy ripe tomatoes, and fat leaves of sweet basil is so good that you'd be crazy not to exploit it as often as possible to make yourself look like a culinary genius. This recipe requires absolutely no effort, save for about 2 minutes of slicing and 2 minutes of toasting. Not in the mood for a sandwich? Ditch the bread, add a handful of your favorite lettuce, and eat this as a salad.

= Best Lunch
497 calories
33 g fat
(8 g saturated)
820 mg sodium
33 g carbohydrates

----
11 g protein
6 g fiber

You'll Need:

1 baguette, sliced in half lengthwise

1 clove garlic, peeled and cut in half

2 large heirloom tomatoes, sliced

4 oz fresh mozzarella, sliced

15–20 fresh basil leaves

Salt and ground black pepper to taste

1 Tbsp olive oil

1 Tbsp balsamic vinegar

How to Make It:

• Preheat the broiler. Broil the baguette, cut sides up, 6 inches from the heat, for about 2 minutes, until the inside is lightly toasted. Rub each half with a half clove of garlic; the crusty bread will release the garlic's essential oils, giving you instant garlic bread.

• Layer the bottom half of the baguette with alternating slices of tomato and mozzarella and with basil leaves. Season evenly with salt and lots of freshly ground black pepper. Finish with a drizzle of olive oil and vinegar, then top with the other baguette half. Cut the whole package into four pieces.

Makes 4 servings

CHEESE
TOTEM POLE

(1 OZ EACH)

FRESH MOZZARELLA
80 calories
6 g fat (4 g saturated)
100 mg sodium

PROVOLONE
100 calories
7 g fat (5 g saturated)
250 mg sodium

MONTEREY
105 calories
9 g fat (5 g saturated)
150 mg sodium

AMERICAN
105 calories
9 g fat (6 g saturated)
185 mg sodium

SWISS
110 calories
8 g fat (5 g saturated)
55 mg sodium

COLBY
110 calories
9 g fat (6 g saturated)
170 mg sodium

CHEDDAR
115 calories
9 g fat (6 g saturated)
180 mg sodium

Not That!

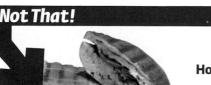

Panera Bread Tomato Mozzarella Hot Panini on Ciabatta
770 calories
29 g fat (10 g saturated)
1,290 mg sodium
96 g carbohydrates

Eat This!

Turkey Reuben

365 calories
14 g fat (4 g saturated)
1,120 mg sodium
38 g carbohydrates

Reubens invariably conjure up the image of a deli sandwich stacked so high with peppery beef you'd need an unhinging snake's jaw just to get your teeth around it—and a generous belt for waistline adjustment in the postprandial aftermath. We've taken the indulgent essence of the Jewish deli staple and distilled it to a sandwich with substance and soul, but without half a day's calories and a day and a half's worth of saturated fat (which is exactly what Applebee's offers with their version).

You'll Need:

¼ cup ketchup

¼ cup olive oil mayonnaise

2 Tbsp relish

Few dashes of Tabasco sauce

Ground black pepper to taste

1 lb turkey pastrami (or, failing that, regular deli-cut turkey)

4 slices low-fat Swiss cheese

8 slices rye bread, toasted

1 cup jarred sauerkraut

How to Make It:

• Combine the ketchup, mayo, relish, and Tabasco in a bowl and mix. Season with a bit of black pepper. Set the dressing aside.

• You can always skip this step and buy a bottle of Russian or Thousand Island dressing, but it's never as good as the homemade stuff.

• Divide the pastrami into four portions, pile on plates, and top each with a slice of cheese.

Microwave briefly, about 30 seconds each, to melt the cheese.

• Lay out four slices of the rye bread on a cutting board. Top each with sauerkraut and then pastrami and cheese. Drizzle with the dressing. Top with the remaining slices of bread.

Makes 4 servings

Plus This!

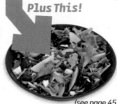

(see page 45)

ETNT Simple Side Salad
170 calories
14 g fat (2 g saturated)
95 mg sodium
10 g carbohydrates

= Best Lunch

535 calories
28 g fat
(6 g saturated)
1,215 mg sodium
48 g carbohydrates

----

26 g protein
6.5 g fiber

SECRET WEAPON

PRIME PASTRAMI

Unfortunately, true beef pastrami comes with a pretty hefty caloric price tag, but on a decadent sandwich like this, turkey pastrami works perfectly. It's laced with all the same spices as the regular stuff, but has about half the calories and fat. Try Jennie-O's lean turkey pastrami on your next Reuben.

Not That!

Applebee's Reuben
1,150 calories
82 g fat
(28 g saturated, 2 g trans)
3,560 mg sodium
49 g carbohydrates

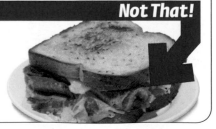

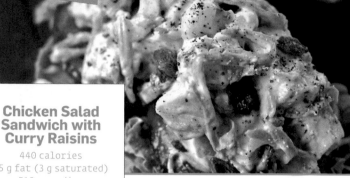

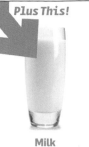

Milk
(1%, 1 cup)
110 calories
2.5 g fat (1.5 g saturated)
108 mg sodium
13 g carbohydrates

Chicken Salad Sandwich with Curry Raisins

440 calories
15 g fat (3 g saturated)
510 mg sodium
38 g carbohydrates

Chicken and salad: two great foods on their own that make for a lousy dish when combined. In fact, chicken and tuna salad sandwiches are consistently the worst options you'll find on a deli menu, be it Subway or your neighborhood sandwich shop. We use a modest amount of olive oil–based mayo, then punch up the flavor with golden raisins and the complex savory notes of curry powder—a hugely addictive yin and yang combination.

=Best Lunch

550 calories
17.5 g fat
(4.5 g saturated)
618 mg sodium
51 g carbohydrates

----

46 g protein
6 g fiber

You'll Need:

3 Tbsp golden raisins

3 cups chopped cooked chicken

2 stalks celery, thinly sliced

½ onion, diced

1 carrot, shredded

½ tsp curry powder

¼ cup olive oil mayonnaise

Salt and ground black pepper to taste

4 large lettuce leaves (romaine, iceberg, or anything else)

8 slices whole grain bread or English muffin halves, toasted

2 medium tomatoes, sliced

How to Make It:

• Cover the raisins with hot water and soak for at least 10 minutes (the water will help the raisins plump up); drain and place in a large bowl. Add the chicken, celery, onion, carrot, curry powder, and mayonnaise. Mix well and season with salt and pepper.

• Place the lettuce leaves on top of four bread slices, then top with tomatoes, chicken salad, and the remaining bread.

Makes 4 servings

SECRET WEAPON

CURCUMIN

Turmeric is the Indian spice that gives curry powder its characteristic yellow hue, and many researchers believe it to be one of nature's most potent cure-alls. The list of benefits that studies have borne out is truly staggering, from helping fight off colon, breast, and skin cancer to reducing inflammation and arthritic symptoms to lowering cholesterol and preventing mental degeneration. Sign us up! To pack more curcumin into your daily diet, try rubbing fish and chicken with it, mixing it with yogurt for a quick sauce or spread, or slathering mustard— also a curcumin vessel—on everything.

Not That!

Boston Market All White Rotisserie Chicken Salad Sandwich

1,040 calories
60 g fat
(9 g saturated, 1 g trans)
1,780 mg sodium
88 g carbohydrates

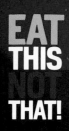

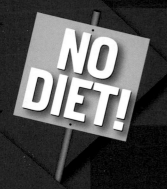
NO
DIET!

CHAPTER 6

Dinner

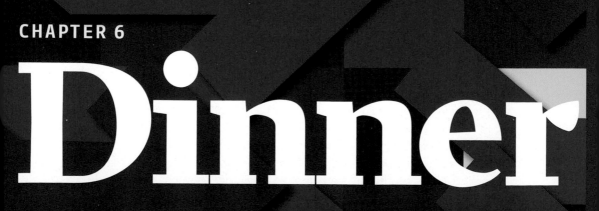

Did you win the Super Bowl today? No? You didn't win the Super Bowl today?

Hmmm

How about an Olympic gold medal—win one of those? No? Not one of those either?

Okay. Perhaps then you performed some other heroic and miraculous feat—saving a family of endangered pandas from a burning zoo, or rescuing a passel of aging cheerleaders who'd been tied to train tracks, or getting a Democrat and a Republican to shake hands with one another. Something like that? No? Okay, then let me ask you a question: Why are you going to Disney World for dinner?

If you're like most Americans, your dinner—night after night after night—is the dietary equivalent of visiting Mickey and Donald. (Often by dining at a place whose name you can conjure by saying "Mickey-Donald" really fast.) For most of us, it's the biggest meal of the day, with about 900 calories for men, and 640 calories for women. The problem with that? It ought to be our smallest meal of the day.

Why? Well, because loading up on calories before you head off on your day's errands makes sense. Loading up on calories before you pass out in front of

Stephen Colbert doesn't. When you eat the majority of your calories before bedtime, your bloodstream is flooded with glucose (sugar), but you have no way to burn that glucose off. So your body has only one option: Store dinner as fat. There are only four things you can do to keep your hefty dinner from winding up around your waistline:

Go to the gym for dessert. It's certainly a possibility—and simply taking a long walk isn't a bad way to burn off a few calories. But an intense workout will actually wake you up, making it harder to fall asleep afterward.

Make mad, passionate, vigorous nookie every night. An hour-long session of lovemaking will burn 100 extra calories, and anything above and beyond standard missionary will burn even more. (Then again, if you're making crazy, wild love for an hour every single night, we should probably be reading your book . . .)

Take up sleepwalking. Or even better, sleep jogging. Sure, there's always the risk of taking a long run off a short pier, but think of the calorie burn!

Eat a smaller, more sensible dinner.

In fact, dinner ought to be no more than maybe 450 calories—about 25 percent smaller than either breakfast or lunch. And if you've followed the advice of *The Eat This, Not That! No-Diet Diet*, that's probably enough. After two big meals and two hearty snacks, your appetite should be only moderate, and your cravings under control. (Besides, you still have dessert to top it all off!) Here are the hallmarks of a sensible dinner.

• *It's got protein.* By now, you've pretty much figured out that earning protein at every meal is key to managing your weight. But just because it's dinnertime doesn't mean there should be a 20-ounce T-bone hanging over the edges of your plate. A single chicken breast or a 4-ounce serving of steak or fish is plenty.

• *It's got vegetables.* Fruits tend to make their appearance at breakfast time and during most snacks. Maybe you got in a serving of greens at lunch, but for the most part, dinner is where vegetables make their entrance. Leafy greens like broccoli, brussels sprouts, spinach, and lettuce-based salads ought to be a part of dinner whenever possible; they're packed with folate, which studies show increases your chances of losing weight. Plus, vegetables tend to be lower in calories than just about any other food, so they're a great way to pack in nutrition while lowering calories.

• *It's got whole grains, beans, or other sources of fiber.*
Slow-burning energy will help keep you full through the evening, and keep you from raiding the icebox at midnight. (Plus, an indulgent dessert will most likely include some refined carbohydrates, and eating whole grains with dinner will help slow the absorption of the sugar, lessening their impact on your belly.)

Eat This!

APPLEBEE'S

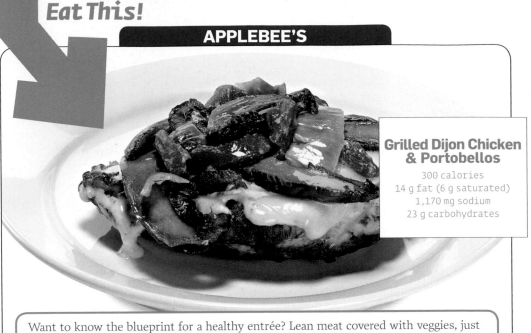

Grilled Dijon Chicken & Portobellos

300 calories
14 g fat (6 g saturated)
1,170 mg sodium
23 g carbohydrates

Want to know the blueprint for a healthy entrée? Lean meat covered with veggies, just like you see here. This chicken is from Applebee's Unbelievably Great Tasting & Under 550 Calories Menu (their name, not ours), and with potatoes and vegetables on the side, it makes for an incredibly balanced dinner. We'd like to see Applebee's go easy with the salt shaker, but until that happens, just cut back your sodium on Applebee's days.

Plus This!

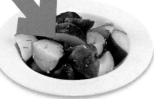

Herbed Steamed Potatoes

105 calories
1 g fat (0 g saturated)
320 mg sodium
19 g carbohydrates

Plus This!

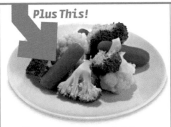

Seasonal Vegetables

45 calories
0 g fat
300 mg sodium
8 g carbohydrates

= Best Dinner

450 calories
15 g fat
(6 g saturated)
1,790 mg sodium
50 g carbohydrates

Perfect post-workout feast! → 6 g fiber
54 g protein

THE TRUE COST OF FREE

THE FREEBIE
SODA,
UNLIMITED REFILLS

THE COST
250 calories
per 20-ounce cup

Each cup has more calories than a Hershey's Milk Chocolate Bar. Drink just two and you've more than doubled the impact of this meal.

Not That!

Crispy Orange Chicken

2,030 calories
80 g fat
(15 g saturated, 1 g trans)
4,480 mg sodium
264 g carbohydrates

ARBY'S

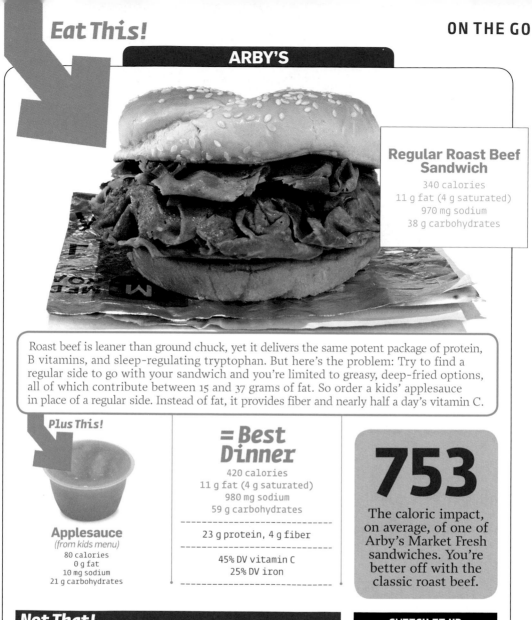

Regular Roast Beef Sandwich
340 calories
11 g fat (4 g saturated)
970 mg sodium
38 g carbohydrates

Roast beef is leaner than ground chuck, yet it delivers the same potent package of protein, B vitamins, and sleep-regulating tryptophan. But here's the problem: Try to find a regular side to go with your sandwich and you're limited to greasy, deep-fried options, all of which contribute between 15 and 37 grams of fat. So order a kids' applesauce in place of a regular side. Instead of fat, it provides fiber and nearly half a day's vitamin C.

Plus This!

Applesauce
(from kids menu)
80 calories
0 g fat
10 mg sodium
21 g carbohydrates

= Best Dinner
420 calories
11 g fat (4 g saturated)
980 mg sodium
59 g carbohydrates
----
23 g protein, 4 g fiber

45% DV vitamin C
25% DV iron

753
The caloric impact, on average, of one of Arby's Market Fresh sandwiches. You're better off with the classic roast beef.

Not That!

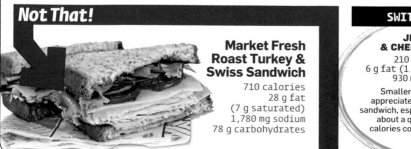

Market Fresh Roast Turkey & Swiss Sandwich
710 calories
28 g fat
(7 g saturated)
1,780 mg sodium
78 g carbohydrates

SWITCH IT UP

JR. HAM & CHEDDAR MELT
210 calories
6 g fat (1.5 g saturated)
930 mg sodium

Smaller appetites will appreciate this 210-calorie sandwich, especially considering about a quarter of these calories come from protein.

Eat This!

ATLANTA BREAD COMPANY

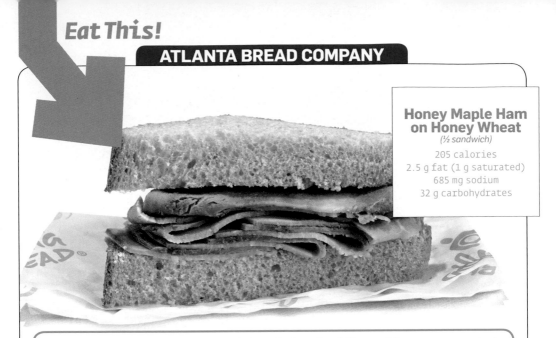

At its best, the half-sandwich, half-salad combo has the ability to chip away at your day's produce quota and pad your belly with protein and fiber without pushing your energy load past the threshold of a healthy dinner. This meal certainly accomplishes those goals, and it does so by avoiding the fatty accoutrements that ruin so many otherwise healthy meals—think bacon, mayonnaise, and oil-based salad dressings.

SANDWICH SELECTOR

CHICKEN SALAD ON SOURDOUGH
440 calories
19 g fat (2 g saturated)

VEGGIE ON NINE GRAIN
500 calories
25 g fat (8 g saturated)

TUNA SALAD ON FRENCH
630 calories
33 g fat (4.5 g saturated)

NY HOT PASTRAMI
660 calories
29 g fat (11 g saturated)

CHICKEN PESTO PANINI
710 calories
26 g fat (9 g saturated)

ABC SPECIAL
750 calories
38 g fat (10 g saturated)

TURKEY BACON RUSTICA
960 calories
56 g fat (19 g saturated)

Plus This!

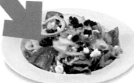

Balsamic Bleu Salad
(½ salad)
165 calories
9 g fat (3 g saturated)
205 mg sodium
17 g carbohydrates

= Best Dinner

370 calories
11.5 g fat
(4 g saturated)
890 mg sodium
49 g carbohydrates

----

26 g protein
5 g fiber

Not That!

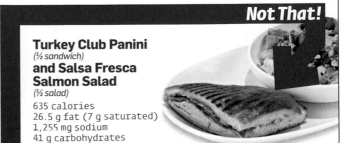

Turkey Club Panini
(½ sandwich)
and Salsa Fresca Salmon Salad
(½ salad)
635 calories
26.5 g fat (7 g saturated)
1,255 mg sodium
41 g carbohydrates

AU BON PAIN

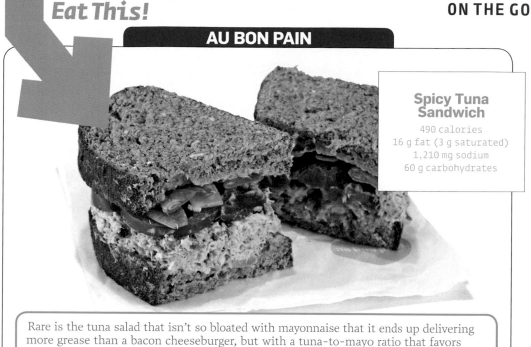

Spicy Tuna Sandwich
490 calories
16 g fat (3 g saturated)
1,210 mg sodium
60 g carbohydrates

Rare is the tuna salad that isn't so bloated with mayonnaise that it ends up delivering more grease than a bacon cheeseburger, but with a tuna-to-mayo ratio that favors protein over fat, Au Bon Pain's version is legit. But what really secures this sandwich a spot on this page is the robust, multigrain bread on which it sits. Along with the snow peas (a great sandwich addition, by the way) it helps give this entrée 11 grams of fiber.

Plus This!

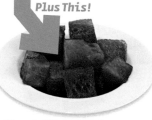

Fresh Watermelon *(8 oz)*
70 calories
0 g fat
0 mg sodium
17 g carbohydrates

= Best Dinner
560 calories
16 g fat (3 g saturated)
1,210 mg sodium
77 g carbohydrates

----

31 g protein, 12 g fiber

85% DV vitamin A, 10% DV calcium,
55% DV vitamin C, 29% DV iron

FOOD COURT

CRIME
Southwest Tuna Wrap
780 calories

PUNISHMENT
1 hour and 35 minutes
hiking with a backpack

Not That!

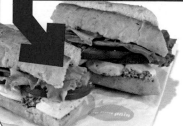

Caprese Sandwich
680 calories
32 g fat (15 g saturated)
1,200 mg sodium
65 g carbohydrates

NUTRITION 101

WATERMELON

Sure, watermelon is 92 percent water, but that other 8 percent is loaded with lycopene, a phytochemical that may protect your heart and help prevent skin damage from exposure to sunlight. Just one 1-inch-thick slab contains as much lycopene as four medium-size tomatoes.

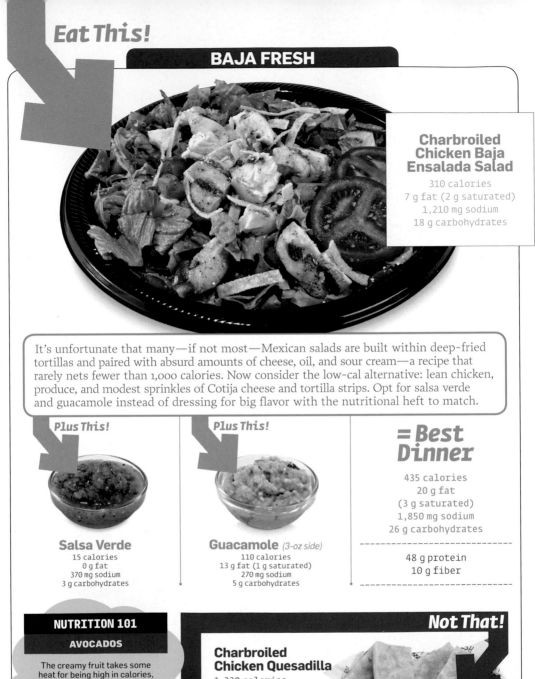

Eat This!

BAJA FRESH

Charbroiled Chicken Baja Ensalada Salad

310 calories
7 g fat (2 g saturated)
1,210 mg sodium
18 g carbohydrates

It's unfortunate that many—if not most—Mexican salads are built within deep-fried tortillas and paired with absurd amounts of cheese, oil, and sour cream—a recipe that rarely nets fewer than 1,000 calories. Now consider the low-cal alternative: lean chicken, produce, and modest sprinkles of Cotija cheese and tortilla strips. Opt for salsa verde and guacamole instead of dressing for big flavor with the nutritional heft to match.

Plus This!

Salsa Verde
15 calories
0 g fat
370 mg sodium
3 g carbohydrates

Plus This!

Guacamole *(3-oz side)*
110 calories
13 g fat (1 g saturated)
270 mg sodium
5 g carbohydrates

= Best Dinner

435 calories
20 g fat
(3 g saturated)
1,850 mg sodium
26 g carbohydrates

----

48 g protein
10 g fiber

NUTRITION 101
AVOCADOS

The creamy fruit takes some heat for being high in calories, but those calories spring primarily from heart-healthy monounsaturated fats. And get this: Half an avocado contains more potassium than a medium banana, 50 percent more fiber than a cup of cooked oatmeal, and a payload of vitamin E.

Not That!

Charbroiled Chicken Quesadilla

1,330 calories
80 g fat
(37 g saturated,
2.5 g trans)
2,590 mg sodium
84 g carbohydrates

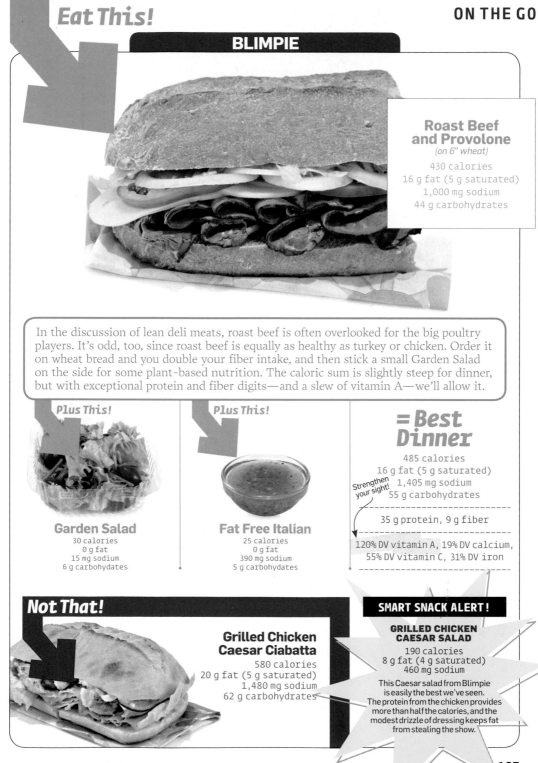

BLIMPIE

Roast Beef and Provolone
(on 6" wheat)
430 calories
16 g fat (5 g saturated)
1,000 mg sodium
44 g carbohydrates

In the discussion of lean deli meats, roast beef is often overlooked for the big poultry players. It's odd, too, since roast beef is equally as healthy as turkey or chicken. Order it on wheat bread and you double your fiber intake, and then stick a small Garden Salad on the side for some plant-based nutrition. The caloric sum is slightly steep for dinner, but with exceptional protein and fiber digits—and a slew of vitamin A—we'll allow it.

Plus This!

Plus This!

= Best Dinner
485 calories
16 g fat (5 g saturated)
1,405 mg sodium
55 g carbohydrates

Strengthen your sight!

----
35 g protein, 9 g fiber

120% DV vitamin A, 19% DV calcium,
55% DV vitamin C, 31% DV iron

Garden Salad
30 calories
0 g fat
15 mg sodium
6 g carbohydates

Fat Free Italian
25 calories
0 g fat
390 mg sodium
5 g carbohydates

Not That!

Grilled Chicken Caesar Ciabatta
580 calories
20 g fat (5 g saturated)
1,480 mg sodium
62 g carbohydrates

SMART SNACK ALERT!

GRILLED CHICKEN CAESAR SALAD
190 calories
8 g fat (4 g saturated)
460 mg sodium

This Caesar salad from Blimpie is easily the best we've seen. The protein from the chicken provides more than half the calories, and the modest drizzle of dressing keeps fat from stealing the show.

Eat This!

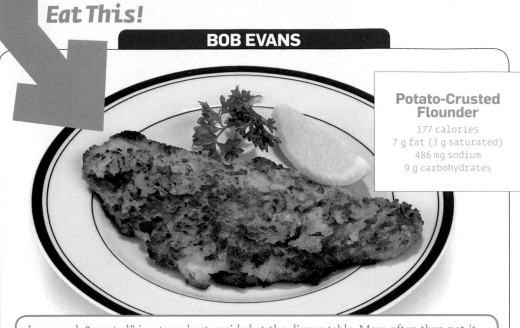

Potato-Crusted Flounder

177 calories
7 g fat (3 g saturated)
486 mg sodium
9 g carbohydrates

In general, "crusted" is a term best avoided at the dinner table. More often than not it indicates a hunk of meat that's been breaded, deep fried, and otherwise stripped of its nutritional merits. This is the exception. Bob's flounder is grilled rather than fried, so it's still a healthy catch. It's typically served with green beans and a baked potato, but to maximize nutrition and minimize calories, swap out the starchy spud for baby carrots.

Plus This!

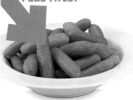

Plus This!

= Best Dinner

325 calories
14 g fat
(6 g saturated)
Low-carb dinner!
1,100 mg sodium
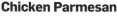
29 g carbohydrates

Glazed Baby Carrots
101 calories
5 g fat (2 g saturated)
99 mg sodium
14 g carbohydrates

Green Beans with Ham
47 calories
2 g fat (1 g saturated)
515 mg sodium
6 g carbohydrates

23 g protein
5 g fiber

NUTRITION 101

BETA-CAROTENE

This antioxidant is responsible for the carrot's orange hue, and it has been linked to diminished risks of cancer and macular degeneration, or age-related vision loss. Once inside the body, beta-carotene is easily converted into vitamin A, which protects your skin and bolsters your immune system.

Not That!

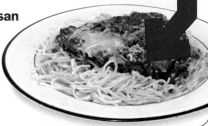

Chicken Parmesan
1,160 calories
55 g fat
(19 g saturated)
2,739 mg sodium
20 g carbohydrates

The Eat This, Not That! No-Diet Cheat Sheets

FISH	CALORIES	FAT (g)	SATURATED (g)	TRANS (g)	SODIUM (mg)	FIBER (g)	PROTEIN (g)	CARBS (g)
1. Red Lobster Seafood Stuffed Flounder (lunch portion)	160	5	1.5	N/A	760	N/A	N/A	6
2. Bob Evans Potato-Crusted Flounder (a la carte)	177	7	3	0	486	0	19	9
3. Ruby Tuesday Creole Catch	196	8	N/A	N/A	383	1	N/A	1
4. Cheesecake Factory Fresh Grilled Mahi Mahi	240	N/A	1	N/A	364	N/A	N/A	2
5. Uno Chicago Grill Baked Haddock (½ serving)	290	17	3	N/A	270	0	27	6
6. Applebee's Weight Watchers Cajun Lime Tilapia	310	6	1.5	0	2,160	9	36	39
7. Romano's Macaroni Grill Snapper "Acqua Pazza"	400	N/A	2.5	N/A	1,420	N/A	N/A	24
8. P.F. Chang's Cantonese Shrimp (full serving)	430	20	4	N/A	1,900	4	42	20
9. Denny's Tilapia Ranchero	450	15	5	0	1,020	4	54	56
10. Ruby Tuesday Trout Almondine	468	30	N/A	N/A	640	2	N/A	3
11. Olive Garden Seafood Brodetto	480	16	3	N/A	2,250	7	N/A	35
12. Chili's GG salmon w/ garlic & herbs	520	16	4	N/A	1,410	5	49	47
13. Outback Atlantic Salmon & Fresh Seasonal Veggies	525	34	11	0	754	4	42	12

Eat This!

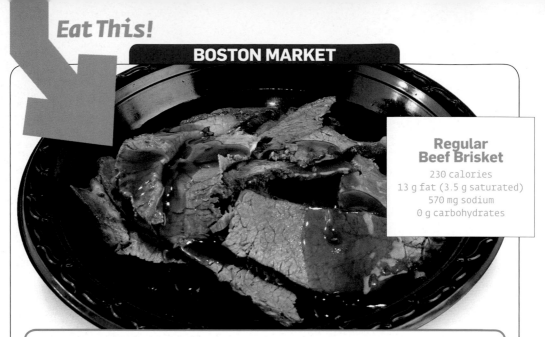

BOSTON MARKET

**Regular
Beef Brisket**
230 calories
13 g fat (3.5 g saturated)
570 mg sodium
0 g carbohydrates

Surviving a meal at Boston Market is simple: Pair lean meat with a couple simple vegetables, and steer your appetite away from calorie-heavy entrées like meat loaf, potpies, and hot Carver sandwiches. This meal combination—lean brisket, green beans, and new potatoes—represents a near-perfect balance of carbohydrates, protein, and fat, with a fistful of fiber to boot. You'd be hard-pressed to cook a healthier dinner yourself.

Plus This!

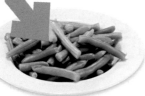

Green Beans
60 calories
3.5 g fat (1.5 g saturated)
180 mg sodium
7 g carbohydrates

Plus This!

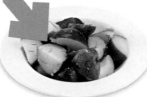

Garlic Dill New Potatoes
140 calories
3 g fat (1 g saturated)
120 mg sodium
24 g carbohydrates

= Best Dinner

430 calories
19.5 g fat
(6 g saturated)
870 mg sodium
31 g carbohydrates

----

33 g protein
6 g fiber

THE TRUE COST OF FREE

**THE FREEBIE
CORNBREAD**

THE COST
200 calories

This complementary touch of Southern comfort is enough to ruin an otherwise healthy meal. Defend yourself by rehearsing this line: "Hold the cornbread." Now put it to practice every time you order at Boston Market.

Not That!

**Regular Meatloaf
with Mashed Potatoes
and Poultry Gravy**
810 calories
43 g fat
(18.5 g saturated,
2 g trans)
2,600 mg sodium
68 g carbohydrates

Eat This!

BURGER KING

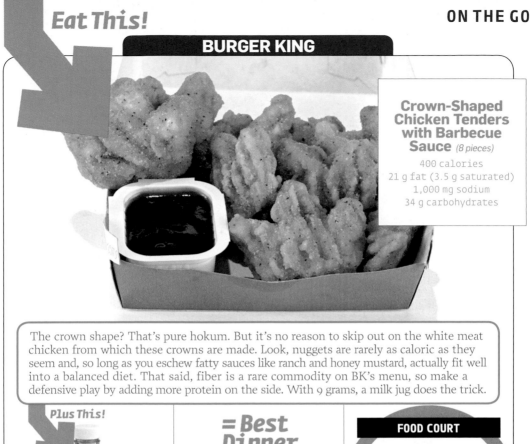

Crown-Shaped Chicken Tenders with Barbecue Sauce *(8 pieces)*
400 calories
21 g fat (3.5 g saturated)
1,000 mg sodium
34 g carbohydrates

The crown shape? That's pure hokum. But it's no reason to skip out on the white meat chicken from which these crowns are made. Look, nuggets are rarely as caloric as they seem and, so long as you eschew fatty sauces like ranch and honey mustard, actually fit well into a balanced diet. That said, fiber is a rare commodity on BK's menu, so make a defensive play by adding more protein on the side. With 9 grams, a milk jug does the trick.

Plus This!

Milk *(fat free, 12 fl oz)*
90 calories
0 g fat
125 mg sodium
13 g carbohydrates

= Best Dinner

490 calories
21 g fat
(3.5 g saturated)
1,125 mg sodium
47 g carbohydrates

-----

27 g protein
0 g fiber

FOOD COURT

CRIME
A.1. Steakhouse XT Burger
970 calories

PUNISHMENT
One full game of rugby from start to finish (that's two 40-minute halves)

Not That!

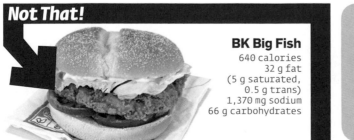

BK Big Fish
640 calories
32 g fat
(5 g saturated,
0.5 g trans)
1,370 mg sodium
66 g carbohydrates

45
Percentage of calories that come from fat in a typical order of french fries.

Eat This!

CALIFORNIA PIZZA KITCHEN

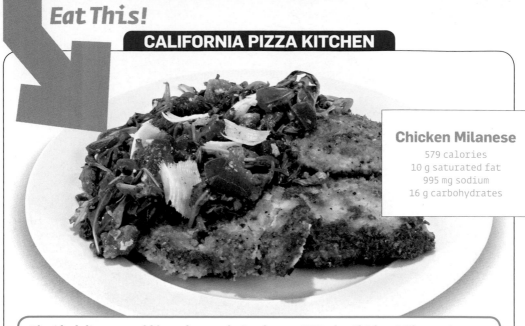

Chicken Milanese
579 calories
10 g saturated fat
995 mg sodium
16 g carbohydrates

The ideal dinner would have fewer calories, but at CPK, the Chicken Milanese is your best shot at avoiding a belly-expanding boatload of fat. The good news? It's a complete meal, with protein and produce already accounted for. That means you can do without a side, but by ordering unsweetened tea, you earn a hit of catechins, antioxidants that bolster your metabolism so you can more quickly slough off those extra dinner calories.

NUTRITION 101
ARUGULA

See the green topping this chicken? That's arugula, and with a big, peppery, mintlike flavor, it just might be the most underutilized of all the leafy greens. Each handful contains generous doses of vitamins A, C, K, and folate, a water-soluble B vitamin that helps battle fatigue and fight depression and plays an essential role in cell regeneration.

Plus This!

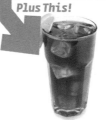

Freshly Brewed Ice Tea
0 calories
0 g fat
0 mg sodium
0 g carbohydrates

= Best Dinner

579 calories
10 g saturated fat
995 mg sodium
16 g carbohydrates
- -
36 g protein
3 g fiber
- -

SWITCH IT UP
MAHI MAHI WITH WOK-STIRRED VEGETABLES
586 calories
4 g saturated
1,591 mg sodium

Outside of a few slices of thin crust pizza or soup and salad, this is your next best option at CPK. Just avoid the spaghettini, which doubles the caloric load.

Not That!

Chicken Marsala
1,412 calories
15 g saturated fat
3,038 mg sodium
113 g carbohydrates

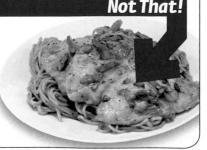

CHEVYS FRESH MEX

Mesquite Grilled Chicken Tacos
(2, without tamalito, beans, or rice)

590 calories
24 g fat (6 g saturated)
1,140 mg sodium
50 g carbohydrates

Chevys is among those restaurants serving portions so egregiously inflated that a 450-calorie dinner—unless you plan to eat beans and salsa—is just out of the question. That said, these tacos deliver a ton of protein, and the side salad is built right into the meal. Stick an unsweetened tea on the side to ratchet your metabolism a few degrees higher. It's not enough to undo an entire dinner, but it's certainly a good place to start.

Plus This!

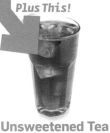

Unsweetened Tea
0 calories
0 g fat
0 mg sodium
0 g carbohydrates

= Best Dinner

590 calories
24 g fat
(6 g saturated)
1,140 mg sodium
50 g carbohydrates

----

40 g protein
3 g fiber

92

Percentage of Chevys dinner entrées that contain more than 2,000 milligrams of sodium.

Not That!

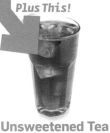

Tostada Salad with Chicken
1,551 calories
94 g fat (37 g saturated)
2,480 mg sodium
50 g carbohydrates

FOOD COURT

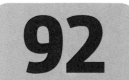

CRIME
Veggie Burrito
1,440 calories

PUNISHMENT
1 hour and 15 minutes running up stairs

Eat This!

CHICK-FIL-A

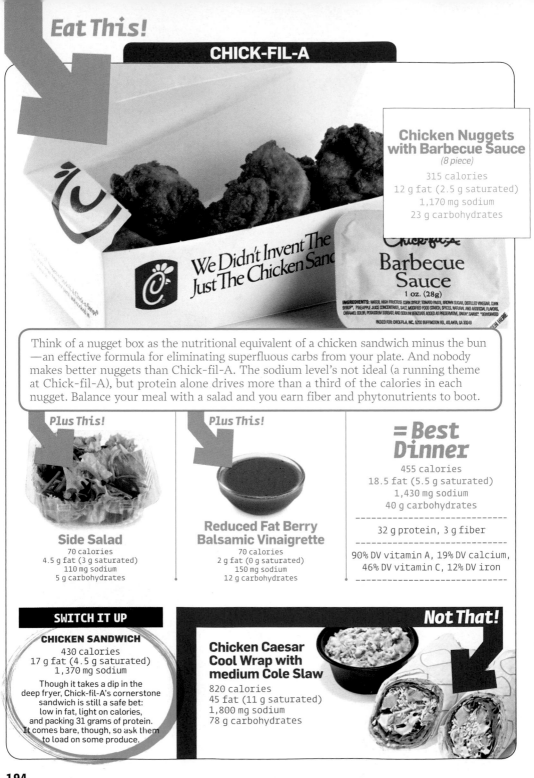

Chicken Nuggets with Barbecue Sauce
(8 piece)

315 calories
12 g fat (2.5 g saturated)
1,170 mg sodium
23 g carbohydrates

Barbecue Sauce
1 oz. (28g)

INGREDIENTS: WATER, HIGH FRUCTOSE CORN SYRUP, TOMATO PASTE, BROWN SUGAR, DISTILLED VINEGAR, CORN SYRUP, PINEAPPLE JUICE CONCENTRATE, SALT, MODIFIED FOOD STARCH, SPICES, NATURAL AND ARTIFICIAL FLAVORS, CARAMEL COLOR, POTASSIUM SORBATE AND SODIUM BENZOATE ADDED AS PRESERVATIVE, ONION, GARLIC. *DEHYDRATED

PACKED FOR CHICK-FIL-A, INC., 5200 BUFFINGTON RD., ATLANTA, GA 30349

Think of a nugget box as the nutritional equivalent of a chicken sandwich minus the bun —an effective formula for eliminating superfluous carbs from your plate. And nobody makes better nuggets than Chick-fil-A. The sodium level's not ideal (a running theme at Chick-fil-A), but protein alone drives more than a third of the calories in each nugget. Balance your meal with a salad and you earn fiber and phytonutrients to boot.

Plus This!

Side Salad
70 calories
4.5 g fat (3 g saturated)
110 mg sodium
5 g carbohydrates

Plus This!

Reduced Fat Berry Balsamic Vinaigrette
70 calories
2 g fat (0 g saturated)
150 mg sodium
12 g carbohydrates

= Best Dinner

455 calories
18.5 fat (5.5 g saturated)
1,430 mg sodium
40 g carbohydrates

----

32 g protein, 3 g fiber

90% DV vitamin A, 19% DV calcium, 46% DV vitamin C, 12% DV iron

----

SWITCH IT UP

CHICKEN SANDWICH
430 calories
17 g fat (4.5 g saturated)
1,370 mg sodium

Though it takes a dip in the deep fryer, Chick-fil-A's cornerstone sandwich is still a safe bet: low in fat, light on calories, and packing 31 grams of protein. It comes bare, though, so ask them to load on some produce.

Not That!

Chicken Caesar Cool Wrap with medium Cole Slaw

820 calories
45 fat (11 g saturated)
1,800 mg sodium
78 g carbohydrates

194

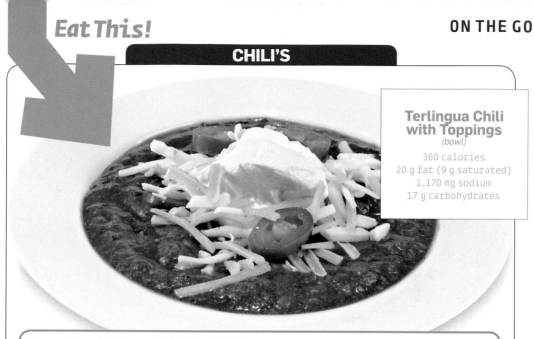

CHILI'S

Terlingua Chili with Toppings
(bowl)

360 calories
20 g fat (9 g saturated)
1,170 mg sodium
17 g carbohydrates

Done right, chili is a veritable hotbed of nutrients, teeming with protein, fiber, and metabolism-boosting antioxidants. At Chili's, it serves another function: It diffuses an otherwise calorie- and sodium-laden menu. Ask your server to drop a few slices of avocado into the bowl and you'll earn extra hits of fiber and monounsaturated fats—two nutrients that increase the hunger-quashing impact of this bowl.

Plus This!

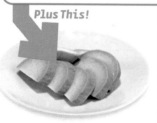

Avocado Slices
80 calories
7 g fat (1 g saturated)
0 mg sodium
4 g carbohydrates

= Best Dinner

440 calories
27 g fat
(10 g saturated)
1,170 mg sodium
21 g carbohydrates

----

30 g protein
8 g fiber

1,672

The average number of calories in a burger at Chili's. That's more than you'd find in three large orders of Burger King Onion Rings.

Not That!

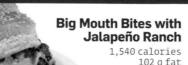

Big Mouth Bites with Jalapeño Ranch
1,540 calories
102 g fat
(28 g saturated)
3,190 mg sodium
88 g carbohydrates

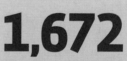

RESTAURANT SURVIVAL GUIDE

ORDER À LA CARTE

Your best bet at nearly any sit down restaurant is to skip the regular menu choices and piece together your own custom-made meal. Nowhere is that strategy more important than at Chili's. Create your own combo with a mix of grilled shrimp, chicken, or sirloin, then tack on a healthy side like black beans or seasonal vegetables. It's one of the only ways to come out unscathed.

Eat This!

CHIPOTLE

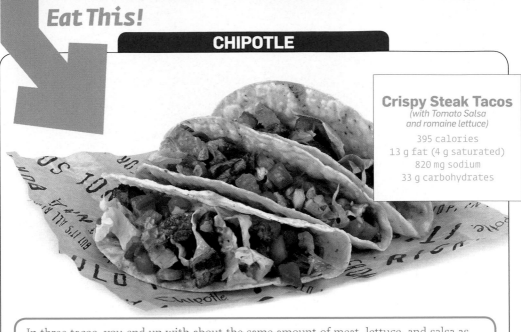

Crispy Steak Tacos
*(with Tomato Salsa
and romaine lettuce)*

395 calories
13 g fat (4 g saturated)
820 mg sodium
33 g carbohydrates

In three tacos, you end up with about the same amount of meat, lettuce, and salsa as you would find in a burrito, but you eliminate sour cream (120 calories), rice (130 calories), and the oversized flour tortilla (290 calories). Total savings: 540 calories. Not bad, right? Now here's a trick to add big flavor and a nutritional cache with no serious caloric strain: Add a scoop of fajita vegetables to each taco. Trust us; you won't regret it.

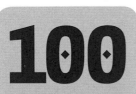

100

The number of calories you eliminate by asking for no cheese on your tacos.

Plus This!

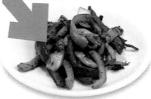

Fajita Vegetables
20 calories
1 g fat (0 g saturated)
170 mg sodium
4 g carbohydrates

= Best Dinner

415 calories
14 g fat
(4 g saturated)
990 mg sodium
37 g carbohydrates

----

34 g protein
3 g fiber

NUTRITION 101

CHILI PEPPERS

The chili's heat is the result of capsaicin, a compound so powerful that many people take it in extract form to battle high blood pressure, poor digestion, inflammation, and headaches. If you can take the heat, maximize the benefits by adding Chipotle's dark red salsa—it's the most chili-dense—to your next taco or salad.

Not That!

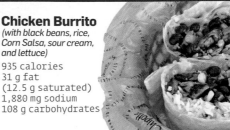

Chicken Burrito
(with black beans, rice, Corn Salsa, sour cream, and lettuce)

935 calories
31 g fat
(12.5 g saturated)
1,880 mg sodium
108 g carbohydrates

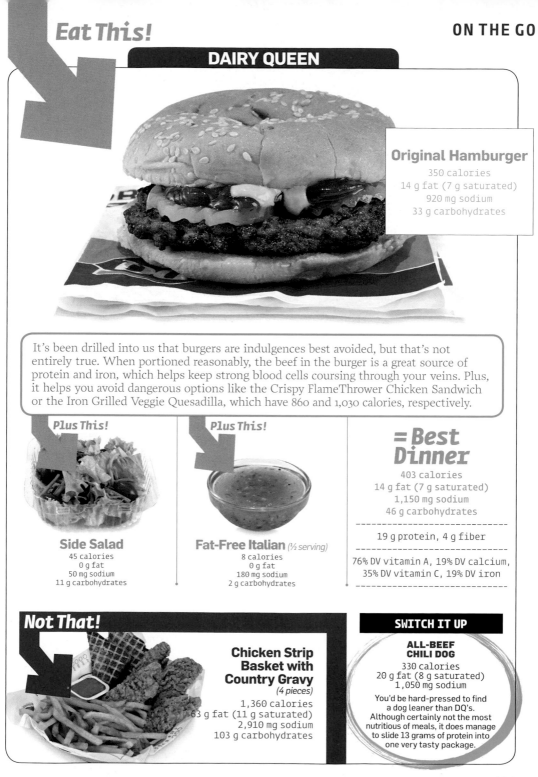

DAIRY QUEEN

Original Hamburger
350 calories
14 g fat (7 g saturated)
920 mg sodium
33 g carbohydrates

It's been drilled into us that burgers are indulgences best avoided, but that's not entirely true. When portioned reasonably, the beef in the burger is a great source of protein and iron, which helps keep strong blood cells coursing through your veins. Plus, it helps you avoid dangerous options like the Crispy FlameThrower Chicken Sandwich or the Iron Grilled Veggie Quesadilla, which have 860 and 1,030 calories, respectively.

Plus This!

Side Salad
45 calories
0 g fat
50 mg sodium
11 g carbohydrates

Plus This!

Fat-Free Italian *(⅓ serving)*
8 calories
0 g fat
180 mg sodium
2 g carbohydrates

= Best Dinner
403 calories
14 g fat (7 g saturated)
1,150 mg sodium
46 g carbohydrates
----
19 g protein, 4 g fiber

76% DV vitamin A, 19% DV calcium,
35% DV vitamin C, 19% DV iron

Not That!

Chicken Strip Basket with Country Gravy
(4 pieces)
1,360 calories
63 g fat (11 g saturated)
2,910 mg sodium
103 g carbohydrates

SWITCH IT UP

ALL-BEEF CHILI DOG
330 calories
20 g fat (8 g saturated)
1,050 mg sodium

You'd be hard-pressed to find a dog leaner than DQ's. Although certainly not the most nutritious of meals, it does manage to slide 13 grams of protein into one very tasty package.

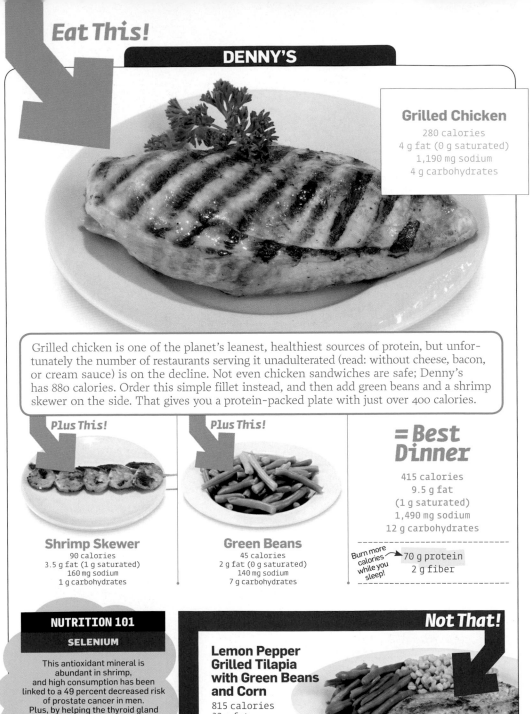

Eat This!

DENNY'S

Grilled Chicken

280 calories
4 g fat (0 g saturated)
1,190 mg sodium
4 g carbohydrates

Grilled chicken is one of the planet's leanest, healthiest sources of protein, but unfortunately the number of restaurants serving it unadulterated (read: without cheese, bacon, or cream sauce) is on the decline. Not even chicken sandwiches are safe; Denny's has 880 calories. Order this simple fillet instead, and then add green beans and a shrimp skewer on the side. That gives you a protein-packed plate with just over 400 calories.

Plus This!

Shrimp Skewer
90 calories
3.5 g fat (1 g saturated)
160 mg sodium
1 g carbohydrates

Plus This!

Green Beans
45 calories
2 g fat (0 g saturated)
140 mg sodium
7 g carbohydrates

= Best Dinner

415 calories
9.5 g fat
(1 g saturated)
1,490 mg sodium
12 g carbohydrates

Burn more calories while you sleep! → 70 g protein
2 g fiber

NUTRITION 101

SELENIUM

This antioxidant mineral is abundant in shrimp, and high consumption has been linked to a 49 percent decreased risk of prostate cancer in men. Plus, by helping the thyroid gland produce hormones, selenium contributes to both cell metabolism and the healthy maintenance of hair and nails.

Not That!

Lemon Pepper Grilled Tilapia with Green Beans and Corn

815 calories
32 g fat
(14 g saturated)
1,950 mg sodium
72 g carbohydrates

Eat This!

DOMINO'S

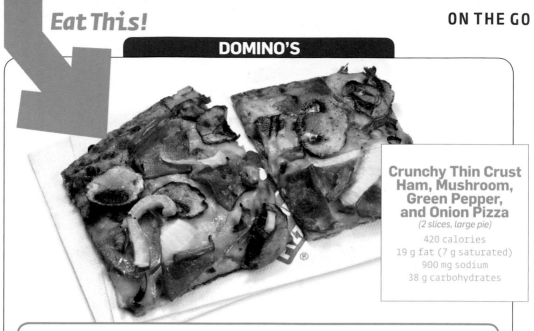

Crunchy Thin Crust Ham, Mushroom, Green Pepper, and Onion Pizza
(2 slices, large pie)
420 calories
19 g fat (7 g saturated)
900 mg sodium
38 g carbohydrates

By topping a thin-crust pie with ham and vegetables, you set the caloric ceiling at just over 400 calories. That alone makes a decent dinner portion, which might have you wondering: Why the side salad? Well, because dinner is a meal best served with loads of vegetables, but even the most produce-packed pie won't satisfy your day's requirements. Plus, by our measure, salad and pizza make one tremendously satisfying duo.

Plus This!

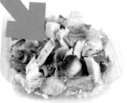

Chicken Caesar Salad
90 calories
3.5 g fat (1.5 g saturated)
290 mg sodium
5 g carbohydrates

= Best Dinner
510 calories
22.5 g fat (8.5 g saturated)
1,190 mg sodium
43 g carbohydrates
----
25 g protein, 4 g fiber

98% DV vitamin A, 29% DV calcium,
52% DV vitamin C, 10% DV iron

61

Number of ingredients in Domino's Cheesy Bread. You could make the same thing at home using five or six ingredients.

Not That!

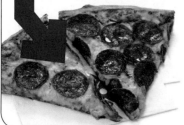

Hand-Tossed Pepperoni Pizza
(2 slices, large pie)
600 calories
25 g fat (11 g saturated)
1,400 mg sodium
68 g carbohydrates

FOOD COURT

CRIME
Italian Sausage and Peppers Sandwich
860 calories

PUNISHMENT
129 laps in an Olympic-size pool

Eat This!

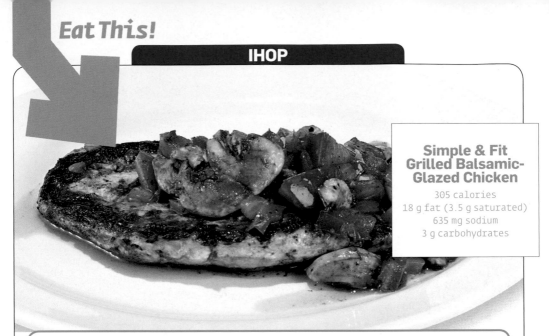

Simple & Fit Grilled Balsamic-Glazed Chicken

305 calories
18 g fat (3.5 g saturated)
635 mg sodium
3 g carbohydrates

IHOP's Simple & Fit section is the saving grace amid the gut bombs and nutritional nightmares that make up the rest of the chain's menu. This Balsamic-Glazed Chicken is the perfect example. Instead of some cheap, oil-based sauce, IHOP employs a coterie of nutritionally stacked vegetables moistened with a drizzle of sweet balsamic glaze. The only thing missing is fiber, and you can pick that up easily with a couple smart sides.

Plus This!

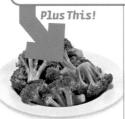

Plus This!

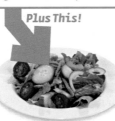

Plus This!

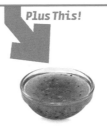

= Best Dinner

440 calories
22 g fat
(3.5 g saturated)
940 mg sodium
25 g carbohydrates

----

39 g protein
8 g fiber

Steamed Broccoli
30 calories
0 g fat
30 mg sodium
6 g carbohydrates

House Salad
90 calories
3 g fat (0 g saturated)
170 mg sodium
15 g carbohydrates

Reduced-Fat Italian
15 calories
1 g fat (0 g saturated)
105 mg sodium
1 g carbohydrates

Not That!

Mediterranean Lemon Chicken with Garlic Bread

930 calories
49 g fat (15 g saturated)
1,600 mg sodium
44 g carbohydrates

Eat This!

KFC

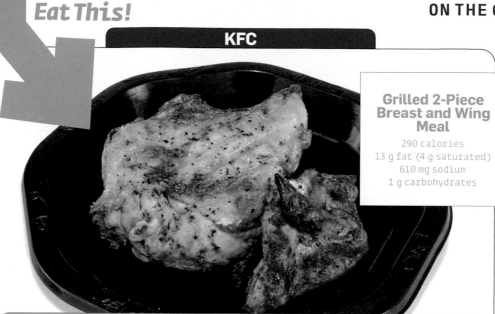

Grilled 2-Piece Breast and Wing Meal

290 calories
13 g fat (4 g saturated)
610 mg sodium
1 g carbohydrates

How important is it to order this meal grilled? Well, consider this: If you order it "extra crispy," you get 410 "extra calories" with your chicken. That's like eating a second dinner made exclusively from breading and fryer fat. So, in other words, grilled chicken is *very* important. The meal comes with two sides, so add green beans and corn on the cob for the most fiber in the fewest calories.

Plus This!

Corn on the Cob *(3")*
70 calories
0.5 g fat (0 g saturated)
0 mg sodium
16 g carbohydrates

Plus This!

Green Beans
20 calories
0 g fat
290 mg sodium
3 g carbohydrates

= Best Dinner

380 calories
13.5 g fat
(4 g saturated)
900 mg sodium
20 g carbohydrates

----

37 g protein
3 g fiber

Not That!

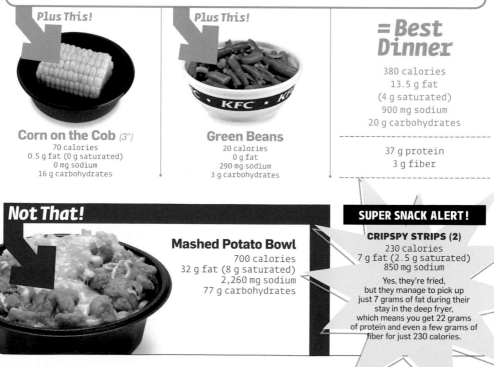

Mashed Potato Bowl
700 calories
32 g fat (8 g saturated)
2,260 mg sodium
77 g carbohydrates

SUPER SNACK ALERT!

CRIPSPY STRIPS (2)
230 calories
7 g fat (2.5 g saturated)
850 mg sodium

Yes, they're fried, but they manage to pick up just 7 grams of fat during their stay in the deep fryer, which means you get 22 grams of protein and even a few grams of fiber for just 230 calories.

Eat This!

MCDONALD'S

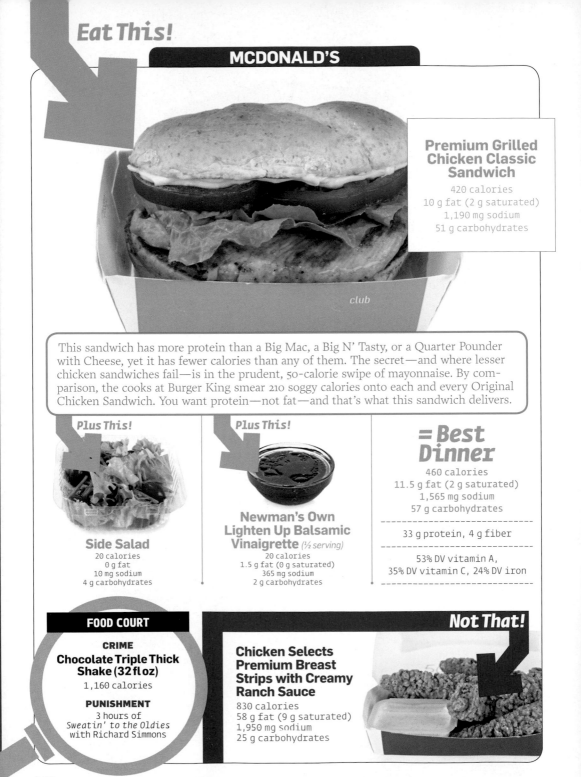

Premium Grilled Chicken Classic Sandwich

420 calories
10 g fat (2 g saturated)
1,190 mg sodium
51 g carbohydrates

club

This sandwich has more protein than a Big Mac, a Big N' Tasty, or a Quarter Pounder with Cheese, yet it has fewer calories than any of them. The secret—and where lesser chicken sandwiches fail—is in the prudent, 50-calorie swipe of mayonnaise. By comparison, the cooks at Burger King smear 210 soggy calories onto each and every Original Chicken Sandwich. You want protein—not fat—and that's what this sandwich delivers.

Plus This!

Side Salad
20 calories
0 g fat
10 mg sodium
4 g carbohydrates

Plus This!

Newman's Own Lighten Up Balsamic Vinaigrette *(½ serving)*
20 calories
1.5 g fat (0 g saturated)
365 mg sodium
2 g carbohydrates

= Best Dinner

460 calories
11.5 g fat (2 g saturated)
1,565 mg sodium
57 g carbohydrates

---

33 g protein, 4 g fiber

53% DV vitamin A,
35% DV vitamin C, 24% DV iron

FOOD COURT

CRIME
Chocolate Triple Thick Shake (32 fl oz)

1,160 calories

PUNISHMENT
3 hours of
Sweatin' to the Oldies
with Richard Simmons

Not That!

Chicken Selects Premium Breast Strips with Creamy Ranch Sauce

830 calories
58 g fat (9 g saturated)
1,950 mg sodium
25 g carbohydrates

OLIVE GARDEN

Venetian Apricot Chicken
(dinner portion)
380 calories
4 g fat (1.5 g saturated)
1,420 mg sodium
32 g carbohydrates

Nine out of ten restaurant sauces are built around some sort of fat, be it cream, butter, or oil. Thankfully the broth- and fruit-based apricot-citrus sauce covering this chicken isn't one of those nine. What's more, the plate comes pre-loaded with lean vegetables, so there's no space for squeezing on anything fried or covered with cheese. On the side, add iced tea; the unique antioxidants, called catechins, help you burn more calories.

Plus This!

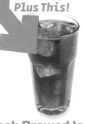

Fresh Brewed Iced Tea
0 calories
0 g fat
0 mg sodium
0 g carbohydrates

= Best Dinner
380 calories
4 g fat (1.5 g saturated)
1,420 mg sodium
32 g carbohydrates

---
8 g fiber

Olive Garden does not disclose protein information.

2,362

Milligrams of sodium in Olive Garden's average dinner-size chicken entrée. That's like pouring a full teaspoon of salt on your meal.

Not That!

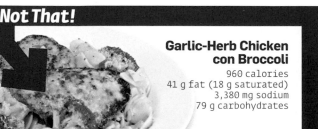

Garlic-Herb Chicken con Broccoli
960 calories
41 g fat (18 g saturated)
3,380 mg sodium
79 g carbohydrates

ETNT DIET STRATEGY
FOOD BEFORE LIQUOR

Drinking on an empty stomach brings on a quicker buzz, which in turn causes you to eat more food. According to a British study, people who drank a juice-based cocktail 30 minutes before mealtime consumed 15 percent more food than people who drank juice only. If you're going to have a drink with dinner, wait until the food arrives.

The Eat This, Not That! No-Diet Cheat Sheets

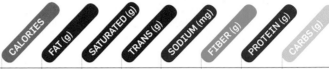

PASTA

		CALORIES	FAT (g)	SATURATED (g)	TRANS (g)	SODIUM (mg)	FIBER (g)	PROTEIN (g)	CARBS (g)
1.	Applebee's Teriyaki Shrimp Pasta	460	9	2	0	3,250	13	31	77
2.	Bob Evans Chicken & Broccoli Alfredo, Savor Size	470	24	9	0	1,157	6	30	35
3.	Olive Garden Capellini Pomodoro	480	11	2	N/A	970	11	N/A	78
4.	Ruby Tuesday Vegetarian Pasta Marinara	487	10	N/A	N/A	1,303	10	N/A	71
5.	Romano's Macaroni Grill Capellini Pomodoro	490	15	2	N/A	960	15	12	76
6.	Red Robin Classic Creamy Mac N' Cheese (w/o sides)	500	23	N/A	N/A	559	3	26	47
7.	Uno Chicago Grill Vermicelli Carbonara (½ serving)	530	28	13	0	860	2	20	52
8.	Red Lobster Shrimp Linguini Alfredo	550	29	10	N/A	1,580	N/A	N/A	41
9.	Fazioli's Spaghetti or Penne Marinara	560	2.5	0	0	970	9	19	111
10.	Bertucci's Lobster Ravioli	640	29	14	N/A	1,740	3	28	64
11.	Sbarro Penne alla Vodka	640	28	N/A	N/A	900	N/A	N/A	N/A
12.	Olive Garden Cheese Ravioli with Marinara Sauce	660	22	11	N/A	1,440	7	N/A	84
13.	California Pizza Kitchen Portobello Mushroom Ravioli with Tomato	718	N/A	10	N/A	1,550	5	21	81

ON THE BORDER

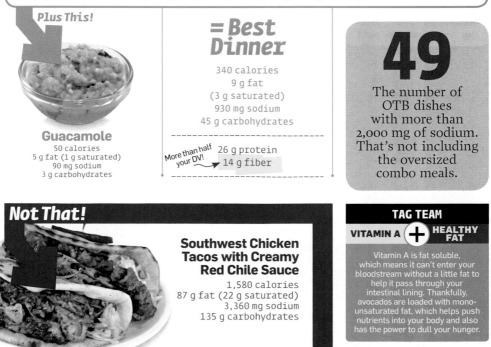

Citrus Chipotle Chicken Salad with Mango Citrus Vinaigrette
290 calories
4 g fat (2 g saturated)
840 mg sodium
42 g carbohydrates

Only one salad on On the Border's menu meets the criteria for a healthy dinner, and this is it. The other four deliver anywhere from 750 to well over 1,000 calories. Fortunately this one's not only within the realm of a nutritious meal, but it's also tremendously tasty. Add a flair of authentic Mexican flavor with a big scoop of guacamole, and the upshot will be a tasty dinner that delivers nearly half your day's fiber intake.

Plus This!

Guacamole
50 calories
5 g fat (1 g saturated)
90 mg sodium
3 g carbohydrates

= Best Dinner
340 calories
9 g fat
(3 g saturated)
930 mg sodium
45 g carbohydrates

More than half your DV! → 26 g protein
14 g fiber

49
The number of OTB dishes with more than 2,000 mg of sodium. That's not including the oversized combo meals.

Not That!

Southwest Chicken Tacos with Creamy Red Chile Sauce
1,580 calories
87 g fat (22 g saturated)
3,360 mg sodium
135 g carbohydrates

TAG TEAM
VITAMIN A + **HEALTHY FAT**

Vitamin A is fat soluble, which means it can't enter your bloodstream without a little fat to help it pass through your intestinal lining. Thankfully, avocados are loaded with mono-unsaturated fat, which helps push nutrients into your body and also has the power to dull your hunger.

Eat This!

OUTBACK STEAKHOUSE

Seared Ahi Tuna
(small)

355 calories
23.5 g fat (2.5 g saturated)
1,661 mg sodium
12 g carbohydrates

This ahi is from the Appetizer menu, but it makes a perfect dinner considering the caloric land mines nestled amidst the actual entrées. Think about it: Hunks of lean tuna served with wasabi vinaigrette, loading your belly with protein and healthy omega-3 fats for a minimal caloric toll. Now bump the fiber up with a side of vegetables, and save yourself the caloric damage by ordering them without the typical wash of butter.

THE TRUE COST OF FREE

THE FREEBIE
Honey Wheat Bushman Bread with Butter

THE COST
467 calories

No sooner is your order in at Outback than the server drops one of these loaves on your table. And although it's unlikely that you'll eat one whole loaf yourself, it's also unlikely that you'll consider the caloric contributions of what you do eat. So here's the score: Each third of this loaf—a couple of thick slices—tacks more than 150 calories onto your meal. It's by no means the worst crime on Outback's menu, but it certainly pushes your meal well outside the realm of nutritional perfection.

Plus This!

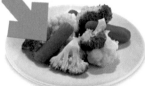

Fresh Seasonal Veggies
(ordered without butter)
49 calories
0.5 g fat (0 g saturated)
49 mg sodium
10 g carbohydrates

= Best Dinner

404 calories
24 g fat
(2.5 g saturated)
1,710 mg sodium
22 g carbohydrates

----

21 g protein
5.5 g fiber

Not That!

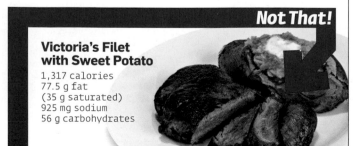

Victoria's Filet with Sweet Potato

1,317 calories
77.5 g fat
(35 g saturated)
925 mg sodium
56 g carbohydrates

Eat This!

P.F. CHANG'S

Spring Rolls with Sweet & Sour Sauce

392 calories
16 g fat (2 g saturated)
752 mg sodium
55 g carbohydrates

The dinner entrées at P.F. Chang's are portioned as if your entire dinner party were planning to share one dish, but rare is the table that doesn't still end up with a full round of orders. Avoid waistline trauma by choosing these Spring Rolls off the restaurant's Starters/Small Plates menu. Sure they're fried, but they're also stuffed with cabbage and carrots, and paired with a side of spinach, they make a very reasonable dinner.

Plus This!

Spinach Stir-Fried with Garlic *(small)*
80 calories
4.5 g fat (1.5 g saturated)
450 mg sodium
5 g carbohydrates

= Best Dinner

472 calories
20.5 g fat
(3.5 g saturated)
1,202 mg sodium
60 g carbohydrates

----

14 g protein
8.5 g fiber

1,015

The average caloric impact of a chicken entrée at P.F. Chang's.

Not That!

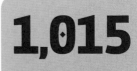

Orange Peel Chicken
999 calories
45 g fat
(9 g saturated)
2,310 mg sodium
14 g carbohydrates

NUTRITION 101

VITAMIN B$_6$

This vitamin plays important roles in protein metabolism, hemoglobin production, and blood sugar regulation. Some studies even suggest that it might help alleviate hangover symptoms. Each half-ounce of garlic has about 10 percent of your recommended daily intake.

Eat This!

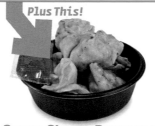

Mongolian Beef
200 calories
7 g fat (1.5 g saturated)
1,000 mg sodium
18 g carbohydrates

This just goes to prove the importance of geography. By appearance alone, it's difficult to tell many of Panda Express's entrées apart, but if you mistakenly order Beijing Beef over this Mongolian bowl, you'll slap an extra 650 calories and 43 grams of fat onto your meal. Make the right choice, however, and you get exactly what you want from on-the-go Chinese food: Lean, flavorful meat blended with a colorful array of A-list vegetables.

Plus This!

Mixed Veggies *(entrée order)*
35 calories
0 g fat
260 mg sodium
7 g carbohydrates

Plus This!

Cream Cheese Rangoons
190 calories
8 g fat (5 g saturated)
180 mg sodium
24 g carbohydrates

= Best Dinner
425 calories
15 g fat
(6.5 g saturated)
1,440 mg sodium
49 g carbohydrates

----

23 g protein
7 g fiber

SWITCH IT UP

MUSHROOM CHICKEN
220 calories
13 g fat (3 g saturated)
780 mg sodium

Slide this lean entrée in place of the veggies and Rangoons for a 420-calorie meal with 34 grams of protein and 5 grams of fiber.

Not That!

Beijing Beef
850 calories
50 g fat (9 g saturated)
1,120 mg sodium
56 g carbohydrates

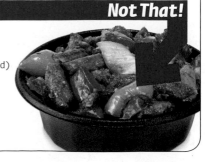

PANERA BREAD

Asian Sesame Chicken Salad with Asian Sesame Vinaigrette
(full portion)

400 calories
20 g fat (3.5 g saturated)
810 mg sodium
31 g carbohydrates

No salad on Panera's menu delivers better nutritional stats than this one. It has 150 fewer calories than the Orchard Harvest Chicken Salad and half the sodium of the Greek Salad, yet still manages to earn about a third of its calories from protein. (Not to mention the fact that we think it's the tastiest salad on the menu.) And the best side? Apple. Compared to a baguette, it has 100 fewer calories and 3 extra grams of fiber.

Plus This!

Apple
80 calories
0 g fat
0 mg sodium
21 g carbohydrates

= Best Dinner

480 calories
20 g fat (3.5 g saturated)
810 mg sodium
52 g carbohydrates

----

31 g protein, 7 g fiber

47% DV vitamin A,
50% DV vitamin C, 22% DV iron

NUTRITION 101
ALMONDS

Almonds are smart snacks—literally. According to researchers at New York-Presbyterian Hospital, just 1 ounce of almonds—like the ones in this salad—boosts your vitamin E level, which in turn improves memory and cognitive performance. Remember that next time your brain needs a jump-start.

Not That!

Half Sierra Turkey Sandwich with Half Greek Salad

670 calories
43 g fat
(10 g saturated)
1,860 mg sodium
48 g carbohydrates

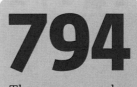

794

The average number of calories in a panini from Panera.

PAPA JOHN'S

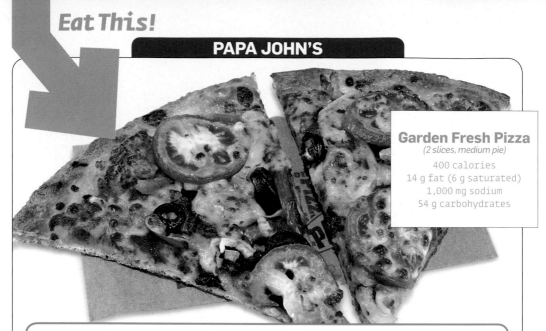

Garden Fresh Pizza
(2 slices, medium pie)

400 calories
14 g fat (6 g saturated)
1,000 mg sodium
54 g carbohydrates

There are two ways pizza can expand your waistline: with thick crust, which can actually double the caloric heft, and with fat-flecked meat toppings. Solve the first problem by ordering thin, and solve the second by steering clear of sausage and pepperoni. You're not missing anything—you still get all the cheesy goodness of the pizza, but you replace nutritionally bankrupt processed meat products with, you know, real nutrition.

NUTRITION 101

OLIVES

Maslinic acid, a compound in olive skins, helps prevent cancerous cell generation and even causes death in colon cancer cells, according to researchers at the University of Granada and the University of Barcelona. That makes a strong case for an olive-topped pie—or a dirty martini for the cocktail-party crowd.

Plus This!

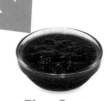

Pizza Sauce
20 calories
1 g fat
230 mg sodium
3 g carbohydrates

= Best Dinner

420 calories
15 g fat (6 g saturated)
1,230 mg sodium
57 g carbohydrates

----

16 g protein, 4 g fiber

12% DV vitamin A, 30% DV calcium, 20% DV vitamin C, 20% DV iron

----

THE TRUE COST OF FREE

THE FREEBIE
Special Garlic Dipping Sauce

THE COST

150 calories and 17 grams of fat per container

It's not the garlic that we take issue with; it's the liquefied butter that delivers more fat in 1 serving than the two slices of pizza on this page.

Not That!

Hawaiian BBQ Chicken Pizza
(2 slices, thin-crust pie)

580 calories
26 g fat (10 g saturated)
1,380 mg sodium
62 g carbohydrates

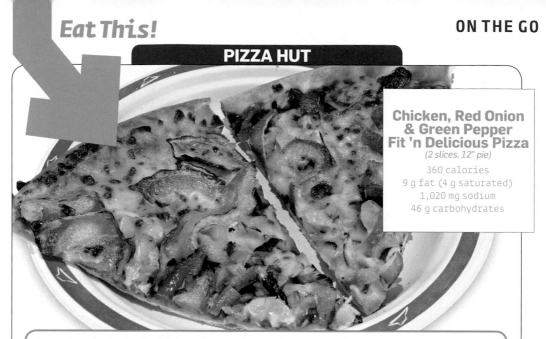

PIZZA HUT

Chicken, Red Onion & Green Pepper Fit 'n Delicious Pizza
(2 slices, 12" pie)
360 calories
9 g fat (4 g saturated)
1,020 mg sodium
46 g carbohydrates

Pizza Hut isn't the healthiest pizza parlor in the country, but it just might have the healthiest menu. Wait, what? Did you read that right? Sure you did. The greater menu isn't so hot, but the chain's Fit 'n Delicious menu—a subset of the regular menu that features low-calorie pies loaded with vegetables and lean meat—puts out some of the best pies we've ever seen. With 12 grams of protein per slice, this one's our favorite.

Plus This!

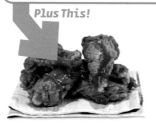

Baked Hot Wings *(2 pieces)*
100 calories
6 g fat (2 g saturated)
430 mg sodium
1 g carbohydrates

= Best Dinner
460 calories
15 g fat
(6 g saturated)
1,450 mg sodium
47 g carbohydrates

---

24 g protein
4 g fiber

1,179

The caloric impact, on average, of a 9-inch Personal PANormous Pizza. That's like eating more than two McDonald's Big Macs.

Not That!

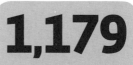

Thin 'N Crispy Cheese Pizza
(2 slices, 14" pie)
520 calories
22 g fat (12 g saturated)
1,480 mg sodium
58 g carbohydrates

NUTRITION 101
BELL PEPPERS

These relatively sweet peppers are veritable treasure troves of nutrients, loading your pizza with respectible hits of vitamins A, K, and B_6. The red ones pack the most potent punch, but even a green pepper provides more than a day's worth of vitamin C.

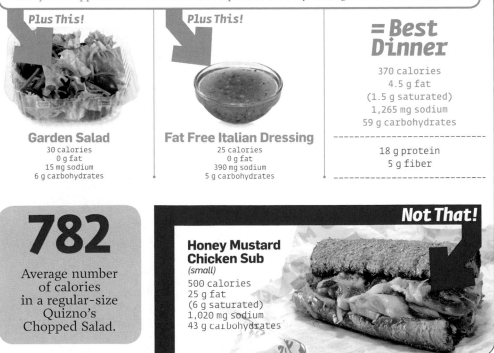

Eat This!

QUIZNO'S

Honey Bourbon Chicken Sub
(small, on 9 Grain Artisan Wheat)

315 calories
4.5 g fat (1.5 g saturated)
860 mg sodium
48 g carbohydrates

Want to order a perfect sandwich from a sub shop? Okay, simple. Start with wheat bread, because it delivers more fiber and nutrients than white. Stuff it with lean meat, like grilled chicken. Then add vegetables, which usher in the antioxidants, and, finally, smear on a light condiment like mustard. In other words, order this sandwich exactly as it appears here. Then make it a perfect meal by adding a salad on the side.

Plus This!

Garden Salad
30 calories
0 g fat
15 mg sodium
6 g carbohydrates

Plus This!

Fat Free Italian Dressing
25 calories
0 g fat
390 mg sodium
5 g carbohydrates

= Best Dinner

370 calories
4.5 g fat
(1.5 g saturated)
1,265 mg sodium
59 g carbohydrates

----

18 g protein
5 g fiber

782

Average number
of calories
in a regular-size
Quizno's
Chopped Salad.

Not That!

Honey Mustard Chicken Sub
(small)

500 calories
25 g fat
(6 g saturated)
1,020 mg sodium
43 g carbohydrates

Eat This!

RED LOBSTER

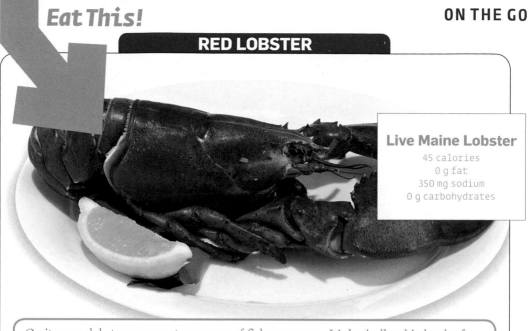

Live Maine Lobster
45 calories
0 g fat
350 mg sodium
0 g carbohydrates

On its own, lobster never put an ounce of flab on anyone. It's basically a big hunk of lean protein. The problem is the sidecar of butter, which is essentially a double shot of fat perched on the edge of your plate. Now, look at the components of this meal, listed below. See any butter? Nope. That's because by making cocktail sauce your dip du jour, you can cut about 300 calories off this meal. Now do that every time you eat lobster.

Plus This!

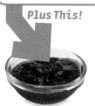

Cocktail Sauce
(1.5 oz)
40 calories
0 g fat
480 mg sodium
9 g carbohydrates

Plus This!

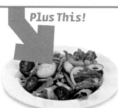

Garden Salad with Balsamic Vinaigrette
170 calories
9 g fat (1 g saturated)
295 mg sodium
13 g carbohydrates

Plus This!

Fresh Broccoli
45 calories
0.5 g fat (0 g saturated)
200 mg sodium
6 g carbohydrates

= Best Dinner
300 calories
9.5 g fat (1 g saturated)
1,325 mg sodium
28 g carbohydrate

Red Lobster does not disclose fiber or protein information.

Not That!

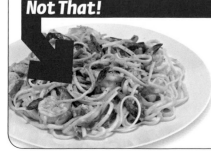

Chef's Signature Lobster and Shrimp Pasta
1,020 calories
50 g fat
(21 g saturated)
2,170 mg sodium
86 g carbohydrates

RESTAURANT SURVIVAL GUIDE

EAT MORE PLANTS

Fruits and vegetables are crucial to weight loss. When Florida researchers tracked the diets of two groups—one overweight and one of normal weight—they discovered that both groups ate approximately the same number of calories. Turns out the thinner group just ate more plant-based foods.

Eat This!

ROMANO'S MACARONI GRILL

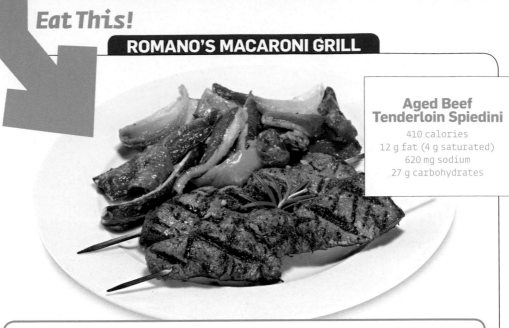

Aged Beef Tenderloin Spiedini
410 calories
12 g fat (4 g saturated)
620 mg sodium
27 g carbohydrates

A spiedini is the Italians' take on a kebob: skewered hunks of protein cooked over an open flame so that the fat can bubble out before it lands on your plate. With the sodium in check and vegetables on the side, this is easily one of the most perfectly balanced restaurant meals in America. Eat it with an extra side of broccoli and you'll still save 550 calories over the Mac Grill's similar-looking Calabrese Strip.

1,520

Number of calories in Mama's Trio. If this is how Mama cooks all her meals, somebody should call Child Services.

Plus This!

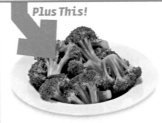

Broccoli
30 calories
0 g fat
90 mg sodium
4 g carbohydrates

= Best Dinner

440 calories
12 g fat
(4 g saturated)
710 mg sodium
31 g carbohydrates

----

52 g protein
10 g fiber

SWITCH IT UP

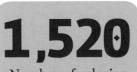

SPIEDINI SELECTION
The Aged Beef Tenderloin is our favorite, but it's certainly not the only meat being skewered at the Mac Grill. Shrimp and chicken make great dinner options, and at 490 calories, the center-cut lamb makes a reasonable lunch. The only one to avoid is the Grilled Salmon Spiedini, which harbors 660 calories and 44 grams of fat.

Not That!

Calabrese Strip
990 calories
64 g fat (23 g saturated)
1,120 mg sodium
34 g carbohydrates

214

RUBY TUESDAY

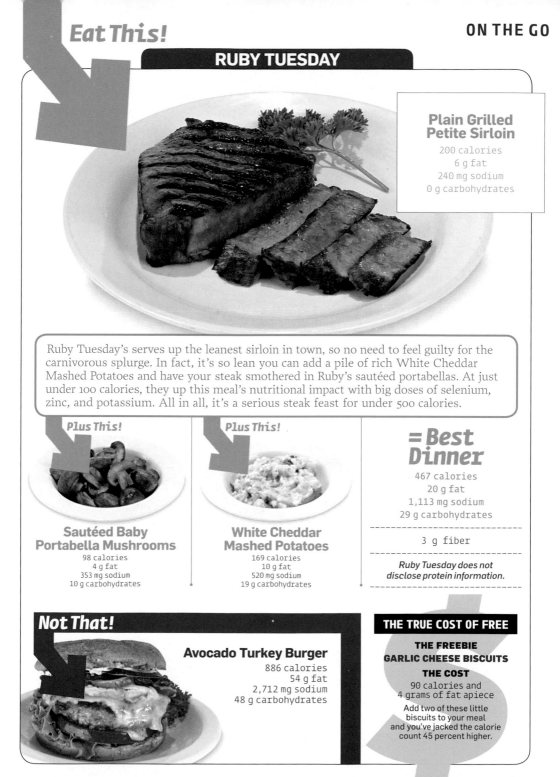

Plain Grilled Petite Sirloin
200 calories
6 g fat
240 mg sodium
0 g carbohydrates

Ruby Tuesday's serves up the leanest sirloin in town, so no need to feel guilty for the carnivorous splurge. In fact, it's so lean you can add a pile of rich White Cheddar Mashed Potatoes and have your steak smothered in Ruby's sautéed portabellas. At just under 100 calories, they up this meal's nutritional impact with big doses of selenium, zinc, and potassium. All in all, it's a serious steak feast for under 500 calories.

Plus This!

Sautéed Baby Portabella Mushrooms
98 calories
4 g fat
353 mg sodium
10 g carbohydrates

Plus This!

White Cheddar Mashed Potatoes
169 calories
10 g fat
520 mg sodium
19 g carbohydrates

= Best Dinner
467 calories
20 g fat
1,113 mg sodium
29 g carbohydrates

----
3 g fiber

Ruby Tuesday does not disclose protein information.

Not That!

Avocado Turkey Burger
886 calories
54 g fat
2,712 mg sodium
48 g carbohydrates

THE TRUE COST OF FREE
THE FREEBIE
GARLIC CHEESE BISCUITS

THE COST
90 calories and
4 grams of fat apiece

Add two of these little biscuits to your meal and you've jacked the calorie count 45 percent higher.

Eat This!

SUBWAY

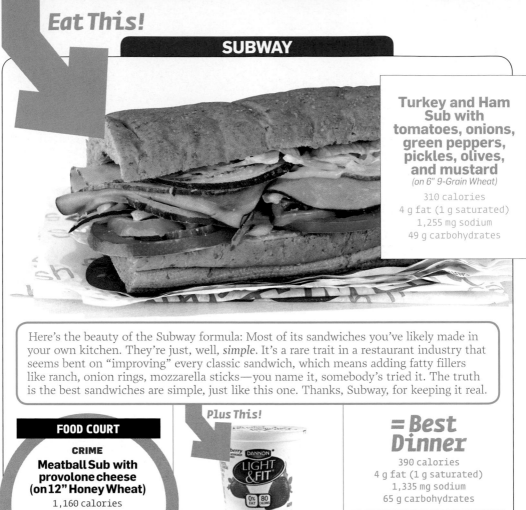

Turkey and Ham Sub with tomatoes, onions, green peppers, pickles, olives, and mustard
(on 6" 9-Grain Wheat)

310 calories
4 g fat (1 g saturated)
1,255 mg sodium
49 g carbohydrates

Here's the beauty of the Subway formula: Most of its sandwiches you've likely made in your own kitchen. They're just, well, *simple*. It's a rare trait in a restaurant industry that seems bent on "improving" every classic sandwich, which means adding fatty fillers like ranch, onion rings, mozzarella sticks—you name it, somebody's tried it. The truth is the best sandwiches are simple, just like this one. Thanks, Subway, for keeping it real.

FOOD COURT

CRIME
Meatball Sub with provolone cheese (on 12" Honey Wheat)

1,160 calories

PUNISHMENT
2 hours spinning a Hula-Hoop without stopping. (Good luck!)

Plus This!

Dannon Light & Fit Yogurt
80 calories
0 g fat
80 mg sodium
16 g carbohydrates

= Best Dinner
390 calories
4 g fat (1 g saturated)
1,335 mg sodium
65 g carbohydrates

---
24 g protein, 5 g fiber

20% DV vitamin C, 21% DV calcium, 25% DV iron

3,466
Milligrams of sodium Americans consume daily, on average, per the Centers for Disease Control.

Not That!

Meatball Marinara
(on 6" white)
570 calories
23 fat
(9 g saturated, 1 g trans)
1,640 mg sodium
70 g carbohydrates

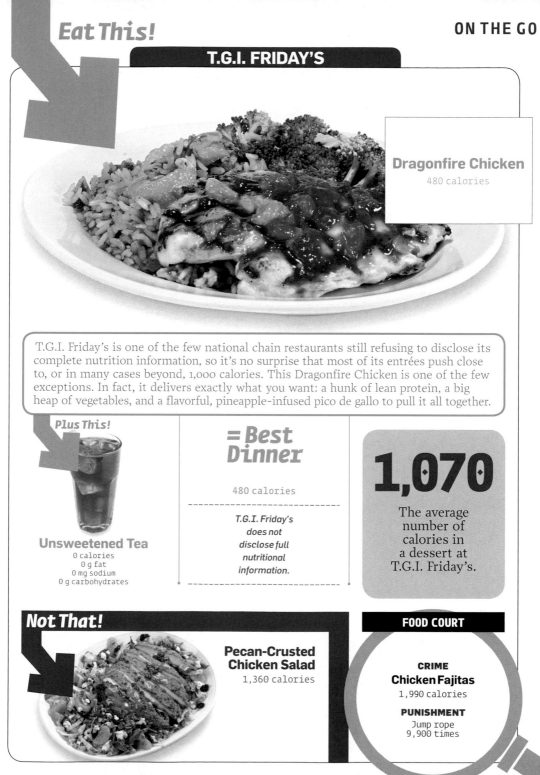

T.G.I. FRIDAY'S

Dragonfire Chicken
480 calories

T.G.I. Friday's is one of the few national chain restaurants still refusing to disclose its complete nutrition information, so it's no surprise that most of its entrées push close to, or in many cases beyond, 1,000 calories. This Dragonfire Chicken is one of the few exceptions. In fact, it delivers exactly what you want: a hunk of lean protein, a big heap of vegetables, and a flavorful, pineapple-infused pico de gallo to pull it all together.

Plus This!

Unsweetened Tea
0 calories
0 g fat
0 mg sodium
0 g carbohydrates

= Best Dinner

480 calories

- - - - - - - - - - - - - - - - - - -

T.G.I. Friday's does not disclose full nutritional information.

- - - - - - - - - - - - - - - - - - -

1,070

The average number of calories in a dessert at T.G.I. Friday's.

Not That!

Pecan-Crusted Chicken Salad
1,360 calories

FOOD COURT

CRIME
Chicken Fajitas
1,990 calories

PUNISHMENT
Jump rope
9,900 times

Eat This!

TACO BELL

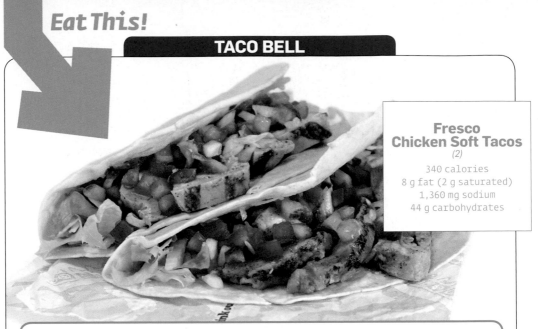

Fresco Chicken Soft Tacos
(2)
340 calories
8 g fat (2 g saturated)
1,360 mg sodium
44 g carbohydrates

Wander south of the border and order a taco; know what you'll get? A tortilla stuffed with nothing more than bare meat and chopped produce, maybe a scoop of guacamole. That's not to say Taco Bell's tacos are authentic, but the Fresco Taco, by ditching the cheese and sauce, is moving in the right direction. The upshot is it's also leaner than its regular counterpart, plus still loaded with protein. Authentic or not, it's definitely healthy.

18

Percentage, on average, by which fast-food restaurants underreport the number of calories in their food, according to researchers from Tufts University. So if you're eating what you think is a 600-calorie burger, there's a good chance the actual toll is north of 700 calories.

Plus This!

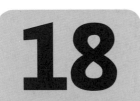

Guacamole
35 calories
3 g fat (0 g saturated)
85 mg sodium
2 g carbohydrates

= Best Dinner

375 calories
11 g fat
(2 g saturated)
1,445 mg sodium
46 g carbohydrates

---

24 g protein
7 g fiber

Not That!

Grilled Stuft Burrito—Chicken
660 calories
24 g fat (7 g saturated)
2,010 mg sodium
77 g carbohydrates

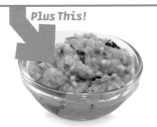

The Eat This, Not That! No-Diet Cheat Sheets

CHICKEN ENTRÉES

		CALORIES	FAT (g)	SATURATED (g)	TRANS (g)	SODIUM (mg)	FIBER (g)	PROTEIN (g)	CARBS (g)
1.	Olive Garden Venetian Apricot Chicken	380	4	1.5	N/A	1,420	8	N/A	32
2.	Romano's Macaroni Grill Grilled Chicken Spiedini	390	9	1.5	N/A	970	7	48	31
3.	Ruby Tuesday Chicken Bella with White Cheddar Mashed Potatoes and Steamed Broccoli	397	15	N/A	N/A	1,526	1	N/A	9
4.	KFC Grilled Chicken Breast and Drumstick with Green Beans & Mashed Potatoes & Gravy	430	16	4.5	N/A	1,510	2	48	22
5.	IHOP Simple & Fit Grilled Balsamic Glazed Chicken	440	22	3.5	N/A	940	8	39	25
6.	Applebee's Grilled Dijon Chicken & Portobellos	450	15	6	N/A	1,790	6	54	30
7.	Boston Market Quarter White Rotisserie Chicken with Fresh Steamed Vegetables and Garlic Dill New Potatoes	520	17	5	N/A	1,060	6	57	32
8.	Red Lobster Maple-Glazed Chicken	570	9	2.5	N/A	1,950	N/A	N/A	62
9.	California Pizza Kitchen Chicken Milanese	579	N/A	10	N/A	995	3	36	16
10.	Chili's Margarita Grilled Chicken (w/ sides)	600	13	3	N/A	1,310	10	49	72
11.	Uno Baked Stuffed Chicken with Steam Broccoli and Whole Grain Brown Rice	610	30	7.5	N/A	1,680	6	60	43
12.	Denny's Fit Fare Sweet & Tangy BBQ Chicken with Vegetables & Tomatoes	640	14	N/A	4	1,430	2	75	56

Eat This!

UNO CHICAGO GRILL

Baked Stuffed Chicken

360 calories
18 g fat (6 g saturated)
1,280 mg sodium
6 g carbohydrates

The word "stuffed" isn't one you typically associate with a healthy dinner, but in this case, it alludes to a profusion of broccoli, spinach, and tomatoes enrobed in just enough feta and mozzarella cheese to lend this meal a touch of indulgence. The sodium's a little high, but that's where the broccoli comes in. Each floret is teeming with potassium, which helps counteract the negative effects of sodium. Gotta love the science of food.

NUTRITION 101

TRYPTOPHAN

The amino acid most blamed for the post-Thanksgiving nap is actually just as abundant in chicken as it is in turkey. And while it won't actually put you to sleep (that'd be the third helping of Thanksgiving stuffing), it will help regulate a normal sleep cycle, boost feel-good chemicals in your brain, and possibly improve the efficiency of your immune system.

Plus This!

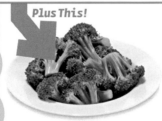

Steamed Broccoli

70 calories
6 g fat (1 g saturated)
360 mg sodium
5 g carbohydrates

= Best Dinner

430 calories
24 g fat (7 g saturated)
1,640 mg sodium
11 g carbohydrates

The complete package!

57 g protein, 5 g fiber

100% DV vitamin A, 44% DV calcium, 200% DV vitamin C

SWITCH IT UP

STEAK ON A STICK

150 calories
5 g fat (2 g saturated)
660 mg sodium

Basically it's a big shish kebab, and it's only served during "snack hours" (4 to 7 p.m. and 10 p.m. to close). If you're there at that time, order two of these for a protein-packed entrée.

Not That!

Baby Back Ribs

1,320 calories
90 g fat (30 g saturated)
1,940 mg sodium
34 g carbohydrates

WENDY'S

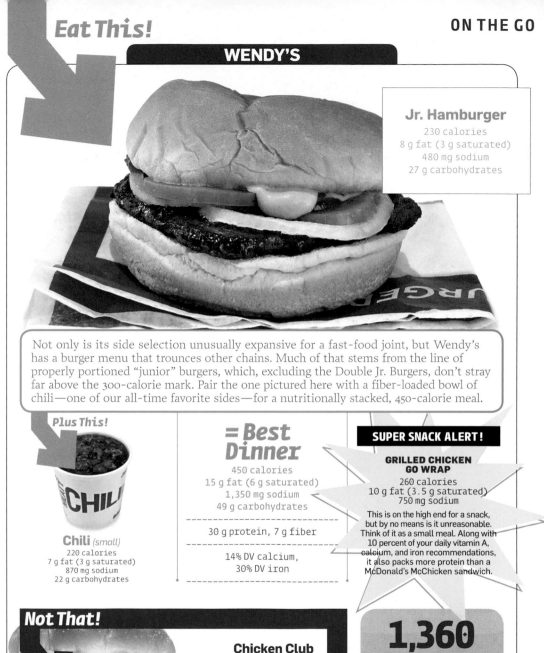

Jr. Hamburger
230 calories
8 g fat (3 g saturated)
480 mg sodium
27 g carbohydrates

Not only is its side selection unusually expansive for a fast-food joint, but Wendy's has a burger menu that trounces other chains. Much of that stems from the line of properly portioned "junior" burgers, which, excluding the Double Jr. Burgers, don't stray far above the 300-calorie mark. Pair the one pictured here with a fiber-loaded bowl of chili—one of our all-time favorite sides—for a nutritionally stacked, 450-calorie meal.

Plus This!

Chili *(small)*
220 calories
7 g fat (3 g saturated)
870 mg sodium
22 g carbohydrates

= Best Dinner
450 calories
15 g fat (6 g saturated)
1,350 mg sodium
49 g carbohydrates

----

30 g protein, 7 g fiber

14% DV calcium,
30% DV iron

SUPER SNACK ALERT!

GRILLED CHICKEN GO WRAP
260 calories
10 g fat (3.5 g saturated)
750 mg sodium

This is on the high end for a snack, but by no means is it unreasonable. Think of it as a small meal. Along with 10 percent of your daily vitamin A, calcium, and iron recommendations, it also packs more protein than a McDonald's McChicken sandwich.

Not That!

Chicken Club
630 calories
31 g fat (10 g saturated)
1,410 mg sodium
55 g carbohydrates

1,360
The number of calories in a Triple Baconator. That's more than you'd find in three medium chocolate Frostys.

Eat This!

Rotisserie chicken
(skin-on breast, 147 grams)

270 calories
12 g fat (3 g saturated)
510 mg sodium
0 g carbohydrates

Typical diet books advise eaters to always remove chicken skin before eating, but this isn't your typical diet book. Sure, you'll save 50 calories by nixing the skin, but most of those calories come from oleic acid, the same heart-healthy, hunger-squashing fat found in olive oil. Skin or no, supermarket rotisserie chickens are valuable allies in the battle of the bulge: inexpensive, delicious, and always available during a busy work week.

Plus This!

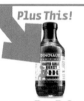

Dinosaur Bar-B-Que Roasted Garlic Honey BBQ Sauce or your favorite barbecue sauce *(2 Tbsp)*
25 calories
0 g fat
155 mg sodium
6 g carbohydrates

Plus This!

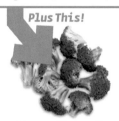

Chopped broccoli
(1 ½ cups)
45 calories
0.5 g fat (0 g saturated)
45 mg sodium
9 g carbohydrates

Plus This!

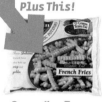

Cascadian Farm Crinkle Cut French Fries
(about 18 pieces)
110 calories
4 g fat (1 g saturated)
10 mg sodium
17 g carbohydrates

= Best Dinner

450 calories
16.5 g fat
Lo-carb feast! (2 g saturated)
720 mg sodium
32 g carbohydrates

----

49 g protein
5.5 g fiber

NUTRITION 101

NIACIN

Chicken and broccoli are both rich sources of niacin, aka vitamin B_3, an essential nutrient that helps your body process carbohydrates into energy. Studies show niacin to be an effective treatment for low HDL cholesterol scores, and a recent study on rats indicates that it might also help treat stroke victims.

Not That!

Fried Chicken Breast
(140 g)
364 calories
18.5 g fat (5 g saturated)
385 mg sodium
12.5 g carbohydrates

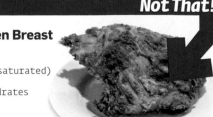

BEST SUPERMARKET SEAFOOD

Supermarket-prepared salmon
(3 oz)
120 calories
5 g fat (1 g saturated)
250 mg sodium
0 g carbohydrates

Precooked seafood from the supermarket deli is just as nutritious as (and a heck of a lot cheaper than) the fish you buy at your local seafood joint. Salmon is ideal, but rainbow trout, mackerel, and striped bass all work well, too. If the fillet looks dry, rub it down with olive oil before warming it in the oven. Then serve it over a bed of quinoa with asparagus for a perfect balance of protein, produce, and complex carbohydrates.

Plus This!

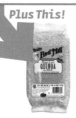

Bob's Red Mill Organic Quinoa
(¼ cup dry)
170 calories
2.5 g fat (0 g saturated)
0 mg sodium
30 g carbohydrates

Plus This!

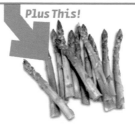

Asparagus *(12 spears)*
40 calories
0 g fat
25 mg sodium
7 g carbohydrates

= Best Dinner
330 calories
7.5 g fat
(1 g saturated)
275 mg sodium
37 g carbohydrates

----

28 g protein
7 g fiber

Not That!

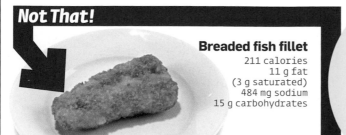

Breaded fish fillet
211 calories
11 g fat
(3 g saturated)
484 mg sodium
15 g carbohydrates

SUPERMARKET SURVIVAL GUIDE

SHOP THE MARGINS

Ever notice how supermarkets place the most nutritionally dense foods—the produce, dairy, and meats—around the perimeter of the store? That's to force you to cover the entire floor and tempt you to make more impulse purchases. Instead, stick to the edges and cut into the aisles only for items you know you need.

BEST TEX-MEX MEAL

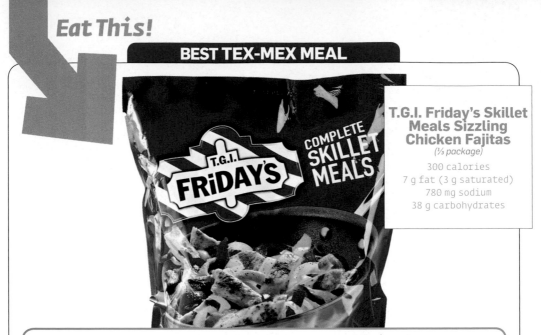

T.G.I. Friday's Skillet Meals Sizzling Chicken Fajitas
(⅓ package)

300 calories
7 g fat (3 g saturated)
780 mg sodium
38 g carbohydrates

If you made fajitas from scratch, they'd probably turn out quite similar to the blend in this bag: chicken, onion, and bell peppers tossed in little oil and served with tortillas. It's a perfectly simple recipe, and we applaud Friday's for resisting the urge to ruin it with some sort of cream-based fusion sauce. Add black beans to boost your fiber and protein intake and a big spoon of creamy, heart-healthy guacamole. You deserve it.

Plus This!

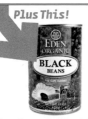

Eden Organic Black Beans
(⅓ cup)
110 calories
1 g fat (0 g saturated)
15 mg sodium
18 g carbohydrates

Plus This!

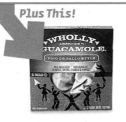

Wholly Guacamole *(2 Tbsp)*
60 calories
5 g fat (1 g saturated)
170 mg sodium
3 g carbohydrates

= Best Dinner

470 calories
13 g fat
(4 g saturated)
965 mg sodium
59 g carbohydrates

----

26 g protein
9 g fiber

STEALTH HEALTH

RED BELL PEPPERS

As it turns out, the red ones are the best peppers for your peepers. The bright color is provided in part by a potent pair of phytonutrients, lutein and zeaxanthin, which have been shown to protect your eyes from macular degeneration. Or, in other words, they keep your vision sharp as you age.

Not That!

Amy's Mexican Casserole Bowl
470 calories
16 g fat (5 g saturated)
780 mg sodium
70 g carbohydrates

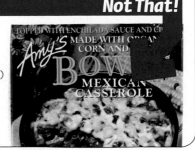

BEST CHICKEN STIR-FRY

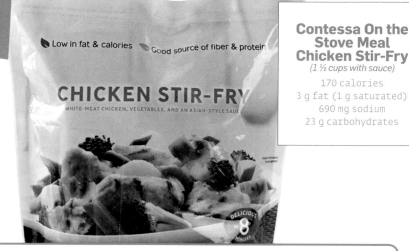

Low in fat & calories   Good source of fiber & protein

CHICKEN STIR-FRY

WHITE-MEAT CHICKEN, VEGETABLES, AND AN ASIAN-STYLE SAUCE

Contessa On the Stove Meal Chicken Stir-Fry
(1 ½ cups with sauce)
170 calories
3 g fat (1 g saturated)
690 mg sodium
23 g carbohydrates

This meal, before you add the sauce that comes with it, has exactly eight ingredients: chicken plus seven different vegetables. That gives you complete protein, complex carbohydrates, and nearly half a day's vision-protecting, skin-smoothing vitamin A. Make it even healthier by replacing the sauce in the bag (it has 12 grams of sugar) with a few splashes of soy sauce, a handful of chopped scallions, and a few twists of black pepper.

Plus This!

Uncle Ben's Whole Grain Brown Ready Rice *(⅓ cup)*
120 calories
1.5 g fat (0 g saturated)
10 mg sodium
19 g carbohydrates

Plus This!

Milk *(1%, 1 cup)*
110 calories
2.5 g fat (1.5 g saturated)
108 mg sodium
13 g carbohydrates

=Best Dinner

400 calories
7 g fat
(2.5 g saturated)
808 mg sodium
55 g carbohydrates

23.5 g protein
5 g fiber

Not That!

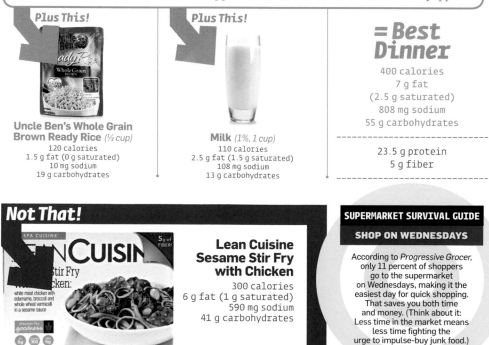

Lean Cuisine Sesame Stir Fry with Chicken
300 calories
6 g fat (1 g saturated)
590 mg sodium
41 g carbohydrates

SUPERMARKET SURVIVAL GUIDE

SHOP ON WEDNESDAYS

According to *Progressive Grocer*, only 11 percent of shoppers go to the supermarket on Wednesdays, making it the easiest day for quick shopping. That saves you both time and money. (Think about it: Less time in the market means less time fighting the urge to impulse-buy junk food.)

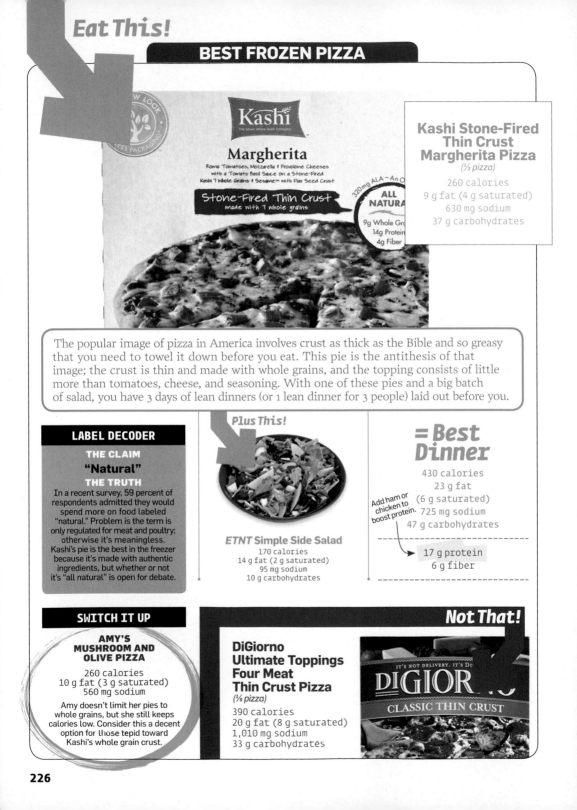

Eat This!

BEST FROZEN PIZZA

Kashi Stone-Fired Thin Crust Margherita Pizza
(⅓ pizza)

260 calories
9 g fat (4 g saturated)
630 mg sodium
37 g carbohydrates

The popular image of pizza in America involves crust as thick as the Bible and so greasy that you need to towel it down before you eat. This pie is the antithesis of that image; the crust is thin and made with whole grains, and the topping consists of little more than tomatoes, cheese, and seasoning. With one of these pies and a big batch of salad, you have 3 days of lean dinners (or 1 lean dinner for 3 people) laid out before you.

LABEL DECODER

THE CLAIM
"Natural"
THE TRUTH
In a recent survey, 59 percent of respondents admitted they would spend more on food labeled "natural." Problem is the term is only regulated for meat and poultry; otherwise it's meaningless. Kashi's pie is the best in the freezer because it's made with authentic ingredients, but whether or not it's "all natural" is open for debate.

Plus This!

***ETNT* Simple Side Salad**
170 calories
14 g fat (2 g saturated)
95 mg sodium
10 g carbohydrates

= Best Dinner

430 calories
23 g fat
(6 g saturated)
725 mg sodium
47 g carbohydrates

Add ham or chicken to boost protein.

17 g protein
6 g fiber

SWITCH IT UP

AMY'S MUSHROOM AND OLIVE PIZZA

260 calories
10 g fat (3 g saturated)
560 mg sodium

Amy doesn't limit her pies to whole grains, but she still keeps calories low. Consider this a decent option for those tepid toward Kashi's whole grain crust.

DiGiorno Ultimate Toppings Four Meat Thin Crust Pizza
(⅙ pizza)

390 calories
20 g fat (8 g saturated)
1,010 mg sodium
33 g carbohydrates

Not That!

BEST QUICK SEAFOOD DINNER

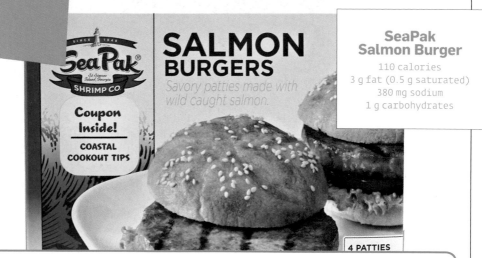

SALMON BURGERS
Savory patties made with wild caught salmon.

SeaPak Salmon Burger
110 calories
3 g fat (0.5 g saturated)
380 mg sodium
1 g carbohydrates

Never had a salmon burger? You don't know what you're missing. Not only is it the most hassle-free vehicle for delivering seafood to your belly, but it's also surprisingly tender and rich. Plus, each burger earns you 680 milligrams of omega-3 fatty acids, and that goes a long way toward keeping your skin, brain, joints, and heart healthy. Melt cheese over the patty and it will taste as indulgent as those beef burgers you crave.

Plus This!

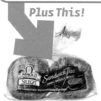

Arnold Select 100% Whole Wheat Sandwich Thins
100 calories
1 g fat (0 g saturated)
230 mg sodium
21 g carbohydrates

Plus This!

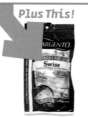

Sargento Reduced Fat Swiss Cheese *(1 slice)*
60 calories
4 g fat (2 g saturated)
30 mg sodium
1 g carbohydrates

Plus This!

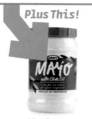

Kraft Mayo with Olive Oil *(1 Tbsp)*
45 calories
4 g fat (0 g saturated)
95 mg sodium
2 g carbohydrates

= Best Dinner

315 calories
12 g fat
(2.5 g saturated)
735 mg sodium
25 g carbohydrates

----

30 g protein
5 g fiber

Not That!

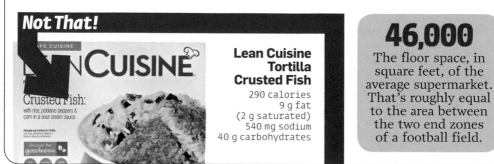

Lean Cuisine Tortilla Crusted Fish
290 calories
9 g fat
(2 g saturated)
540 mg sodium
40 g carbohydrates

46,000
The floor space, in square feet, of the average supermarket. That's roughly equal to the area between the two end zones of a football field.

Eat This!

BEST ADD-MEAT MEAL

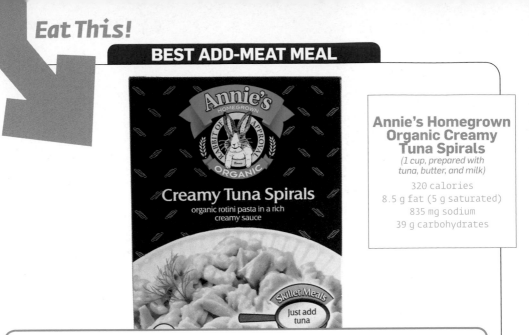

Annie's Homegrown Organic Creamy Tuna Spirals
(1 cup, prepared with tuna, butter, and milk)

320 calories
8.5 g fat (5 g saturated)
835 mg sodium
39 g carbohydrates

This box bests the competition by avoiding nefarious ingredients like hydrogenated oil and MSG (we're looking at you, Tuna Helper). That said, it isn't exactly a complete meal—it suffers from a serious lack of green. That's where the broccoli comes in. Steam a cup and stir it into the Spirals. Your portion not only doubles, but also develops 2 days' worth of vitamins C and K, half a day's vitamin A, and a quarter of your folate.

Plus This!

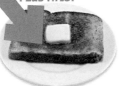

Nature's Own Double Fiber Wheat Bread *(1 slice toasted, with a pat of butter and a pinch of garlic salt)*
85 calories
4.5 g fat (2.5 g saturated)
290 mg sodium
13 g carbohydrates

Plus This!

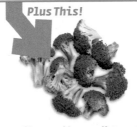

Chopped broccoli *(1 cup)*
30 calories
0 g fat (0 g saturated)
30 mg sodium
6 g carbohydrates

= Best Dinner

435 calories
13 g fat
(7.5 g saturated)
1,155 mg sodium
58 g carbohydrates

Perfectly balanced dinner!
27.5 g protein
9.5 g fiber

Not That!

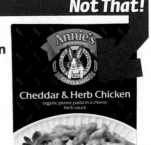

Annie's Organic Cheddar & Herb Chicken
(1 cup prepared)

450 calories
24 g fat (7 g saturated)
863 mg sodium
44 g carbohydrates

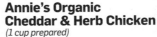

BEST BAGGED SEAFOOD MEAL

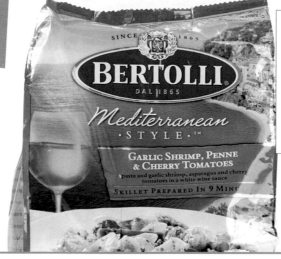

Bertolli Garlic Shrimp, Penne & Cherry Tomatoes
(½ package)

340 calories
11 g fat (1 g saturated)
740 mg sodium
42 g carbohydrates

The shrimp in this bag is small in stature only. In nutritional terms, it's gargantuan. Each crustacean loads your body with selenium, a mineral that reduces joint pain; tryptophan, an amino acid that promotes a calm mind; and vitamin D, a nutrient that battles fatigue and helps your body absorb calcium. And unlike some of Bertolli's other bagged meals, this one manages to deliver the goods while keeping the fat toll in check.

Plus This!

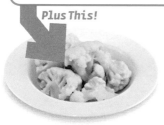

Chopped cauliflower *(1 cup)*
25 calories
0.5 g fat (0 g saturated)
30 mg sodium
5.5 g carbohydrates

= Best Dinner

365 calories
11.5 g fat
(1 g saturated)
770 mg sodium
47.5 g carbohydrates

----

15 g protein
7 g fiber

2009

The year in which Americans began spending more money eating out than they did preparing meals in their own homes. In fact, total food dollars spent on out-of-home foods have increased 97 percent over the past 40 years.

Not That!

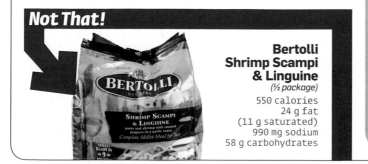

Bertolli Shrimp Scampi & Linguine
(½ package)
550 calories
24 g fat
(11 g saturated)
990 mg sodium
58 g carbohydrates

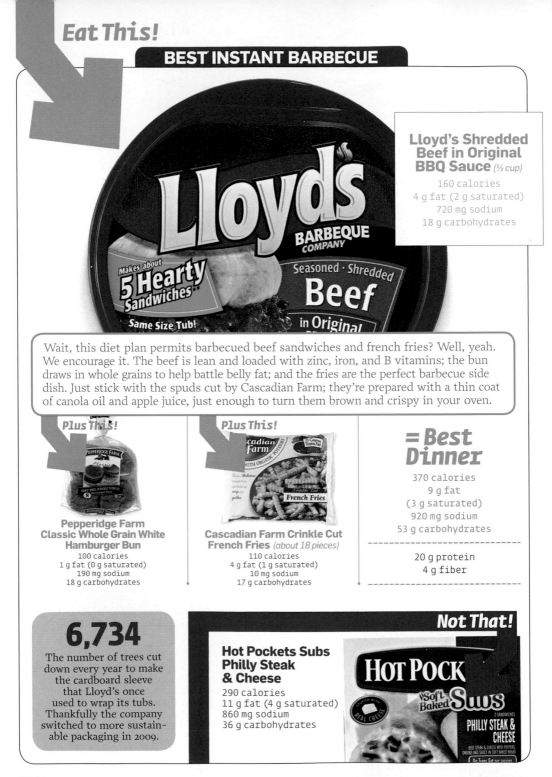

Eat This!

BEST INSTANT BARBECUE

Lloyd's Shredded Beef in Original BBQ Sauce (½ cup)
160 calories
4 g fat (2 g saturated)
720 mg sodium
18 g carbohydrates

Wait, this diet plan permits barbecued beef sandwiches and french fries? Well, yeah. We encourage it. The beef is lean and loaded with zinc, iron, and B vitamins; the bun draws in whole grains to help battle belly fat; and the fries are the perfect barbecue side dish. Just stick with the spuds cut by Cascadian Farm; they're prepared with a thin coat of canola oil and apple juice, just enough to turn them brown and crispy in your oven.

Plus This!

Pepperidge Farm Classic Whole Grain White Hamburger Bun
100 calories
1 g fat (0 g saturated)
190 mg sodium
18 g carbohydrates

Plus This!

Cascadian Farm Crinkle Cut French Fries (about 18 pieces)
110 calories
4 g fat (1 g saturated)
10 mg sodium
17 g carbohydrates

= Best Dinner
370 calories
9 g fat
(3 g saturated)
920 mg sodium
53 g carbohydrates

----

20 g protein
4 g fiber

6,734
The number of trees cut down every year to make the cardboard sleeve that Lloyd's once used to wrap its tubs. Thankfully the company switched to more sustainable packaging in 2009.

Not That!

Hot Pockets Subs Philly Steak & Cheese
290 calories
11 g fat (4 g saturated)
860 mg sodium
36 g carbohydrates

BEST BAGGED BEEF MEAL

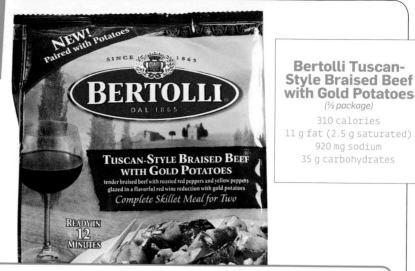

Bertolli Tuscan-Style Braised Beef with Gold Potatoes
(½ package)

310 calories
11 g fat (2.5 g saturated)
920 mg sodium
35 g carbohydrates

Is any meal more comforting than steak and potatoes? We think not. Yet despite the air of indulgence, it's actually a perfectly healthy dinner—loaded with protein and energy-producing B vitamins. Add a serving of peas to boost your intake of more than a dozen vital nutrients and pour yourself a glass of red wine. Yes, there's room for alcohol in this "diet," especially when it comes with red wine's huge dose of antioxidants.

Plus This!

Plus This!

= Best Dinner

470 calories
11.5 g fat
(2.5 g saturated)
930 mg sodium
48.5 g carbohydrates

22.5 g protein
8 g fiber

Green peas *(½ cup)*
60 calories
0.5 g fat (0 g saturated)
5 mg sodium
10.5 g carbohydrates

Red wine *(4 oz)*
100 calories
0 g fat (0 g saturated)
5 mg sodium
3 g carbohydrates

Not That!

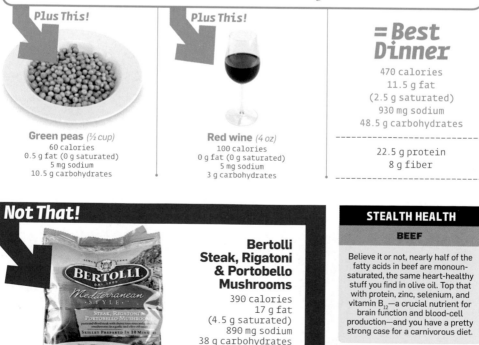

Bertolli Steak, Rigatoni & Portobello Mushrooms

390 calories
17 g fat
(4.5 g saturated)
890 mg sodium
38 g carbohydrates

STEALTH HEALTH

BEEF

Believe it or not, nearly half of the fatty acids in beef are monoun-saturated, the same heart-healthy stuff you find in olive oil. Top that with protein, zinc, selenium, and vitamin B_{12}—a crucial nutrient for brain function and blood-cell production—and you have a pretty strong case for a carnivorous diet.

Eat This!

Honey-Mustard Salmon

with Parmesan Asparagus

360 calories
16 g fat (6 g saturated)
400 mg sodium
13 g carbohydrates

Many Americans view fresh fish as restaurant fare, best left to professionals to skillfully prepare. But when you leave the fish cooking to "professionals" at places like Outback, T.G.I. Friday's, and Applebee's, your hopes for a healthy dinner may be sunk. Why blow the cash and the heavy caloric toll on a meal you can prepare at home in less time than it takes to order out? Plus, if you ever hope to get a kid to eat fish, the 3-minute sauce that's part of this dish (and goes great on shrimp, scallops, and chicken, as well) is the key.

You'll Need:

1 Tbsp butter

1 Tbsp brown sugar

2 Tbsp Dijon mustard

1 Tbsp honey

1 Tbsp soy sauce

½ Tbsp olive oil

Salt and ground black pepper to taste

4 salmon fillets (6 oz each)

Parmesan Asparagus (see Perfect Sides recipe on page 237)

How to Make It:

• Preheat the oven to 400°F. Combine the butter and brown sugar in a bowl and microwave for 30 seconds, until they have melted together. Stir in the mustard, honey, and soy sauce.

• Heat the oil in an ovenproof skillet over high heat. Season the salmon with salt and pepper and add to the pan flesh side down. Cook for 3 to 4 minutes until fully browned and then flip. Brush with half of the glaze and place the pan in the oven until the salmon is firm and flaky (but before white fat begins to form on the surface), about 5 minutes. Remove, brush with more of the honey-mustard mixture, and serve with the quinoa.

Makes 4 servings

Plus This!

Quinoa
(¼ cup cooked)
55 calories
1 g fat (0 g saturated)
5 mg sodium
10 g carbohydrates

= Best Dinner

415 calories
17 g fat
(6 g saturated)
405 mg sodium
23 g carbohydrates

----

41 g protein
3.5 g fiber

MASTER THE TECHNIQUE

PERFECTING FISH

The single most important skill you need when cooking fish is judging doneness. Chefs use a simple trick to get it right every time: Insert the tip of a knife or metal skewer into the center of the fillet. Remove it and touch it to the base of your thumb. If it's warm, the fish is done.

Not That!

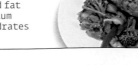

California Pizza Kitchen Ginger Salmon

979 calories
8 g saturated fat
2,299 mg sodium
74 g carbohydrates

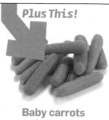

Baby carrots
(about 9)
30 calories
0 g fat
65 mg sodium
7 g carbohydrates

Italian Panini
with Provolone, Peppers, and Arugula
350 calories
12 g fat (4 g saturated)
1,010 mg sodium
38 g carbohydrates

Typically, Italian hoagies—towering creations of fatty meat, cheese, and oil—pack about 1,000 calories apiece, but our version takes the same classic flavors and turns them into a crispy, melted panini. We promise you won't miss the bulky bread, the mound of meats, or the excess 650 calories.

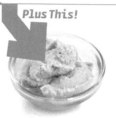

Hummus
(2 Tbsp)
50 calories
3 g fat (0.5 g saturated)
115 mg sodium
4.5 g carbohydrates

You'll Need:

- 8 slices sourdough bread
- 4 slices provolone
- ½ red onion, very thinly sliced
- ½ cup jarred roasted red peppers
- 4 cups arugula
- 8 slices reduced-fat spicy salami
- 8 oz sliced ham
- 1 Tbsp olive oil

How to Make It:

• Lay four slices of the bread on a cutting board. Cover each with a provolone slice, then top with onion, peppers, and arugula. Layer the salami and ham over the arugula and top with the remaining four slices of bread.

• Heat ½ tablespoon of the oil in a grill pan or large cast-iron skillet over medium-low heat. Add the sandwiches, being careful not to crowd, and weigh them down with something (if cooking individually, a teakettle partly filled with water works nicely; if cooking together, a few cans in a large pasta pot will do the trick). Cook for 3 to 4 minutes, until the bottoms have toasted nicely and the cheese has begun to melt. Remove the weight, flip, reapply the weight, and cook for another 3 to 4 minutes. Cut the sandwiches on the diagonal and serve with the baby carrots and hummus.

Makes 4 servings

=*Best Dinner*
430 calories
15 g fat
(4.5 g saturated)
1,190 mg sodium
49.5 g carbohydrates

27.5 g protein
6.5 g fiber

SECRET WEAPON
ROASTED PEPPERS

Not many foods pack so much flavor and nutrition into so few calories. Aside from the playful sweetness they add to your sandwich, they also impart massive shots of vitamins A and C, and they do this in no more than about 10 calories per serving.

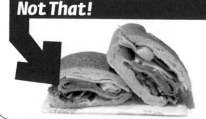

Not That!

Panera Bread Italian Combo on Ciabatta
1,040 calories
45 g fat (17 g saturated, 1 g trans)
3,080 mg sodium
95 g carbohydrates

Eat This!

Plus This!
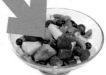

(see page 41)

ETNT Fruit Salad
(½ cup)
40 calories
0 g fat
0 mg sodium
10 g carbohydrates

Grilled Cheese
with Sautéed Mushrooms

340 calories
12 g fat (6 g saturated)
570 mg sodium
36 g carbohydrates

To most people, grilled cheese means a few Kraft Singles sandwiched between slices of Wonder Bread. As comforting as it may be, the standard take offers only a glimpse of grilled cheese's full potential. A better grilled cheese needs substance, something to turn it from a high-calorie snack into a low-calorie meal. That's why this recipe calls in piles of mushrooms and caramelized onions. The result is a sandwich simple enough to be a quick meal for one, and sophisticated enough to be a cozy dinner for two.

= Best Dinner

380 calories
12 g fat
(6 g saturated)
570 mg sodium
46 g carbohydrates

- - - - - - - - - - - - - - - - - -

22.5 g protein
6 g fiber

- - - - - - - - - - - - - - - - - -

MEAL MULTIPLIER

GRILLED CHEESE GALORE
Is there anything as satisfying as a crispy, melty grilled cheese? If you doubt us, try one of these gourmet grilled cheeses on for size:

• Artichoke hearts, sundried tomatoes, pesto, mozzarella
• Jack, cream cheese, jalapeños, crushed Fritos
• Cheddar, sliced apple, and crumbled bacon
• Mascarpone, Nutella, sliced banana

You'll Need:

½ Tbsp olive oil

2 cups cremini mushrooms, sliced

Salt and ground black pepper to taste

8 slices rye bread

2 cups shredded Swiss cheese

1 cup Caramelized Onions (see page 241)

½ Tbsp fresh thyme leaves (optional)

2 Tbsp softened butter

How to Make It:

• Heat the olive oil in a skillet over medium heat. Add the mushrooms and cook for about 6 minutes, until caramelized. Season with salt and pepper.

• Lay four slices of the bread on a cutting board. Dividing half of the cheese equally between the sandwiches, top the bread with it, then with a quarter each of the onions and mushrooms. Add the thyme (if using) and the remaining cheese. Top with the remaining slices of rye. Spread the softened butter on both sides of the sandwiches.

• Heat a large cast-iron or nonstick skillet over medium-low heat. Add the sandwiches, working in batches if you must, and cook for 5 to 6 minutes per side, until fully toasted and golden brown.

Makes 4 servings

Not That!

Cheesecake Factory Grilled Cheese

1,050 calories
31 g saturated fat
1,714 mg sodium
51 g carbohydrates

Eat This!

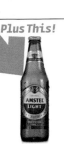

Amstel Light
95 calories
0 g fat
5 mg sodium
5 g carbohydrates

Turkey Sloppy Joes
340 calories
11 g fat (2.5 g saturated)
820 mg sodium
38 g carbohydrates

The best part about sloppy joes is that everything you need is likely already in your pantry and spice cabinet, gathering dust, waiting for a chance to shine. Open a can, measure out a few spices (if you have children, employ them as your sous chefs), and you'll have a crowd-pleasing dinner on the table in about 15 minutes.

= Best Dinner
435 calories
11 g fat
(2.5 g saturated)
825 mg sodium
43 g carbohydrates

- - - - - - - - - - - - - - - - - - - -

27 g protein
6 g fiber

- - - - - - - - - - - - - - - - - - - -

You'll Need:
½ Tbsp olive oil

1 large onion, diced

1 green bell pepper, diced

1 lb lean ground turkey

1½ cups tomato sauce

2 Tbsp tomato paste

2 Tbsp brown sugar

1 Tbsp red wine vinegar

1 Tbsp Worcestershire sauce

½ Tbsp chili powder

10–12 shakes of

Tabasco or other hot sauce

Salt and ground black pepper to taste

4 whole wheat or sesame buns, split and toasted

How to Make It:
• Heat the oil in a large skillet over medium heat. Add the onion and bell pepper and cook for 2 minutes, until softened. Add the turkey and cook, using a spoon to break up the meat, until the turkey is lightly browned. Add the tomato sauce, tomato paste, sugar, vinegar, Worcestershire, chili powder, and hot sauce and season with salt and black pepper.

• Simmer for 10 minutes, until the liquid has reduced and the sauce fully coats the meat. Divide the mixture among the buns.
Makes 4 servings

STEALTH HEALTH
CANNED TOMATO SAUCE

Generally speaking, whole foods are your best vehicles for nutrients, but canned tomatoes might be one of the few exceptions. The processing that takes place to go from tomato to sauce increases the bioavailability of lycopene, a powerful antioxidant that battles cancer, protects your skin from sun damage, and helps preserve your vision. Researchers believe that the extra lycopene results from cell walls being broken down, which releases the antioxidant from the tissue of the tomato. That doesn't mean you should swear off fresh tomatoes, but it wouldn't hurt to keep a few cans stocked in your cupboard.

Not That!

Subway Meatball Marinara Sandwich (6")
580 calories
23 g fat
(9 g saturated, 1 g trans)
1,530 mg sodium
70 g carbohydrates

235

Eat This!

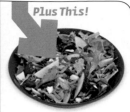

Plus This!

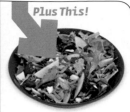

(see page 41)

ETNT Simple
Side Salad
170 calories
14 g fat (2 g saturated)
95 mg sodium
10 g carbohydrates

Loaded Pizza
300 calories
14 g fat (6 g saturated)
780 mg sodium
29 g carbohydrates

Ordering a supreme pizza for delivery is an open invitation for caloric calamity. Best-case scenario, you're looking at 250 calories a slice; worst case, 500 or more. Here, we use Boboli's Whole Wheat Thin Crust shell as a low-cal, fiber-rich base. We then load the pizza with a team of nutritional all-stars (red peppers, artichokes, fresh basil) and a goodly amount of turkey pepperoni. Torn deli ham or Canadian bacon would also work great here in place of the pepperoni.

= Best Dinner
470 calories
28 g fat
(8 g saturated)
875 mg sodium
39 g carbohydrates

----

22 g protein
5 g fiber

You'll Need:
1 Boboli 100% Whole Wheat Thin Pizza Crust (12")

1 cup tomato-basil pasta sauce (we like Muir Glen)

2 cups shredded part-skim mozzarella

15 slices turkey pepperoni

½ cup sliced onion

½ cup chopped jarred roasted red peppers

½ cup chopped green olives

2 cloves garlic, minced

½ tsp red pepper flakes

1 jar (6 oz) artichoke hearts, drained

1 cup fresh basil leaves (optional)

How to Make It:
• Preheat the oven to 400°F. Cover the crust with the sauce and then the cheese. Sprinkle with the pepperoni, onion, roasted peppers, olives, garlic, pepper flakes, and artichokes.

• Bake for 12 to 15 minutes, until the cheese is bubbling. Top with the basil (if using) and serve immediately.
Makes 4 servings

SECRET WEAPON
HORMEL TURKEY PEPPERONI
Pepperoni slices are like little discs of obesity, waiting to infuse every bite with ungodly amounts of fat, calories, and sodium. Too bad they're America's pizza topping of choice. Thankfully, Hormel has made this turkey version as well, which has half the calories of the pork stuff.

MEAL MULTIPLIER
Pizza is made for improvisation. Start with a prebaked crust (or split English muffins, which work great for mini pizzas) and try one of these unconventional combinations:

• Pesto, goat cheese, and sundried tomato
• Barbecue sauce, gouda, rotisserie chicken, and cilantro
• Fresh fig, ricotta, prosciutto, and arugula

Not That!

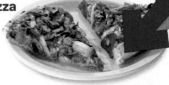

Pizza Hut Supreme Pan Pizza
(2 slices, large pie)
840 calories
46 g fat (16 g saturated)
1,840 mg sodium
76 g carbohydrates

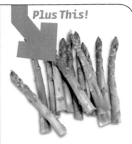

Asparagus
(4 spears)
40 calories
0 g fat
25 mg sodium
7 g carbohydrates

Chicken Parmesan

340 calories
11 g fat (4 g saturated)
670 mg sodium

Chicken parm normally suffers from a glut of oil, cheese, and carb-heavy spaghetti as the base. We slice calories by 60 percent without sacrificing its indulgent essence.

= Best Dinner

380 calories
11 g fat
(4 g saturated)
695 mg sodium
25 g carbohydrates

Protein power! 42 g protein
4 g fiber

You'll Need:

4 boneless, skinless chicken breast halves (4–6 oz each)

½ tsp salt

½ tsp black pepper

2 egg whites, lightly beaten

1 cup bread crumbs, preferably panko

2 Tbsp grated Parmesan

½ Tbsp Italian seasoning

1 Tbsp olive oil

1 cup tomato sauce

4 oz shredded part-skim mozzarella

Fresh basil leaves (optional)

How to Make It:

• Preheat the broiler. Cover the chicken breasts with parchment paper or plastic wrap and, using a meat mallet or a heavy-bottomed pan, pound the chicken until it is uniformly ¼" thick. Season with the salt and pepper.

• Place the egg whites in a shallow bowl. Mix the bread crumbs, Parmesan, and Italian seasoning on a large plate. Dip each breast into the egg, then into the crumb mixture, patting the crumbs so they fully cover the chicken.

• Heat the oil in a large skillet over medium heat. Cook the chicken for 3 to 4 minutes on the first side. (The crust should be browned.) Cook for another 2 to 3 minutes, then transfer to a baking sheet.

• Spoon the tomato sauce over the chicken, then top with the cheese and place underneath the broiler for 2 to 3 minutes or until the cheese is melted. Serve garnished with basil (if using).

Makes 4 servings

PERFECT SIDES

PARMESAN ASPARAGUS

Preheat the oven to 400°F. Snap off the woody bottoms of the asparagus spears (they'll break naturally at the point where the tough, fibrous part ends and the softer, tasty stuff begins) and toss with enough olive oil to lightly coat them, salt and pepper, and a good grating of Parmesan cheese. Lay them out on a baking sheet and roast until the spears turn tender and the cheese is lightly browned, which should be about 12 minutes. Before serving, squeeze a lemon over the top.

Not That!

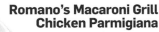

Romano's Macaroni Grill Chicken Parmigiana

850 calories
11 g saturated fat
1,700 mg sodium

Eat This!

Chicken Marsala
390 calories
9 g fat (2 g saturated)
520 mg sodium
28 g carbohydrates

Chicken Marsala is another delicious Italian creation that has suffered at the hands of corporate cooks. Which is why this is a recipe worth mastering at home, not just so you can save 500 or more calories over dinner, but because it's an easy way to show off for your next round of dinner guests.

You'll Need:

4 boneless, skinless chicken breasts, pounded to a uniform ¼" thickness

Salt and ground black pepper to taste

1 cup flour

1 Tbsp olive oil

2 oz prosciutto, sliced into thin strips

8 oz cremini mushrooms, stems removed and sliced

¾ cup Marsala wine

¾ cup low-sodium chicken broth

¼ cup chopped fresh parsley

How to Make It:

• Season the chicken with pinches of salt and pepper. Place the flour in a shallow bowl and add the chicken; coat evenly, shaking off any excess flour.

• Heat the oil in a large nonstick pan or cast-iron skillet over medium heat. Cook the chicken (don't overcrowd the pan; cook in two batches if need be) for 3 to 4 minutes per side, until golden brown on the outside and cooked all the way through. Transfer to a serving platter and keep warm.

• Add additional oil to the pan if needed, then sauté the prosciutto for 1 to 2 minutes, until it starts to crisp up. Add the mushrooms and continue sautéing until well browned. Stir in the Marsala and broth, scraping to release any browned bits stuck to the bottom of the pan. Cook until the liquid has reduced to about ½ cup. Season the sauce with salt and pepper, add the parsley to it, and pour it over the chicken.

Makes 4 servings

Plus This!

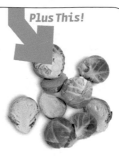

Brussels sprouts
(1 cup cooked)
55 calories
1 g fat (0 g saturated)
200 mg sodium
11 g carbohydrates

=Best Dinner
445 calories
10 g fat
(2 g saturated)
720 mg sodium
39 g carbohydrates

----

40 g protein
5 g fiber

PERFECT SIDES

SAUTÉED BRUSSELS SPROUT

Halve sprouts and cook in a large sauté pan (don't crowd!) with olive oil and chopped garlic. When tender, add a cup of peeled, cubed apple pieces and a handful of pine nuts. Sauté for another few minutes and season with salt and pepper.

Not That!

Romano's Macaroni Grill Chicken Marsala (dinner portion)
810 calories
35 g fat (12 g saturated fat)
1,110 mg sodium
61 g carbohydrates

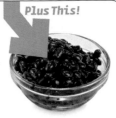

Plus This!

Black beans
(½ cup)
115 calories
0.5 g fat (0 g saturated)
205 mg sodium
20.5 g carbohydrates

Coffee-Rubbed Steak

270 calories
15 g fat (6 g saturated)
600 mg sodium
1 g carbohydrates

= Best Dinner

385 calories
15.5 g fat
(6 g saturated)
805 mg sodium
21.5 g carbohydrate

----

35 g protein
2 g fiber

Coffee and steak might seem like an unlikely partnership, but the flavor of beef is actually heightened by the robust notes of java. This dish would be perfect with grilled vegetables and a side of black or pinto beans. Or, if you like, heat up a few corn tortillas and pass them out so everyone can make their own tacos. Either way, be sure to let the beef rest before cutting; slice into it too early and all the hot juices will bleed onto your cutting board instead of being reabsorbed by the meat.

You'll Need:

½ Tbsp finely ground coffee or espresso

½ Tbsp chili powder

Salt and ground black pepper to taste

1 lb flank or skirt steak

Your favorite jarred or fresh salsa

1 lime, quartered

How to Make It:

• Heat a grill, stovetop grill pan, or cast-iron skillet until very hot. Combine the coffee grounds with the chili powder and a few generous pinches of salt and pepper in a small bowl. Rub the spice mixture all over the steak. Cook the beef for 3 to 4 minutes per side, depending on the thickness, until it is slightly firm but still yielding.

• Let the steak rest for at least 5 minutes, then slice thinly against the grain of the meat. Serve with a big scoop of pico de gallo and a wedge of lime on each plate.

Makes 4 servings

SECRET WEAPON

FLANK STEAK

You'd be hard-pressed to find a cut of meat with a better flavor-to-calorie ratio than this humble hunk of beef. Long and flat and shot through with beefy flavor, flank is perfect for taking on aggressive marinades and spice rubs. Try soaking it in a mixture of orange juice, garlic, cilantro, and chipotle pepper, then grilling it quickly over high heat. The result is the perfect meat for fajitas and steak tacos. Just be sure to slice it width-wise, against the grain of connective fibers that run the length of the meat, to avoid having a chewy piece of beef.

Not That!

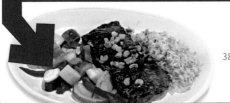

On the Border Carne Asada
970 calories
38 g fat (15 g saturated)
1,830 mg sodium
105 g carbohydrates

Eat This!

Grilled Chili Relleno

360 calories
16 g fat (6 g saturated)
400 mg sodium
31 g carbohydrates

Traditionally, chiles rellenos require a staggering amount of work: roasting, peeling, stuffing, dipping, and deep-frying. Rather than going through all that labor, just cut off the peppers' tops, scoop in the stuffing, and pop them on the grill (or in a 450°F oven). You'll save about 90 minutes of prep work, 20 minutes of cleanup, and a few hundred calories per pepper.

You'll Need:

2 ears fresh corn, shucked

½ Tbsp canola oil

8 oz cooked shrimp, chopped into ½" pieces

½ can (14–16 oz) black beans, rinsed and drained

1 cup shredded Monterey Jack cheese

Juice of 1 lime

½ cup chopped fresh cilantro

½ tsp ground cumin

Salt and ground black pepper to taste

8 poblano peppers

Salsa (optional)

How to Make It:

• Stand each ear of corn up on a cutting board and run your knife along the cob to remove the kernels. Heat the oil in a large nonstick pan over medium heat. Add the corn kernels and cook for about 5 minutes, until lightly toasted. Remove from the heat, then add the shrimp, beans, cheese, lime juice, cilantro, cumin, salt, and black pepper.

• Preheat a grill, grill pan, or 450°F oven.

Remove the tops of the peppers and scoop out the seeds. Use a spoon to stuff the shrimp mixture into each pepper cavity, being careful not to overfill.

• Cook on the grill or in the oven until the skins have lightly blistered and the flesh has softened, about 10 to 15 minutes. Serve with a bit of salsa, if you like.

Makes 4 servings

= Best Dinner

460 calories
16 g fat
(6 g saturated)
405 mg sodium
34 g carbohydrates

----

27 g protein
9 g fiber

SWITCH IT UP

PEPPER SWAP

Not a fan of heat? No problem. Poblano peppers are mildly spicy, but for some that may be too much. Simply follow the exact same recipe, but sub in large green or red bell peppers. Since bells are larger than poblanos, plan on serving just one per person.

Not That!

On the Border Cheese-Stuffed Chile Relleno with Ranchero Sauce *(2)*

1,340 calories
114 g fat (10 g saturated)
2,360 mg sodium
52 g carbohydrates

Eat This!

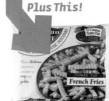

**Cascadian Farm
Crinkle Cut
French Fries**
(about 18 pieces)
110 calories
4 g fat (1 g saturated)
10 mg sodium
17 g carbohydrates

The Ultimate Burger
320 calories
12 g fat (6 g saturated)
710 mg sodium
28 g carbohydrates

It is nearly impossible to find a burger at a sit-down restaurant with fewer than 1,000 calories. Blame the high-fat meat and heavy condiments. Here, we start with ground brisket, which is relatively lean but packed with big burger flavor (ask your butcher to grind it fresh for you), then cover it in sweet caramelized onions and peppery arugula. We think it makes for a fine burger.

= Best Dinner
430 calories
16 g fat
(7 g saturated)
720 mg sodium
45 g carbohydrates

----
34 g protein
5 g fiber

You'll Need:

10 oz ground sirloin

10 oz ground brisket

1 tsp salt

1 tsp freshly cracked pepper

4 hamburger buns (preferably Martin's Potato Rolls), toasted

2 cups arugula

½ cup Caramelized Onions (see Secret Weapon to the right)

How to Make It:

• Heat a grill or stovetop grill pan until hot. Combine the sirloin, brisket, salt, and pepper in a bowl and gently mix. Form into 4 patties. Caution: Overworking the meat or packing your patties too tightly can make tough burgers.

• Cook the burgers for 2 to 3 minutes and flip. Cook on the other side for another 2 to 3 minutes, until nicely charred on the outside but still medium-rare to medium within. (The center of the patty should be firm but easily yielding—like a Nerf football.)

• After you remove the burgers, toast the buns briefly. Divide the arugula among the buns and top with the burgers and onions.

Makes 4 servings

SECRET WEAPON

CARAMELIZED ONIONS

Properly caramelized onions take time, but make up a big batch and have them on hand for smothering burgers, covering sandwiches, and topping juicy hunks of grilled steak or fish. Cook at least 3 large red onions (remember, they'll shrink down as the water cooks out) in a large pot with a bit of butter over a very low flame. Add a generous pinch of salt, which will help draw the moisture out. Cover the pot, removing the lid every 3 or 4 minutes to stir the onions. Cook for at least 20 minutes, or up to 45, depending on how sweet you like your onions.

Not That!

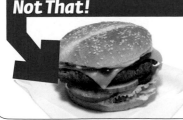

Carl's Jr. The Original Six Dollar Burger
890 calories
54 g fat (20 g saturated)
2,040 mg sodium
59 g carbohydrates

Eat This!

Turkey Chili
330 calories
6 g fat (1 g saturated)
490 mg sodium
29 g carbohydrates

We've never been shy about professing our undying affection for chili. Go lean by using ground turkey and build flavor with spices, beer, and a bit of chocolate.

You'll Need:

1 Tbsp canola oil

1 large onion, chopped

2 cloves garlic, minced

1 tsp ground cumin

½ tsp dried oregano

¼ cup chili powder

⅛ tsp ground cinnamon

2 bay leaves

2 lb lean ground turkey

2 Tbsp tomato paste

1 oz dark chocolate or 1 Tbsp cocoa powder

1 bottle or can (12 oz) dark beer

1 Tbsp chopped chipotle pepper

1 can (28 oz) whole peeled tomatoes

1 can (14 oz) white beans, rinsed and drained

1 can (14 oz) pinto beans, rinsed and drained

Salt and ground black pepper to taste

Hot sauce or cayenne

pepper to taste

Chopped onions, shredded cheese, lime wedges, sour cream (optional)

How to Make It:

• Heat the oil in a large pot over medium heat. Add the onion and garlic and cook until the onion is translucent, about 5 minutes. Add the cumin, oregano, chili powder, cinnamon, and bay and cook for another 2 to 3 minutes, until the spices are very fragrant.

• Add the turkey and tomato paste and cook, stirring constantly, until the turkey is no longer pink. Add the chocolate, beer, chipotle, and tomatoes, squeezing each tomato between your fingers before adding it so that it's still chunky but not whole. Turn down the heat and simmer for 45 minutes.

• Add the beans and season with salt and black pepper. Taste; if you like your chili hotter, add your favorite hot sauce or a few pinches of cayenne. Serve topped with your choice of garnishes.

Makes 6 servings

Plus This!

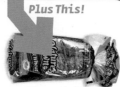

Nature's Own Double Fiber Wheat Bread
(1 slice toasted, with a pat of butter and a pinch of garlic salt)
85 calories
4.5 g fat (2.5 g saturated)
290 mg sodium
13 g carbohydrates

Plus This!

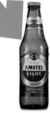

Amstel Light
95 calories
0 g fat
5 mg sodium
5 g carbohydrates

= Best Dinner
510 calories
10.5 g fat
(3.5 g saturated)
785 mg sodium
47 g carbohydrates

----

43 g protein
10 g fiber

Not That!

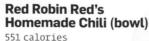

Red Robin Red's Homemade Chili (bowl)
551 calories
32 g fat
1,329 mg sodium
26 g carbohydrates

Plus This!

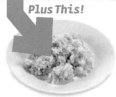

Quinoa
(¼ cup cooked)
55 calories
1 g fat (0 g saturated)
5 mg sodium
10 g carbohydrates

Grilled Mahi Mahi
280 calories
15 g fat (2.5 g saturated)
390 mg sodium
2 g carbohydrates

What do you get when you combine moist, meaty grilled halibut with a garlicky, herb-strewn sauce? A restaurant-quality dinner for half the price and a quarter the calories.

Plus This!

Red wine
(4-oz glass)
100 calories
0 g fat
5 mg sodium
3 g carbohydrates

You'll Need:

¾ cup chopped fresh parsley

¼ cup chopped fresh mint (optional)

Juice of 1 lemon

¼ cup olive oil + more for grilling

2–3 anchovy fillets, minced

2 Tbsp capers, rinsed and chopped

2 cloves garlic, finely minced

Pinch of red pepper flakes

Ground black pepper to taste

4 mahi mahi fillets, or another firm white fish like halibut, sea bass, or swordfish (about 6 oz each)

Salt to taste

How to Make It:

• Preheat a grill. Make sure the grate is clean and oiled.

• Combine the parsley, mint if using, lemon juice, olive oil, anchovies, capers, garlic, and pepper flakes in a mixing bowl. Season with black pepper. Set the salsa verde aside.

• Rub the fish fillets with a thin layer of oil, then season all over with salt and black pepper. Place the fillets on the grill skin side down and grill for 5 minutes, until the skin is lightly charred and crisp and pulls away freely (if you mess with the fish before it's ready to flip, it's likely to stick). Flip and cook on the other side for 2 to 3 minutes longer, until the fish flakes on gentle pressure from your fingertip. Serve the fillets with the salsa spooned over the top.

Makes 4 servings

= *Best Dinner*

435 calories
16 g fat
(2.5 g saturated)
400 mg sodium
15 g carbohydrates

----

35 g protein
2.5 g fiber

PERFECT SIDES

GARLIC SPINACH

Cook two cloves of garlic and a pinch of red pepper flakes in olive oil until fragrant. Add two boxes of defrosted frozen spinach and cook for 5 minutes. Season with salt and pepper.

Not That!

Cheesecake Factory Mahi Mahi Mediterranean
1,210 calories
23 g saturated fat
1,992 mg sodium

Eat This!

Bloody Mary Skirt Steak

270 calories
11 g fat (4.5 g saturated)
450 mg sodium
8 g carbohydrates

As delicious as a Bloody Mary is as a drink, it makes an even better marinade. That's because the mix of sweet and salty from the tomato juice, the heat from the horseradish and Tabasco, and the acid from the lemon work together to both tenderize and energize an otherwise normal piece of beef. This marinade could do magic on chicken and pork as well, but the bold flavors of a Bloody seem to pair best with a hunk of grilled beef. Serve with roasted potatoes for a near-perfect meal. (We're betting it makes a pretty good hangover remedy, too!)

You'll Need:

2 cups tomato juice (Spicy Hot V8 works best)

2 Tbsp jarred prepared horseradish

4 cloves garlic, minced

Juice of 1 lemon

½ Tbsp Worcestershire sauce

10–15 shakes of Tabasco sauce

Ground black pepper to taste

1 lb skirt or flank steak

How to Make It:

• Combine the tomato juice, horseradish, garlic, lemon juice, Worcestershire, Tabasco, and pepper in a baking dish and use a whisk to thoroughly mix. Add the steak and turn to coat. Cover with plastic wrap. Marinate in the refrigerator for at least 2 hours or up to 12.

• Preheat a grill. Pour off the marinade and discard. Use a paper towel to pat most of the marinade from the steak. When the grill is very hot, add the steak and cook for 3 to 4 minutes per side until medium rare. Let the meat rest for at least 5 minutes before cutting it into thin slices against the grain of the meat.

Makes 4 servings

Plus This!

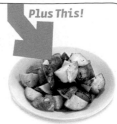

Roasted red potatoes
(1 cup diced)
135 calories
0 g fat
20 mg sodium
29.5 g carbohydrates

= Best Dinner

405 calories
11 g fat
(4.5 g saturated)
470 mg sodium
37.5 g carbohydrates

35.5 g protein
3.5 g fiber

PERFECT SIDES

HERB-ROASTED POTATOES

Preheat oven to 400°F. Cut 2 pounds red potatoes into ½-inch chunks and toss with ½ Tbsp fresh or 1 tsp dried rosemary, plus a generous drizzle of olive oil and salt and pepper. Roast until the flesh is soft and lightly browned, about 25 minutes.

Not That!

Outback 10 oz Ribeye with House Salad and Honey Mustard Dressing

1,234 calories
98 g fat (42 g saturated)
1,260 mg sodium
31 g carbohydrates

244

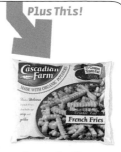

**Cascadian Farm
Crinkle Cut
French Fries**
(about 18 pieces)
110 calories
4 g fat (1 g saturated)
10 mg sodium
17 g carbohydrates

Seared Scallops
with White Beans and Spinach

280 calories
7 g fat (2.5 g saturated)
360 mg sodium
27 g carbohydrates

Scallops rarely end up on the American dinner table and we can't figure out why. They're a tremendous source of lean protein and super-easy to cook, and they stack up well with bold and subtle flavors alike. Learn to properly sear a scallop (see sidebar below) and you'll be won over.

You'll Need:

2 strips bacon, chopped into small pieces

½ red onion, minced

1½ cans white beans (14 oz each), rinsed and drained

Salt and black pepper to taste

1 Tbsp butter

Juice of 1 lemon

How to Make It:

• Heat a medium saucepan over low heat.

Cook the bacon until it has begun to crisp. Add the onion and garlic; sauté until the onion is soft and translucent, 2 to 3 minutes. Add the white beans and spinach and simmer until the beans are hot and the spinach is wilted. Keep warm.

• Heat a large cast-iron skillet or sauté pan over medium-high heat. Blot the scallops dry with a paper towel and season

with salt and pepper on both sides. Add the butter and the scallops to the pan and sear the scallops for 2 to 3 minutes per side, until deeply caramelized.

• Before serving, add the lemon juice to the beans. Season with salt and pepper. Divide the beans among 4 warm bowls or plates and top with scallops.

Makes 4 servings

= Best Dinner

390 calories
11 g fat
(3.5 g saturated)
370 mg sodium
44 g carbohydrates

----

28 g protein
7 g fiber

MASTER THE TECHNIQUE

SEAR FACTOR

Scallops are only slightly more difficult to cook than toast, assuming you follow a few basic rules. First, preheat a pan with a bit of olive oil over high heat. Next, use paper towels to blot the scallops dry (if there is moisture on the surface, they'll steam rather than caramelize). Season with salt and pepper and, when the oil is lightly smoking, add to the pan. Cook, undisturbed, for 2 to 3 minutes per side, until a golden crust has developed.

Not That!

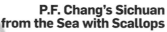

P.F. Chang's Sichuan from the Sea with Scallops

885 calories
45 g fat (9 g saturated)
3,690 mg sodium
78 g carbohydrates

Eat This!

Grilled Steak Tacos

250 calories
7 g fat (1.5 g saturated)
310 mg sodium
23 g carbohydrates

Taco night normally means ground beef and a package of mysterious spices, but instead you can have two salsa-strewn, guac-slathered steak tacos for just 250 calories. Hard to believe, especially when two restaurant tacos routinely pack nearly four times that amount, but this just goes to underscore the importance of taking to the kitchen.

You'll Need:

2 chipotle peppers in adobo sauce

1 cup orange juice

1 tsp ground cumin

2 cloves garlic

2 cups chopped fresh cilantro + more for garnish

1 lb flank steak

½ tsp salt

½ tsp ground black pepper

8 corn tortillas

¼ cup guacamole

Salsa

1 red onion, minced

2 limes, quartered

How to Make It:

• Combine the chipotle peppers, orange juice, cumin, garlic, and cilantro in a blender and puree. Place the steak and marinade in a resealable plastic bag and refrigerate for 30 minutes or up to 8 hours.

• Remove the steak from the marinade. Season with salt and black pepper. Heat a grill, grill pan, or cast-iron skillet over high heat until hot. Cook the steak for 3 to 4 minutes per side (for medium rare).

• Heat the tortillas until warm and pliable. It's best to do this on a hot grill or in a cast-iron skillet, but in a pinch, wrap the tortillas together in damp paper towels and microwave for 45 seconds.

• Slice the steak across the grain into thin pieces and divide among the tortillas. Top each with guacamole, salsa, onion, extra cilantro, and a squirt of lime juice.

Makes 4 servings

Plus This!

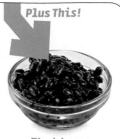

Black beans
(½ cup)
115 calories
0.5 g fat (0 g saturated)
205 mg sodium
20.5 g carbohydrates

Plus This!

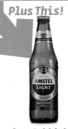

Amstel Light
95 calories
0 g fat
5 mg sodium
5 g carbohydrates

= Best Dinner
460 calories
7.5 g fat
(1.5 g saturated)
520 mg sodium
48.5 g carbohydrates

----

32 g protein
11 g fiber

Not That!

Chevys Mesquite Grilled Steak Tacos

1,110 calories
44 g fat (13 g saturated)
2,490 mg sodium
124 g carbohydrates

246

Plus This!

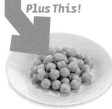

Spicy chickpeas
(¼ cup cooked)
65 calories
1 g fat (0 g saturated)
100 mg sodium
11 g carbohydrates

Plus This!

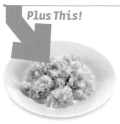

Quinoa
(¼ cup cooked)
55 calories
1 g fat (0 g saturated)
5 mg sodium
10 g carbohydrates

Lamb with Tzatziki
260 calories
15 g fat (4 g saturated)
390 mg sodium
4 g carbohydrates

Lamb has long been a second-class citizen in American households, a meat you turn to maybe once a year when you've grown tired of chicken and beef. Too bad, since lamb is not only jam-packed with flavor and easy to cook, but also surprisingly lean when you work with the right cuts. This yogurt-based tzatziki pairs perfectly with grilled chicken, pork, and salmon, as well.

You'll Need:

1 cucumber, peeled, halved, and seeded

1 cup plain Greek-style yogurt (we like Fage Total 2%)

Juice of 1 lemon

2 Tbsp olive oil

2 cloves garlic, finely minced

2 tsp minced fresh dill

Salt and ground black pepper to taste

4 loin or shoulder lamb chops (about 4 oz each)

How to Make It:

• Preheat a grill. Grate the cucumber with a cheese grater, then use your (clean!) hands to wring out all the excess water. Combine the cucumber with the yogurt, lemon juice, 1 tablespoon of the olive oil, garlic, dill, and a goodly pinch of salt and pepper. Set the tzatziki aside.

• Rub the lamb with the remaining tablespoon of olive oil, then season all over with salt and pepper. Grill, turning once, until a meat thermometer inserted into the deepest part of a chop reads 135°F, 10 to 12 minutes, depending on the thickness of the cut. Serve with the tzatziki.

Makes 4 servings

= Best Dinner
380 calories
17 g fat
(4 g saturated)
495 mg sodium
25 g carbohydrates

33.5 g protein
4.5 g fiber

PERFECT SIDES

SPICY CHICKPEAS

Saute two cloves of garlic and a few pinches of chili flakes in olive oil until fragrant, then stir in canned, drained chicken and cook until heated through.

Not That!

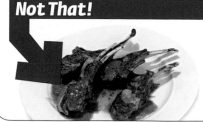

Outback New Zealand Rack of Lamb
1,303 calories
112 g fat (58 g saturated)
1,473 mg sodium
5 g carbohydrates

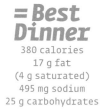

Eat This!

(see Perfect Sides recipe on page 238)

Brussels sprouts
(1 cup cooked)
55 calories
1 g fat (0 g saturated)
200 mg sodium
11 g carbohydrates

Plus This!

Roast Pork Loin
Porchetta-Style with Lemony White Beans
350 calories
10 g fat (3 g saturated)
410 mg sodium
18 g carbohydrates

Pork may have a reputation for being fatty, but a pork loin has about the same amount of fat as a boneless, skinless chicken breast. Plus, we think it's twice as flavorful, especially when rubbed with this heady mix of garlic, fennel, rosemary, and orange.

= Best Dinner
405 calories
11 g fat
(3 g saturated)
610 mg sodium
29 g carbohydrates

----
48 g protein
10 g fiber

STEALTH HEALTH

BRUSSELS SPROUTS
Along with broccoli and cabbage, brussels sprouts are members of the cruciferous family of vegetables, which makes them cancer-fighting heroes and excellent sources of folate. The more folate you have in your diet, the lower your risk of obesity, heart disease, stroke, cognitive impairment, Alzheimer's, and depression.

You'll Need:

3 cloves garlic, minced

Grated zest of 2 oranges

1 Tbsp fennel seeds

1½ Tbsp chopped fresh rosemary

1 Tbsp olive oil

1 pork loin (2 lb), preferably with a small rim of fat still attached

Salt and black pepper to taste

2 cans (16 oz each) cannellini, Great Northern, or white kidney beans, rinsed and drained

Juice of 1 lemon

How to Make It:

• Preheat the oven to 450°F. On a cutting board, combine the garlic, orange zest, fennel seeds, and 1 tablespoon of the rosemary.

Run your knife repeatedly through the mix until it begins to take on a pastelike consistency. Scoop it up into a bowl and add the olive oil. Season the pork with salt and pepper, then rub it all over with the paste. At this point, you can cook it immediately or marinate the loin for up to 4 hours in the refrigerator for deeper flavor.

• Lay the pork in a roasting pan and roast for 25 to 30 minutes (depending on the thick-

ness of the loin), until an instant-read thermometer inserted into the middle reads 150° to 155°F. Remove from the oven and allow to rest for 10 minutes before slicing.

• While the pork rests, combine the beans, lemon juice, and the remaining ½ tablespoon of rosemary in a saucepan and cook until warm all the way through. Season with salt and pepper. Serve slices of the pork over the beans.

Makes 6 servings

Not That!

IHOP Savory Pork Chops with onion rings
1,240 calories
57 g fat (12 g saturated)
1,440 mg sodium
111 g carbohydrates

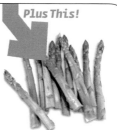

(see Perfect Sides recipe on page 237)

Asparagus
(4 spears)
40 calories
0 g fat (0 g saturated)
25 mg sodium
7 g carbohydrates

Blackened Tilapia
with Garlic-Lime Butter
300 calories
14 g fat (6 g saturated)
510 mg sodium
1 g carbohydrates

Ever eaten any blackened food that wasn't delicious? Neither have we. Consider it a bonus that blackening is actually an incredibly healthy way of cooking, giving the fish or meat a body armor of potent disease-fighting antioxidants in the form of tantalizing spices. Try this same blackening technique with chicken breasts, pork chops, or thin cuts of steak like flank and skirt.

= Best Dinner
340 calories
14 g fat
(6 g saturated)
535 mg sodium
8 g carbohydrates

----

49 g protein
4 g fiber

You'll Need

2 Tbsp butter, softened at room temperature

2 Tbsp chopped fresh cilantro

2 cloves garlic, finely minced

1 tsp lime zest + juice of 1 lime

1 Tbsp canola oil

4 tilapia fillets (6 oz each)

1 Tbsp store bought blackening spice

How to Make It:

• Combine the butter, cilantro, garlic, lime zest, and lime juice in a small mixing bowl and stir to thoroughly blend. Set aside.

• Heat the oil in a large cast-iron skillet or sauté pan over high heat. Rub the tilapia all over with the blackening spice. When the oil in the pan is lightly smoking, add the fish and cook, undisturbed, for 3 to 4 minutes on the first side, until the spice rub is dark and crusty. Flip and continue cooking for 1 to 2 minutes more, until the fillets flake on gentle pressure from your finger.

• Transfer the fish to four serving plates and immediately top each with a bit of the flavored butter.

Makes 4 servings

MASTER THE TECHNIQUE

FLAVORED BUTTERS

Butter has a bad reputation, but don't dismiss it so easily. A small pat of butter can help your body absorb fat-soluble nutrients and make a meal feel more filling in your belly. Take it one step further, though, by mixing softened butter with any of the following flavorful, nutrient-dense ingredients. Then, spoon a bit over a piece of grilled meat or your next baked potato.

• Sundried tomatoes and chopped olives
• Chopped garlic, scallion, and jalapeño
• Fresh grated ginger, lime zest, and a drizzle of soy sauce

Not That!

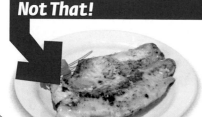

Denny's Lemon Pepper Grilled Talapia
640 calories
27 g fat (14 g saturated)
1,190 mg sodium
39 g carbohydrates

Eat This!

Red wine
(4-oz glass)
100 calories
0 g fat
5 mg sodium
3 g carbohydrates

Orecchiette with Broccoli Rabe and Turkey Sausage

345 calories
8 g fat (1.5 g saturated)
410 mg sodium
53 g carbohydrates

Order a bowl of restaurant pasta at your own peril. Our nutritional analysis shows that the average bowl of pasta from a chain restaurant well exceeds 1,000 calories. The trick to making pasta a viable home meal is to invert the ratio of toppings to noodles, filling your bowl with more vegetables and lean protein and fewer quick-burning carbohydrates. It might not be the Italian way, but it makes for a delicious solution to the pasta problem.

= Best Dinner

445 calories
8 g fat
(1.5 g saturated)
415 mg sodium
56 g carbohydrates

----

21 g protein
5.5 g fiber

You'll Need:

1 bunch broccoli rabe, bottom 1" removed

10 oz orecchiette pasta

½ Tbsp olive oil

2 links uncooked turkey or chicken sausage, casings removed

4 cloves garlic, minced

¼ tsp red pepper flakes

¾ cup low-sodium chicken stock

Salt and ground black pepper to taste

Pecorino, Romano, or Parmesan cheese

How to Make It:

• Bring a large pot of salted water to a boil. Drop in the broccoli rabe and cook for 3 minutes. Use tongs to remove the greens and chop them into ½" pieces. Return the water to a boil. Cook the pasta until al dente.

• While the pasta cooks, heat the olive oil in a large skillet over medium heat. Add the sausage and cook until lightly browned, about 5 minutes, then add the garlic and pepper flakes and sauté for another 3 minutes. Stir in the broccoli rabe and stock and lower the heat to a simmer. Season with salt and black pepper.

• Drain the pasta and toss it immediately into the pan with the sausage and greens. If the mixture looks dry, use a bit of the pasta cooking water to loosen it up. Serve immediately with freshly grated cheese.

Makes 4 servings

SECRET WEAPON

BROCCOLI RABE

This leafy vegetable is like a cross between spinach and broccoli, with a slightly bitter note and a robust package of nutrients. Add it to your arsenal: Cook for 3 minutes in salted, boiling water, drain, then saute in olive oil with garlic and red pepper flakes for another 3 to 5 minutes. Squeeze a lemon over the top.

Not That!

Ruby Tuesday Chicken & Broccoli Pasta

1,564 calories
96 g fat
2,811 mg sodium
87 g carbohydrates

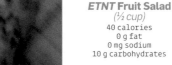

(see page 41)

Plus This!

ETNT Fruit Salad
(½ cup)
40 calories
0 g fat
0 mg sodium
10 g carbohydrates

Plus This!

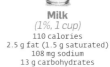

Milk
(1%, 1 cup)
110 calories
2.5 g fat (1.5 g saturated)
108 mg sodium
13 g carbohydrates

Chicago Dogs
250 calories
9 g fat (3.5 g saturated)
1,020 mg sodium
30 g carbohydrates

Hot dogs have long had a reputation for being unhealthy street corner fare, but when done right (lean beef, plenty of healthy condiments), a dog can actually be a reasonable meal with fewer than half the calories found in an average hamburger. Nobody does dogs better than Chicagoans (sorry, New York), who pack their buns with a garden's worth of produce.

You'll Need:

4 reduced-fat all-beef dogs (we like anything from Applegate Farms)

4 poppy seed hot dog buns

Yellow mustard

Relish

1 small yellow onion, minced

1 large beefsteak tomato, cut into wedges

4 pickle spears

8 jarred sport peppers

Celery salt

How to Make It:

• Bring a medium pot of water to a boil. Turn the heat to low, add the hot dogs, and cook for 5 minutes, until heated all the way through. Alternatively, you can grill the dogs until lightly charred all over.

• Dump out all but a few inches of the water and place a steamer basket in the pot. Steam the buns until warm and very soft.

• Place a dog in each bun, then arrange the toppings in the following order: mustard, relish, onion, a few tomato wedges, pickle spear, 2 sport peppers, and a pinch of celery salt.

Makes 4 servings

Best Dinner
400 calories
11.5 g fat
(5 g saturated)
1,128 mg sodium
53 g carbohydrates
- - - - - - - - - - - - - - - - - -
19.5 g protein
5 g fiber
- - - - - - - - - - - - - - - - - -

SWITCH IT UP

MEXICAN DOGS
The flavors of Mexico also inspire an excellent dog. Try it out: Swap out the accoutrements in this recipe for pico de gallo, guacamole, pickled jalapeños, and lightly charred scallions (a grill or hot skillet both do the job).

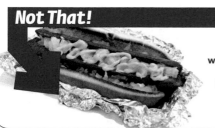

Not That!

Five Guys Hot Dog
with mustard, relish, and onions
570 calories
35 g fat (15.5 g saturated)
1,271 mg sodium
47 g carbohydrates

Snacks

CHAPTER 7

NO DIET!

The best way to lose weight quickly is to snack between meals.

Stop squinting. No, you read that right: The best way to lose weight quickly is to snack between meals.

Sure, it runs counter to some commonsense knowledge about weight loss, but before you doubt our words of wisdom, do us a favor. Drive to your local big-box store. Stand in the middle of the place. Take a look around. You see all those pudgy people? Almost every one of them believes that the best way to lose weight is to avoid snacking between meals.

So how's that working out for them?

In a world where two out of three women and three out of four men are either overweight or obese, it's time we take a look at some of the commonsense knowledge about weight loss and realize that while it might be common, it most certainly doesn't make any sense.

Not eating between meals means letting your energy store get low, which means hunger, blood sugar crashes, cravings, over-ordering, overeating, bloating, more sugar crashes, fatigue, more overeating, more fatigue, and the inevitable final munchie attack just as Stewart's passing the baton to Colbert.

Snacking between meals, however, means keeping hunger at bay, keeping your blood sugar even, eating more sensible meals, and enjoying high energy levels all through the day. The key is knowing how to recognize a sensible snack:

• It helps break up long stretches between meals.
It doesn't count as a smart snack if you eat lunch at 2 and have a cookie at 2:30. Snacking is like comedy—timing is everything. If lunch is at 2 and dinner is at 7, snack time ought to be around 4:30.

• It helps fill in the nutrients you missed at mealtime.
You should always be asking yourself, "Am I eating enough fruits and vegetables? Am I getting enough calcium from dairy foods?" If you had to skimp on one of your meals, snack time is the time to get your body back in balance.

• It's got protein, fiber, or both.
Peanut butter on whole grain crackers, baked chips with bean dip, a hunk of cheese and an apple—the perfect snack will have a boost of protein and as much fiber as you can pack in.

THE SNACK MATRIX

Hundred-calorie snack packs are the hottest thing in the packaged food industry since the hot sauce wars of '87. But while they may provide a decent defense against portion distortion, nearly all of them are total junk. Oreos, Chips Ahoy!, Cheetos—these heavily processed nutritional vortexes are built primarily around sugars and starches, fast-digesting, nutritionally vacuous carbohydrates that rain terror on your body.

See, when your stomach's empty, and you fill it with 100 calories of junk-food carbohydrates, your blood receives a near-instant jolt of glucose. If you happen to be in the middle of a jog, your muscles might suck that sugar up and convert it into footfalls. But if you're driving, sitting at your desk, or lounging poolside in Palm Springs, that sugar will be stored for later use. And how does your body store energy? With fat.

Luckily, there are more than a few ways to combine protein, fiber, and healthy fats—the nutrients that temper your snack's glucose jolt to a trickle and take a legitimate bite out of your hunger. Here, we've created a range of two-piece snack combinations, one part relying on a healthy vehicle like fresh fruit and whole wheat crackers, the other being a tasty topper with real nutritional benefits. Each component adds up to 100 calories and, with the help of plastic bags and containers, is no less portable than the 100-calorie packs you find in the impulse aisle.

More than anything, this matrix shows you how to build a great-tasting combo loaded with the foundations of sound snacking, and that's the secret to converting your body from a fat-storage to a fat-burning machine.

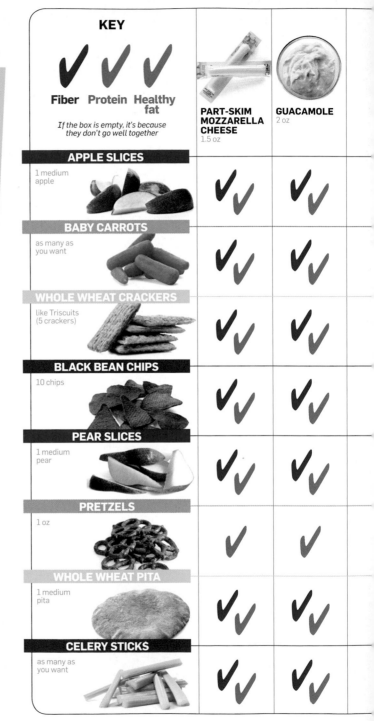

KEY

Fiber   Protein   Healthy fat

If the box is empty, it's because they don't go well together

	PART-SKIM MOZZARELLA CHEESE 1.5 oz	GUACAMOLE 2 oz
APPLE SLICES 1 medium apple	✔✔	✔✔
BABY CARROTS as many as you want	✔✔	✔✔
WHOLE WHEAT CRACKERS like Triscuits (5 crackers)	✔✔	✔✔
BLACK BEAN CHIPS 10 chips	✔✔	✔✔
PEAR SLICES 1 medium pear	✔✔	✔✔
PRETZELS 1 oz	✔	✔
WHOLE WHEAT PITA 1 medium pita	✔✔	✔✔
CELERY STICKS as many as you want	✔✔	✔✔

SALSA as much as you can handle	DARK CHOCOLATE 1 square	HAM, TURKEY, OR ROAST BEEF 4 slices	LOW-FAT COTTAGE CHEESE ¾ cup	PEANUT BUTTER 1 Tbsp	HUMMUS ¼ cup	TUNA, IN WATER ½ can
	✔✔	✔✔	✔✔	✔✔	✔✔	✔✔
✔		✔✔	✔✔	✔✔	✔✔	✔✔
✔		✔✔	✔✔	✔✔	✔✔	✔✔
✔		✔✔	✔✔	✔✔	✔✔	✔✔
	✔✔	✔✔	✔✔	✔✔	✔✔	✔✔
✔	✔	✔	✔	✔✔	✔✔	✔✔
✔		✔✔	✔✔	✔✔	✔✔	✔✔
✔		✔✔	✔✔	✔✔	✔✔	✔✔

16 Instant Hunger-Squashing Snacks

Congratulations. With two snacks now part of your daily routine, you've just earned 730 new eating opportunities this year. Now use the suggestions here to make the most of it. Not only do they pack a mean nutritional punch, but they also taste pretty dang delicious.

1 Spread the inside of a pita half with a thick layer of hummus and top with sliced tomato, onion, lettuce, and a few squirts of hot sauce.

2 Wrap slices of melon or cantaloupe with good prosciutto or Spanish ham.

3 Pop a bag of plain popcorn. Remove from the bag and toss with chopped rosemary, freshly grated parmesan cheese, and a drizzle of olive oil.

4 Lay out slices of prosciutto or other thinly sliced ham. Mix chopped olives and sun-dried tomatoes with fresh ricotta, then place a spoonful into the center of the prosciutto slices. Wrap like a burrito.

5 Peel a mango and cut it into spears. Top with fresh lime juice and chili powder.

6 Thread hunks of watermelon, cherry tomatoes, pieces of fresh mozzarella, and leaves of basil on wooden skewers.

Ants on a log: Slather celery with smooth or chunky peanut butter. Dot with raisins.

8

Lay a slice of Swiss cheese on a cutting board. Top with a slice of deli turkey and a spoonful of hummus or guacamole. Wrap like a jelly roll and eat.

9

Boil or microwave a few cups of frozen edamame until tender. Drain and toss with a light coating of sesame oil, soy sauce, and red pepper flakes.

10

Combine a can of tuna with your favorite salsa. Use Triscuits for scooping.

11

Toss a combination of nuts—pecans, almonds, peanuts, cashews—with chili powder, black pepper, and a pinch of cayenne. Roast in a 400°F oven for 10 minutes, until warm and toasty.

12

Pop a bag of popcorn. While it's still hot, toss with half a tablespoon of melted butter, a tablespoon of sugar, and half a teaspoon of cinnamon.

13

Green eggs and ham: Split a hard-boiled egg in half, top with a spoonful of prepared pesto, then wrap each half with a slice of deli ham or turkey.

14

Pave a slice of toasted wheat bread with peanut butter and banana slices. Top with a drizzle of honey.

15

Stuff cherry peppers or bottled Peppadew peppers with soft goat cheese or mini balls of fresh mozzarella.

16

Lightly butter a slice of toasted wheat or pumpernickel bread and top with thick slices of tomato, coarse sea salt, and fresh cracked pepper. Unbeatable in summer.

THE 50 BEST

SNACK FOODS

IN AMERICA

Tsunamis don't make rivers. They make destruction. No, if Mother Nature wants to cut a new river across the face of the earth, she must supply a slow, steady stream of water to strategically erode one narrow swath of land into a channel. And the same is true with calories: You need a slow, steady supply to wear down the flab that's stretched out across your belly.

To supply those calories, you need snacks. Problem is, if your snack is a tsunami—too big or nutritionally hostile—then you'll create, well, destruction. To that end, we've put together a list of the healthiest snacks in the supermarket. Let the erosion commence.

BARS

1. BEST FIBER BAR

Fiber One Chewy Bars Oats & Peanut Butter

Per bar:
150 calories,
4.5 g fat,
10 g sugars,
3 g protein, 9 g fiber

With about a third of your day's recommended fiber intake, this is the ideal snack for those days when your produce and whole grain intake are below par.

3. BEST PROTEIN BAR

Atkins Advantage Peanut Butter Granola Bar

Per bar:
200 calories,
7 g fat, 1 g sugars,
17 g protein,
6 g fiber

This bar has more protein than two Crunchy Beef Tacos from Taco Bell, plus a fifth of your day's fiber. That's enough to stop hunger in its tracks.

2. BEST ALL-NATURAL BAR

Lärabar Pecan Pie

Per bar:
220 calories,
14 g fat, 19 g sugars,
3 g protein, 4 g fiber

It's a lot of sugar, but every gram of it comes from natural dates, and other than that, there are only two ingredients in this bar: pecans and almonds. It's like trail mix compressed into a neat, easy-to-carry package.

4. BEST HEALTHY-FAT BAR

Kind Plus Almond Cashew + Omega-3

Per bar:
150 calories,
9 g fat, 14 g sugars,
4 g fiber,
4 g protein

Almonds and cashews bring in a major haul of monounsaturated fats, and the flaxseed rounds it out with omega-3s. That's a lot of nutrition for such a tiny package.

5. BEST FRUIT-FILLED BAR

Kashi TLC Soft-Baked Snack Bars Ripe Strawberry

Per bar:
110 calories,
3 g fat, 9 g sugars,
2 g protein,
3 g fiber

The fruity interior provides a fresh burst of sweetness, and the whole-grain exterior counters it with a nutty flavor that reminds you you're still eating real food.

7. BEST VEGETABLE JUICE

V8 100% Vegetable Juice, Low Sodium

Per 8 fl oz:
50 calories, 0 g fat,
140 mg sodium,
2 g protein,
2 g fiber

Each cup counts as two servings of vegetables, making this a wise beverage to drink in the wake of a produce-less lunch. Hey, gotta squeeze in those veggies however you can.

9. BEST PROTEIN SHAKE

EAS AdventEdge Carb Control Ready-to-Drink French Vanilla

Per 11 fl oz:
110 calories,
3 g fat, 0 g sugars,
17 g protein

This is a near-perfect load of post-workout protein. Maximize your gym time by tossing one of these in your gym bag and guzzling it on your way out the door.

10. BEST CHILI

Kettle Cuisine Three Bean Chili

Per container:
220 calories,
3.5 g fat,
450 mg sodium,
11 g protein,
13 g fiber

No food is better than chili for bringing together fiber and protein in such a flavor-loaded package. This one earns our love by combining three different beans with four different peppers.

12. BEST OVERALL SOUP

Campbell's Select Harvest Light Italian-Style Vegetable Soup

Per cup:
50 calories,
0 g fat,
480 mg sodium,
3 g protein,
4 g fiber

This is as light as soup gets. You can slurp the whole veggie-loaded can for 100 calories and not worry about serving-size overload.

6. BEST CHOCOLATE BAR

Lärabar Chocolate Chip Brownie

Per bar:
200 calories,
9 g fat, 4 g protein,
5 g fiber

This bar has only six ingredients, and every one of them is something you likely have or have had in your own kitchen. That makes it a rarity among the heavily processed foods populating the shelves of the supermarket.

8. BEST FRUIT SMOOTHIE

Bolthouse Farms Berry Boost

Per 8 oz:
130 calories,
1 g fat, 0 g protein,
4 g fiber

With no added sugar, this is one of the lowest-calorie bottles in the cooler. Thank the mix of blackberries, boysenberries, blueberries, and raspberries for their help in contributing big flavor, a boatload of antioxidants, and 5 days' worth of vitamin C.

11. BEST LEGUME-BASED SOUP

Health Valley Organic Split Pea & Carrots Soup (40% Less Sodium)

Per cup:
120 calories, 0 g fat,
480 mg sodium,
7 g protein, 7 g fiber

This can's ingredient statement reads like a vegan shopping list: split peas, carrots, potatoes, and lentils, all of which are organic. Even if you eat both servings in the can, you still fall within the caloric range of a healthy snack.

13. BEST CHICKEN SOUP

Campbell's Select Harvest Healthy Request Mexican Style Chicken Tortilla Soup

Per cup:
130 calories,
2 g fat,
410 mg sodium,
8 g protein,
2 g fiber

This Mexican-Style Chicken Tortilla Soup has a bigger flavor kick—and about 45 percent less sodium—than the more common varieties of chicken noodle.

CANNED AND FROZEN SNACKS

14. BEST FROZEN SNACK

Cedarlane Garden Vegetable Enchiladas

Per enchilada: 140 calories, 3 g fat, 9 g protein, 3 g fiber

Each enchilada has a quarter of your day's vitamin A and 20 percent of your daily calcium. The package comes with two servings, so eat one as a snack or add a side salad and eat both as lunch.

16. BEST PIZZA SNACK

Lean Pockets Whole Grain Supreme Pizza

Per pocket: 220 calories, 6 g fat, 10 g protein, 4 g fiber

These inverted pizzas deliver commendable hits of protein, fiber, and calcium. Plus they have more than a hundred fewer calories than similar flavors of Hot Pockets.

15. BEST MEAT-SUBSTITUTE SNACK

Morningstar Farms Meal Starters Chik'n Strips

Per 12 strips: 140 calories, 3.5 g fat, 23 g protein, 1 g fiber

With faux-chicken there's no need to pull out a frying pan. Just zap them in the microwave and serve with ketchup or barbecue sauce for a protein-loaded snack you can eat at your desk.

17. BEST FROZEN FINGER FOOD

Alexia Mushroom Bites

Per 5 pieces: 110 calories, 4 g fat, 3 g protein, 2 g fiber

Lightly breaded and cooked in olive oil, Alexia's mushrooms are loaded with both healthy fats and B vitamins, the latter of which converts carbohydrates into energy to keep your metabolism humming along smoothly.

CEREALS AND BREADS

18. BEST SWEETENED CEREAL

Kashi Whole Wheat Biscuits, Cinnamon Harvest

Per 2 oz (28 biscuits): 180 calories, 6 g protein, 5 g fiber

Aside from the touch of cane juice, the only ingredients are whole wheat and cinnamon. The wheat delivers protein and fiber, and the cinnamon helps counteract the cane juice's impact on blood sugar.

20. BEST OATMEAL

Quaker Weight Control Instant Oatmeal, Cinnamon

Per packet: 160 calories, 3 g fat, 7 g protein, 6 g fiber

Don't confine oatmeal to the breakfast table. A bowl of instant oats makes a perfect snack. Each packet has only 1 gram of sugar, an impressive 20 percent of your day's fiber, and thanks to the whey protein powder, a healthy array of amino acids.

19. BEST GRANOLA

Kashi GoLean Crisp! Toasted Berry Crumble

Per ¾ cup: 100 calories, 4 g fat, 9 g protein, 8 g fiber

Big-flavor add-ins like cranberries and blueberries allow Kashi to keep the fat and sugar levels below those of other granolas on the market. Pour some over a cup of Greek yogurt for a sweet and hearty snack.

21. BEST SNACK BREAD

Pepperidge Farm Swirl 100% Whole-Wheat Cinnamon with Raisins

Per slice: 80 calories, 1 g fat, 3 g protein, 2 g fiber

Cinnamon toast is usually little more than sugar and starch, a decadent duo with love-handle repercussions. Go with the whole wheat variety and you can snack without the guilt, even if you opt for a second slice.

PANTRY SNACKS

22. BEST WHOLE WHEAT CRACKER

Triscuit Original

Per 6 crackers: 120 calories, 4.5 g fat, 19 g carbohydrates, 3 g fiber

To make crackers, you need only two ingredients: wheat and oil. That, plus a dash of salt, is all Nabisco uses in the Triscuit formula. You won't find a better, more robust cracker anywhere.

23. BEST FLAVORED CRACKER

Wheat Thins Fiber Selects 5-Grain Crackers

Per 13 crackers: 120 calories, 4.5 g fat, 22 g carbohydrates, 5 g fiber

The mix of whole wheat, rolled oats, barley, and flaxseed lends these crackers a massive hit of fiber, and the touch of refined flour prevents them from tasting like chaff.

24. BEST POTATO CHIPS

Food Should Taste Good Sweet Potato Tortilla Chips

Per 12 chips:
140 calories,
6 g fat,
18 g carbohydrates,
3 g fiber, 2 g protein

Part chip, part cracker, and all good. These nibbles provide 20 percent of your daily dose of vitamin A, and they're gluten-free.

26. BEST PRETZELS

Newman's Own Organics Spelt Pretzels

Per 20 pretzels:
120 calories,
1 g fat,
23 g carbohydrates,
4 g protein,
4 g fiber

Spelt is a grain related to wheat but with more fiber and protein, and the fact that it's organic is just a bonus. Pair these with a hunk of cheddar to rope even more protein into your snack break.

28. BEST VEGETABLE DIPPERS

Earthbound Farm Organic Mini Peeled Carrots with Ranch Dip

Per package:
90 calories, 8 g fat,
5 g carbohydrates,
1 g protein,
1 g fiber

These baby carrots come with just enough ranch to kick up the flavor without burdening you with a nutritionally nullifying load of fat, and each serving has 130 percent of your day's recommended vitamin A.

29. BEST PLAIN YOGURT

Fage Total 2% Greek Yogurt

Per 7-ounce container:
130 calories,
4.5 g fat,
15 g protein

Greek yogurt has more than double the protein of standard American-style yogurt. Make it a simple parfait by adding fruit, nuts, seeds, or granola.

31. BEST COTTAGE CHEESE

Fiber One Lowfat Cottage Cheese with Fiber

Per ½ cup:
80 calories, 2 g fat,
10 g protein,
5 g fiber

Cottage cheese is famous for its abundant supply of complete protein, but the 5 grams of fiber come from the addition of a natural plant compound called inulin. Top your curds with canned or fresh fruit for an ultra-sweet snack (or dessert!).

25. BEST VEGETABLE CHIPS

Terra Exotic Harvest Vegetable Chips

Per oz
(about 16 chips):
130 calories,
6 g fat,
16 g carbohydrates,
2 g protein,
3 g fiber

This fun mix of carrots, blue potatoes, and kabocha squash boasts 40 percent less fat than potato chips and enough fiber to take the edge off your hunger. (Plus they look pretty on the chip 'n' dip platter.)

27. BEST POPCORN

Orville Redenbacher's Smart Pop! Gourmet Popping Corn (94% Fat-Free) Mini Bags

Per bag (popped):
100 calories,
1.5 g fat,
21 g carbohydrates,
3 g fiber, 3 g protein

The mini bags serve a dual function: They keep you from overeating and they do away with the need for a popcorn bowl. Keep a few bags tucked into your desk at work, and a fiber-rich snack will never be far from reach.

30. BEST FLAVORED YOGURT

Chobani Nonfat Blueberry Greek Yogurt

Per 6-oz container:
140 calories,
0 g fat, 14 g protein

Often what yogurt processors call "fruit" is actually artificially colored high-fructose corn syrup with just a touch of actual plant matter. Chobani's delivers real blueberry, and sugar plays a mere supporting role.

32. BEST CHEESE

Horizon Organic Mozzarella String Cheese

Per stick:
80 calories,
5 g fat, 8 g protein

Each stick has a fifth of your day's calcium intake, and Horizon keeps the fat down by using part-skim milk. The creaminess of the cheese pairs particularly well with an apple, and the duo just so happens to make one perfect snack-size portion.

33. BEST SPREADABLE CHEESE

The Laughing Cow Light Mozzarella, Sun-Dried Tomato & Basil

Per wedge:
35 calories, 2 g fat, 2 g protein

Keep one of these cheese wheels in the office fridge to fight on-the-job hunger. Spread a couple wedges over whole wheat crackers and you hit both major benchmarks of satiety: protein and fiber.

35. BEST PORTABLE EGG

Eggology Cage Free Hardboiled Eggs

Per egg:
70 calories, 4 g fat, 6 g protein

These are natural eggs, cooked, peeled, and ready to eat. Make a complete snack by spreading hummus on whole wheat toast and slicing the hard-boiled egg over the top.

36. BEST PEANUT BUTTER

Smucker's Natural Chunky Peanut Butter

Per 2 Tbsp:
200 calories, 16 g fat, 7 g protein, 2 g fiber

You'll find no added oils, sweeteners, or fillers in this jar—just peanuts and salt. Stay within the snack-size calorie range by eating one tablespoon with crackers or two tablespoons with baby carrots or celery.

38. BEST SWEET SPREAD

Peanut Butter & Co. Dark Chocolate Dreams

Per 2 Tbsp: 170 calories, 13 g fat, 7 g sugars, 6 g protein, 2 g fiber

Peanut Butter & Co. makes this delecta-ble spread with peanut butter, cocoa, and vanilla, basically providing all the indulgence of Nutella without Nutella's glut of added sugar. Pair a scoop with a banana for an incredibly tasty and surprisingly healthy snack.

40. BEST GUACAMOLE

Wholly Guacamole

Per 2 Tbsp:
60 calories, 5 g fat, 1 g protein, 2 g fiber

With so many faux-guacamoles at the supermarket, it's important to find one good brand and stick to it. So let us intro-duce you to Wholly, the supermarket's most reliable purvey-or of authentic, avocado-based guac. Oils, starches, and artificial colors are nowhere to be found in this package.

34. BEST CHOCOLATE MILK

Organic Valley Lowfat Chocolate Milk

Per 8 fl oz:
150 calories, 2.5 g fat, 9 g protein

Chocolate milk is the perfect drinkable snack before you head in for a workout. The sugar fuels your muscles for maximum power, and the protein helps rebuild them afterward.

37. BEST ALTERNATIVE NUT BUTTER

MaraNatha Creamy & Roasted Almond Butter

Per 2 Tbsp:
190 calories, 16 g fat, 7 g protein, 4 g fiber

Almond butter has more heart-healthy monounsaturated fatty acids than peanut butter, and it's just as convenient. Try smearing some over apple slices for a tasty blend of sweet and savory.

39. BEST HUMMUS

Sabra Sun Dried Tomato Hummus

Per 2 Tbsp:
60 calories, 5 g fat, 1 g protein, 1 g fiber

If you don't already keep hummus stocked in your fridge, add it to your shopping list right now. The creamy puree of chickpeas and sesame seeds carries a balanced mix of protein, fiber, and healthy fat, and it pairs well with just about anything you can dip.

41. BEST FRUIT SNACK

Peeled Snacks Much-Ado-About Mango

Per bag:
120 calories,
28 g carbohydrates,
2 g protein,
2 g fiber

Think of Peeled Snacks' Much-Ado-About-Mango like a Fruit Roll-Up for adults. It contains no added sugars or artificial ingredients, just organic mango. That's how each bag ends up with nearly a third of your day's vitamin A.

43. BEST SHELL-ON NUTS

Everybody's Nuts! European Roast Pistachios

Per ½ cup:
170 calories,
14 g fat, 6 g protein,
2 g fiber

We're not sure how they got the vinegar flavor inside the shell, but we do know it's totally addictive. Good thing the shells prevent you from wolfing them down too quickly.

45. BEST NUT MIX

Planters NUTrition Heart Healthy Mix

Per oz: 170 calories,
15 g fat, 6 g protein,
3 g fiber

Inside this can is an awesome blend of heart-protecting peanuts, almonds, pecans, pistachios, hazelnuts, and walnuts. Consider it a great base for homemade trail mix.

47. BEST SEASONED NUTS

Sahale Snacks Southwest Cashews

Per ¼ cup:
140 calories,
10 g fat,
5 g protein,
1 g fiber

Sahale hit upon an insanely flavorful recipe with these cashews. They're slow roasted with cheddar and Monterey Jack cheese, paprika, and two varieties of chili powder. Yeah, they're good.

49. BEST JERKY

Jack Link's Premium Cuts Original Beef Jerky

Per oz: 80 calories,
1 g fat, 15 g protein

No snack on the planet offers such a reliable dose of protein in a more convenient package. Consider this your best option on days when you're too busy to be bothered with snack-time complications.

42. BEST CHOCOLATE-COVERED FRUIT

Sunsweet Chocolate PlumSweets

Per 14 pieces:
120 calories,
6 g fat, 13 g sugars,
1 g protein,
2 g fiber

Per serving Sunsweet's plums have half as much sugar as Raisinets, and because they're coated in dark (instead of milk) chocolate, they boast a greater antioxidant boon.

44. BEST SEEDS

Eden Organic Pumpkin Seeds

Per ¼ cup:
200 calories,
16 g fat,
10 g protein,
5 g fiber

Not only are they loaded with protein and fiber, but pumpkin seeds are also one of the world's best sources of magnesium, a mineral that helps strengthen bones and improve blood circulation.

46. BEST PACKAGED TRAIL MIX

Eden Organic Wild Berry Mix-Nuts, Seeds & Berries

Per 3 Tbsp:
150 calories,
8 g fat, 5 g protein,
4 g fiber

No time to blend your own mix? Fine, this one carries an anti-oxidant powerhouse of raisins, cranberries, wild blueberries, almonds, and seeds. That makes it simul-taneously chewy, crunchy, and sweet.

48. BEST CHOCOLATE-COVERED NUTS

Emerald Cocoa Roast Almonds, Dark Chocolate

Per ¼ cup:
150 calories,
13 g fat, 1 g sugars,
6 g protein,
3 g fiber

This snack tastes like candy but has all the nutritional kick of an almond. Plus, since each serving has only 1 gram of sugar, you'll incur no candy-splurging penalties.

50. BEST TUNA SNACK

Bumble Bee Sensations Sundried Tomato & Basil Tuna Medley

Per 6 oz:
220 calories,
8 g fat,
4 g carbohydrates,
32 g protein

This little dish pads your belly with more protein than a Burger King Whopper, but it does so with fewer than a third as many calories. Eat it straight out of the container or dump it over some greens for a simple tuna salad.

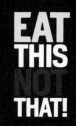

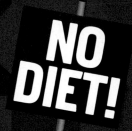
NO
DIET!

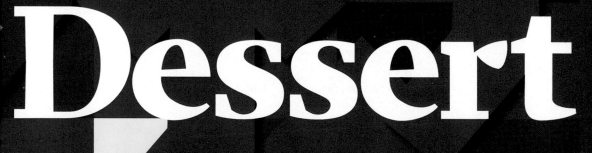

CHAPTER 8

Dessert

What do Darth Vader, King Kong, Hannibal Lecter, and an ice cream sundae all have in common?

They're all destructive, havoc-wreaking villains. But if you look deeper, you discover that they all have a good side, as well.

Kong may have made a mess of Midtown Manhattan, but his animal rage was driven by his love for Fay Ray. Sure, Lord Vader wanted to destroy the Jedi, but when push came to shove, he put Skywalker first. And Dr. Lecter really just wanted to help Clarice Starling get ahead, while also snacking on an occasional chunk of human liver. (Cannibalism or no cannibalism, can't we all just get along?)

The same is true of the ice cream sundae sitting in your dish. Sure, it's packed with fat and sugar, and it has more calories than perhaps you might like. But look deeper into that bowl: The ice cream provides calcium, which binds to fatty acids in the digestive tract, blocking their absorption. And a ½ cup of vanilla ice cream gives you 17 milligrams of choline, which can lower levels of homocysteine—an amino acid that restricts bloodflow—by 8 percent, according to USDA research. That means lower risks of stroke and heart disease. Also on that sundae? Probably some nuts (fiber, vitamins, minerals, protein, and heart-healthy fat), and maybe some dried fruit (more fiber, vitamins, and minerals).

So it is with dessert: If you can look at your after-dinner treat as an opportunity to add something more than just calories, you're on your way to a healthier (and more indulgent) diet. Fruits, nuts, and ice cream, as well as dark chocolate, ought to be a regular part of your diet; they all provide healthy, good-for-you nutrients while making you feel as though you're cheating. (It's the equivalent of meeting your wife or husband in a hotel room and playing "the traveling salesman and the cocktail waitress.")

But before you go ahead and order off that little mini menu in the center of the table, ask yourself a few questions:

Did I eat well throughout the day?

If the answer's yes, then you should indulge. Indeed, studies show that each time you turn down temptation, it actually makes it harder to make the right choice the next time around.

Is there at least one nutritionally beneficial element here?

Cakes and cookies are generally nonstarters if they're just sitting there alone on a plate. But if there's a bit of ice cream or another protein source, some kind of fruit or vegetable, or perhaps some nuts popping up in there, then it probably makes sense to say yes.

Is there someone cute at the table that I can share this with?

A sensible dessert should have only as many calories as your typical snack— no more than 250 per serving. For almost every dessert at almost every restaurant in America, that means you're sharing.

Eat This!
AU BON PAIN

English Toffee Cookie *(1)*
250 calories
14 g fat (6 g saturated)
17 g sugars

English toffee is a sweet, buttery, almond-infused confection—a bit like alcohol-free nibs of amaretto —and it makes for one super-tasty cookie. As a rule of thumb, cookies always beat out cake and pie when you're looking for a sweet fix at a café or coffee shop.

Not That!

Crumb Cake
720 calories
40 g fat
(17 g saturated)
42 g sugars

Eat This!
BASKIN-ROBBINS

BRight Choices Fat-Free Vanilla Frozen Yogurt
(4-oz scoop with half a banana)
200 calories
0 g fat
31 g sugars

Not much on Baskin's menu meets the criteria of a modest dessert. The lightest sundae has more than 600 calories, and most surpass 900. This yogurt, however, is safe, and you can punch up the flavor by asking for a sliced banana on top. The chain keeps them on hand for the Banana Splits.

Not That!

Brownie Sundae
920 calories
47 g fat
(22 g saturated)
97 g sugars

Eat This!
BEN & JERRY'S

Cherry Garcia Ice Cream
(½ cup)
200 calories
11 g fat (8 g saturated)
20 g sugars

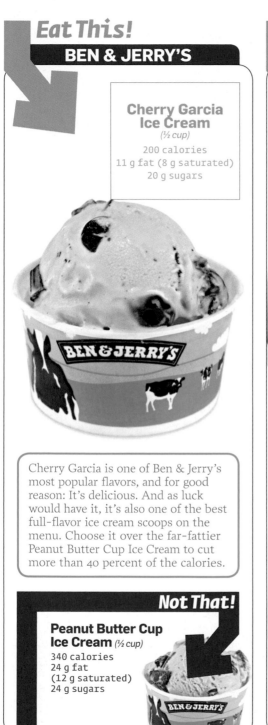

Cherry Garcia is one of Ben & Jerry's most popular flavors, and for good reason: It's delicious. And as luck would have it, it's also one of the best full-flavor ice cream scoops on the menu. Choose it over the far-fattier Peanut Butter Cup Ice Cream to cut more than 40 percent of the calories.

Not That!

Peanut Butter Cup Ice Cream *(½ cup)*
340 calories
24 g fat
(12 g saturated)
24 g sugars

Eat This!
BOB EVANS

Vanilla Ice Cream
(2.8-oz scoop with a fruit dish)
169 calories
6 g fat (4 g saturated)
23 g sugars

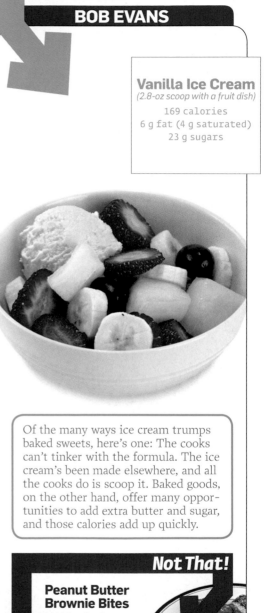

Of the many ways ice cream trumps baked sweets, here's one: The cooks can't tinker with the formula. The ice cream's been made elsewhere, and all the cooks do is scoop it. Baked goods, on the other hand, offer many opportunities to add extra butter and sugar, and those calories add up quickly.

Not That!

Peanut Butter Brownie Bites
1,024 calories
49 g fat
(13 g saturated)
96 g sugars

Eat This!
BURGER KING

Funnel Cake Sticks with icing
(9 pieces)

300 calories
11 g fat (3 g saturated)
30 g sugars

A funnel cake ordered from a fairground purveyor pushes close to 600 calories. That doesn't make BK's "healthy," but in purely relative terms, the fried bread sticks are quite the caloric bargain. Even with icing dip, they have fewer than half the calories of a small Oreo BK Sundae Shake.

Not That!

Oreo BK Sundae Shake—Chocolate
(small)

650 calories
21 g fat
(15 g saturated)
89 g sugars

Eat This!
CHEESECAKE FACTORY

Chocolate Ice Cream
("kid"-size scoop with fresh strawberries)

270 calories
7 g saturated fat
33 g carbohydrates

Too proud to order a kid-size scoop? Get over it. The smallest "adult" scoop has well over twice the calories, and the Specialty Desserts menu ranges from 950 to 1,670 calories (that's per dish!). And really, this desssert straddles the line between decadence and prudence beautifully.

Not That!

Tiramisu

950 calories
33 g saturated fat
74 g carbohydrates

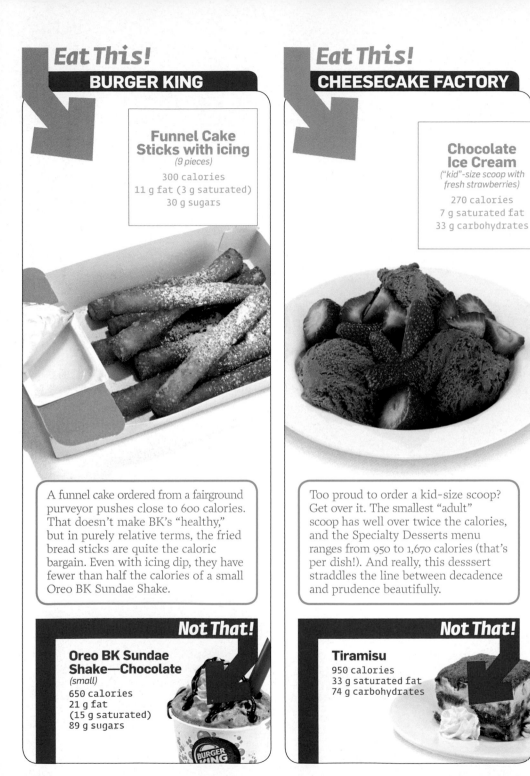

Eat This!
CHICK-FIL-A

Icedream
170 calories
4 g fat (2 g saturated)
25 g sugars

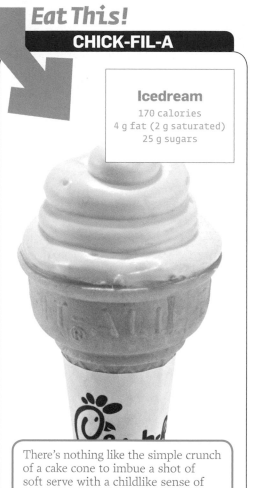

There's nothing like the simple crunch of a cake cone to imbue a shot of soft serve with a childlike sense of indulgence. That's fine too, considering the cone itself has no more than about 20 calories. Consider the Icedream the perfect bookend to one of Chick fil-A's lean sandwiches.

Not That!
Peppermint Chocolate Chip Milkshake
(small)
610 calories
23 g fat
(13 g saturated)
89 g sugars

Eat This!
COLD STONE CREAMERY

Tart and Tangy Plain Yogurt
(Like It size with walnuts)
270 calories
13 g fat (1 g saturated)
24 g sugars

At a mere 140 calories, the Like It sized Tart and Tangy Yogurt is the ideal base for a healthy topping of your choice. Fruit works fine, but walnuts usher in fiber and healthy fats, both of which work to keep your blood sugar in a healthy range as you indulge your sweet tooth.

Not That!
Oreo Crème Ice Cream
(Like It size)
440 calories
31 g fat
(14 g saturated)
38 g sugars

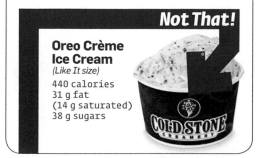

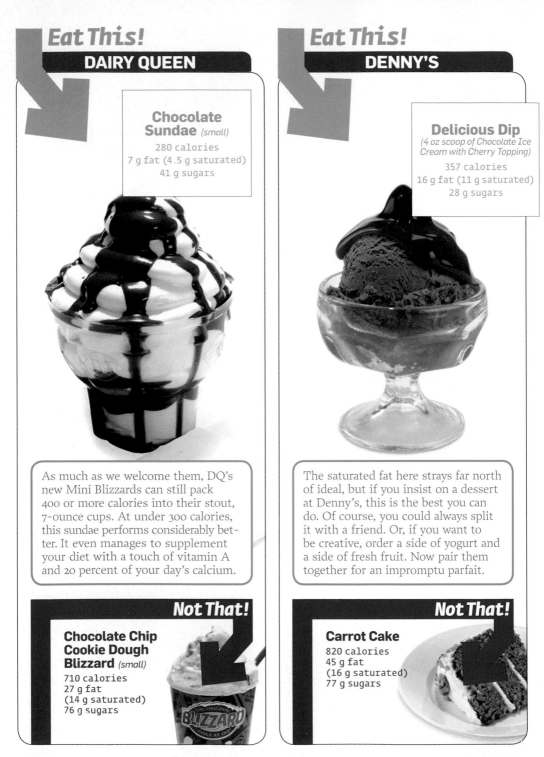

Chocolate Sundae *(small)*

280 calories
7 g fat (4.5 g saturated)
41 g sugars

Delicious Dip
(4 oz scoop of Chocolate Ice Cream with Cherry Topping)

357 calories
16 g fat (11 g saturated)
28 g sugars

As much as we welcome them, DQ's new Mini Blizzards can still pack 400 or more calories into their stout, 7-ounce cups. At under 300 calories, this sundae performs considerably better. It even manages to supplement your diet with a touch of vitamin A and 20 percent of your day's calcium.

The saturated fat here strays far north of ideal, but if you insist on a dessert at Denny's, this is the best you can do. Of course, you could always split it with a friend. Or, if you want to be creative, order a side of yogurt and a side of fresh fruit. Now pair them together for an impromptu parfait.

Not That!

Chocolate Chip Cookie Dough Blizzard *(small)*

710 calories
27 g fat
(14 g saturated)
76 g sugars

Not That!

Carrot Cake

820 calories
45 g fat
(16 g saturated)
77 g sugars

Eat This!
HÄAGEN-DAZS

Zesty Lemon Sorbet *(½ cup)*

120 calories
0 g fat
27 g sugars

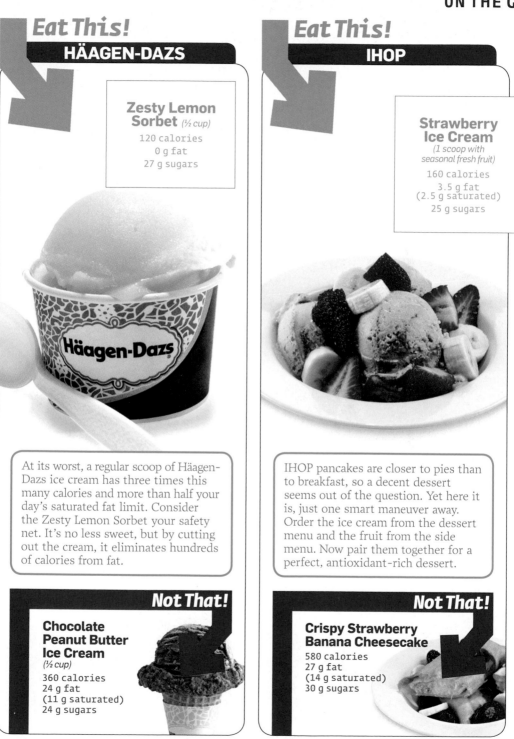

At its worst, a regular scoop of Häagen-Dazs ice cream has three times this many calories and more than half your day's saturated fat limit. Consider the Zesty Lemon Sorbet your safety net. It's no less sweet, but by cutting out the cream, it eliminates hundreds of calories from fat.

Not That!

Chocolate Peanut Butter Ice Cream
(½ cup)

360 calories
24 g fat
(11 g saturated)
24 g sugars

Eat This!
IHOP

Strawberry Ice Cream
(1 scoop with seasonal fresh fruit)

160 calories
3.5 g fat
(2.5 g saturated)
25 g sugars

IHOP pancakes are closer to pies than to breakfast, so a decent dessert seems out of the question. Yet here it is, just one smart maneuver away. Order the ice cream from the dessert menu and the fruit from the side menu. Now pair them together for a perfect, antioxidant-rich dessert.

Not That!

Crispy Strawberry Banana Cheesecake

580 calories
27 g fat
(14 g saturated)
30 g sugars

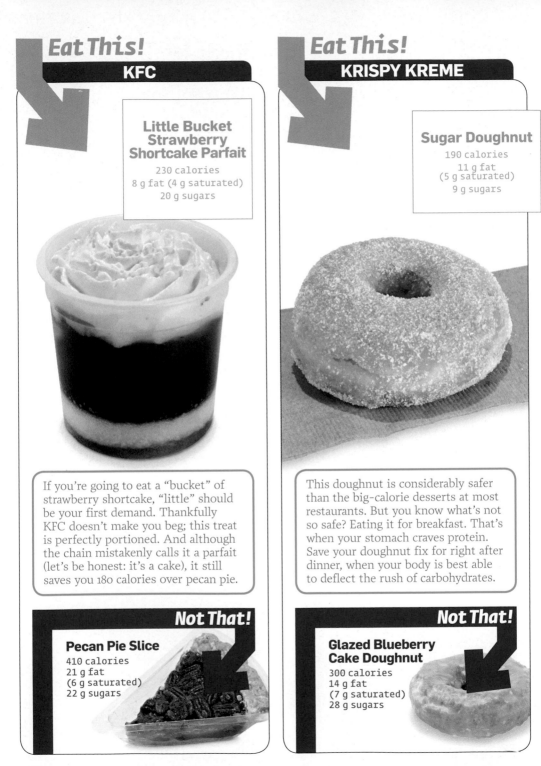

Eat This!
KFC

Little Bucket Strawberry Shortcake Parfait
230 calories
8 g fat (4 g saturated)
20 g sugars

If you're going to eat a "bucket" of strawberry shortcake, "little" should be your first demand. Thankfully KFC doesn't make you beg; this treat is perfectly portioned. And although the chain mistakenly calls it a parfait (let's be honest: it's a cake), it still saves you 180 calories over pecan pie.

Not That!

Pecan Pie Slice
410 calories
21 g fat
(6 g saturated)
22 g sugars

Eat This!
KRISPY KREME

Sugar Doughnut
190 calories
11 g fat
(5 g saturated)
9 g sugars

This doughnut is considerably safer than the big-calorie desserts at most restaurants. But you know what's not so safe? Eating it for breakfast. That's when your stomach craves protein. Save your doughnut fix for right after dinner, when your body is best able to deflect the rush of carbohydrates.

Not That!

Glazed Blueberry Cake Doughnut
300 calories
14 g fat
(7 g saturated)
28 g sugars

Eat This!
MCDONALD'S

Vanilla Reduced-Fat Ice Cream Cone
(with sundae peanuts)

195 calories
7 g fat (2.5 g saturated)
18 g sugars

Eat This!
OLIVE GARDEN

Strawberry & White Chocolate Cream Cake Dolcini

210 calories
11 g fat (6 g saturated)
27 g carbohydrates

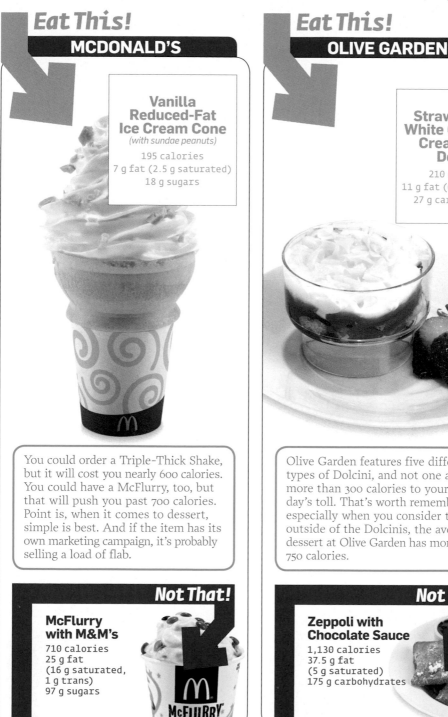

You could order a Triple-Thick Shake, but it will cost you nearly 600 calories. You could have a McFlurry, too, but that will push you past 700 calories. Point is, when it comes to dessert, simple is best. And if the item has its own marketing campaign, it's probably selling a load of flab.

Olive Garden features five different types of Dolcini, and not one adds more than 300 calories to your day's toll. That's worth remembering, especially when you consider that outside of the Dolcinis, the average dessert at Olive Garden has more than 750 calories.

Not That!
McFlurry with M&M's

710 calories
25 g fat
(16 g saturated,
1 g trans)
97 g sugars

Not That!
Zeppoli with Chocolate Sauce

1,130 calories
37.5 g fat
(5 g saturated)
175 g carbohydrates

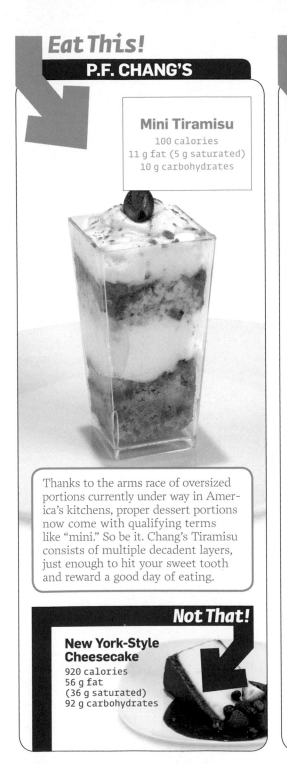

Thanks to the arms race of oversized portions currently under way in America's kitchens, proper dessert portions now come with qualifying terms like "mini." So be it. Chang's Tiramisu consists of multiple decadent layers, just enough to hit your sweet tooth and reward a good day of eating.

In terms of healthy dining, Red Lobster's Fresh Fish menu is second to none. Too bad the same can't be said for the dessert menu. The lightest item has 520 calories, and the worst, the Chocolate Wave, has nearly 1,500. Instead, order off the kids' menu. This sundae is just what you want.

Eat This!

RUBY TUESDAY

**Berry Good
Yogurt Parfait**

162 calories
3 g fat
26 g carbohydrates

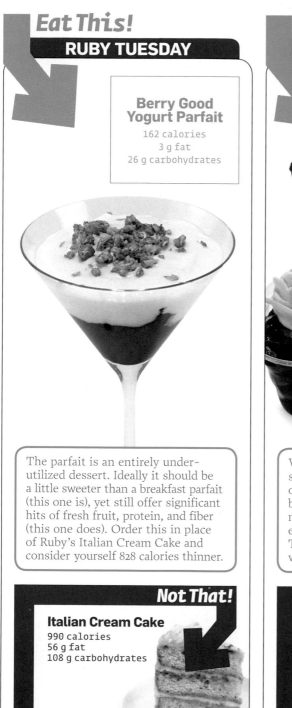

The parfait is an entirely under-utilized dessert. Ideally it should be a little sweeter than a breakfast parfait (this one is), yet still offer significant hits of fresh fruit, protein, and fiber (this one does). Order this in place of Ruby's Italian Cream Cake and consider yourself 828 calories thinner.

Not That!

Italian Cream Cake

990 calories
56 g fat
108 g carbohydrates

Eat This!

SONIC

**Junior
Banana Split**

200 calories
6 g fat (4.5 g saturated)
22 g sugars

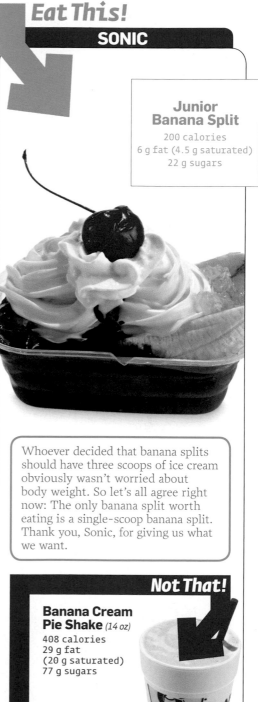

Whoever decided that banana splits should have three scoops of ice cream obviously wasn't worried about body weight. So let's all agree right now: The only banana split worth eating is a single-scoop banana split. Thank you, Sonic, for giving us what we want.

Not That!

**Banana Cream
Pie Shake** *(14 oz)*

408 calories
29 g fat
(20 g saturated)
77 g sugars

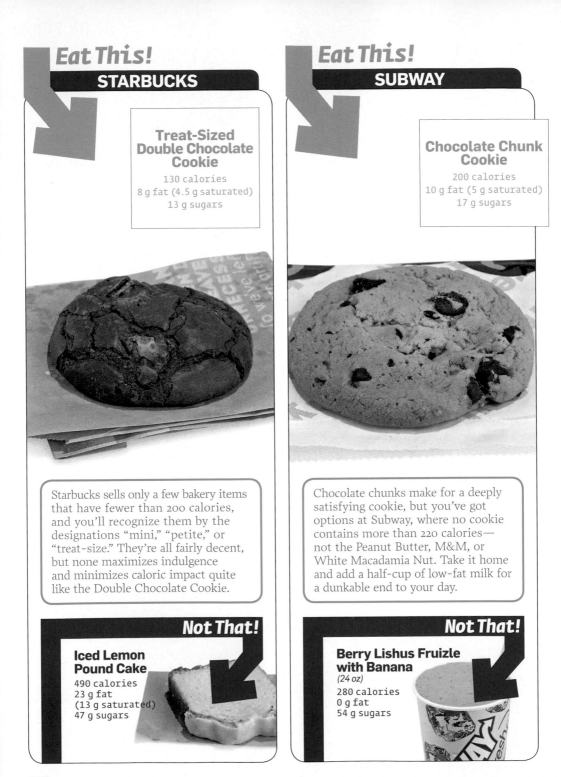

**Treat-Sized
Double Chocolate
Cookie**

130 calories
8 g fat (4.5 g saturated)
13 g sugars

Starbucks sells only a few bakery items that have fewer than 200 calories, and you'll recognize them by the designations "mini," "petite," or "treat-size." They're all fairly decent, but none maximizes indulgence and minimizes caloric impact quite like the Double Chocolate Cookie.

Not That!

**Iced Lemon
Pound Cake**

490 calories
23 g fat
(13 g saturated)
47 g sugars

**Chocolate Chunk
Cookie**

200 calories
10 g fat (5 g saturated)
17 g sugars

Chocolate chunks make for a deeply satisfying cookie, but you've got options at Subway, where no cookie contains more than 220 calories— not the Peanut Butter, M&M, or White Macadamia Nut. Take it home and add a half-cup of low-fat milk for a dunkable end to your day.

Not That!

**Berry Lishus Fruizle
with Banana**
(24 oz)

280 calories
0 g fat
54 g sugars

Eat This!
UNO CHICAGO GRILL

Mini Granny Smith All American
320 calories
14 g fat (8 g saturated)
31 g sugars

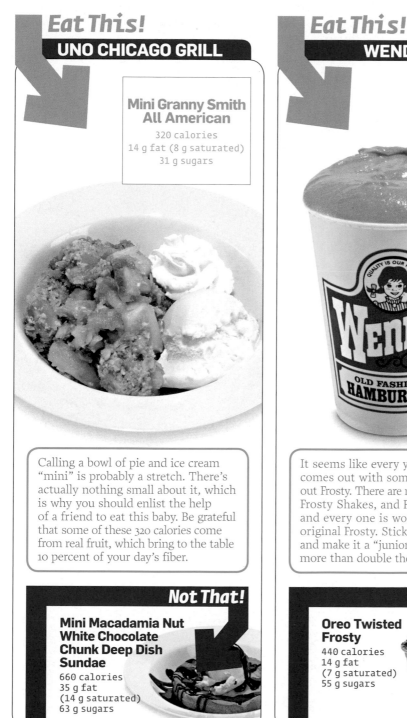

Calling a bowl of pie and ice cream "mini" is probably a stretch. There's actually nothing small about it, which is why you should enlist the help of a friend to eat this baby. Be grateful that some of these 320 calories come from real fruit, which bring to the table 10 percent of your day's fiber.

Not That!
Mini Macadamia Nut White Chocolate Chunk Deep Dish Sundae
660 calories
35 g fat
(14 g saturated)
63 g sugars

Eat This!
WENDY'S

Jr. Original Chocolate Frosty
150 calories
4 g fat (2.5 g saturated)
22 g sugars

It seems like every year Wendy's comes out with some new, tricked-out Frosty. There are now Frosty Floats, Frosty Shakes, and Frosty-cinos, and every one is worse than the original Frosty. Stick to the classic, and make it a "junior." The small has more than double the calories.

Not That!
Oreo Twisted Frosty
440 calories
14 g fat
(7 g saturated)
55 g sugars

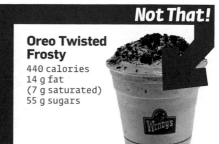

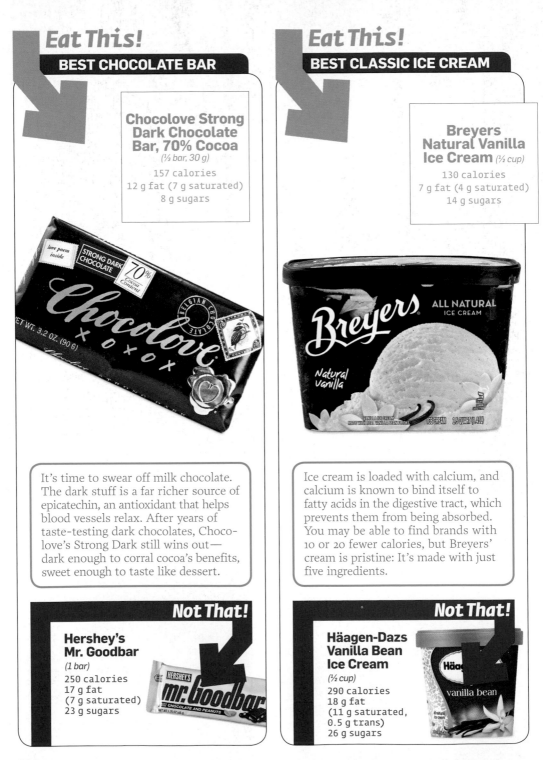

Eat This!

Chocolove Strong Dark Chocolate Bar, 70% Cocoa
(⅓ bar, 30 g)

157 calories
12 g fat (7 g saturated)
8 g sugars

It's time to swear off milk chocolate. The dark stuff is a far richer source of epicatechin, an antioxidant that helps blood vessels relax. After years of taste-testing dark chocolates, Chocolove's Strong Dark still wins out— dark enough to corral cocoa's benefits, sweet enough to taste like dessert.

Not That!

Hershey's Mr. Goodbar
(1 bar)
250 calories
17 g fat
(7 g saturated)
23 g sugars

Eat This!

BEST CLASSIC ICE CREAM

Breyers Natural Vanilla Ice Cream *(½ cup)*

130 calories
7 g fat (4 g saturated)
14 g sugars

Ice cream is loaded with calcium, and calcium is known to bind itself to fatty acids in the digestive tract, which prevents them from being absorbed. You may be able to find brands with 10 or 20 fewer calories, but Breyers' cream is pristine: It's made with just five ingredients.

Not That!

Häagen-Dazs Vanilla Bean Ice Cream
(½ cup)
290 calories
18 g fat
(11 g saturated,
0.5 g trans)
26 g sugars

Eat This!

BEST SWIRLED ICE CREAM

**Breyers
All Natural
Vanilla Fudge
Twirl** *(½ cup)*

130 calories
6 g fat (3.5 g saturated)
15 g sugars

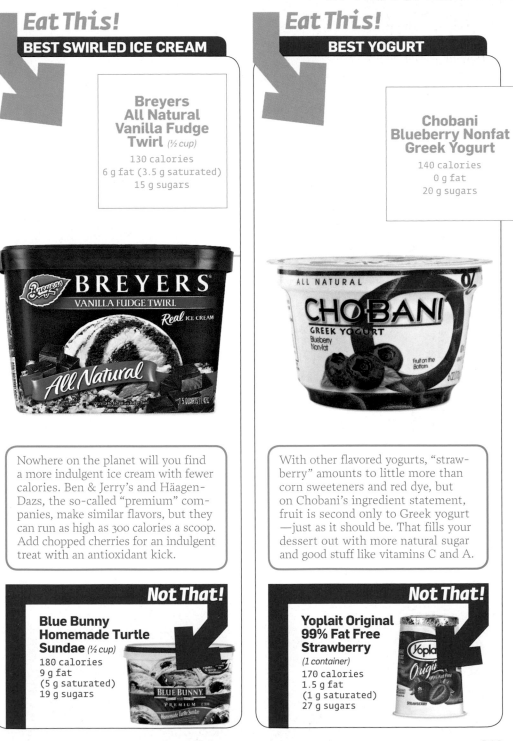

Nowhere on the planet will you find a more indulgent ice cream with fewer calories. Ben & Jerry's and Häagen-Dazs, the so-called "premium" companies, make similar flavors, but they can run as high as 300 calories a scoop. Add chopped cherries for an indulgent treat with an antioxidant kick.

Not That!

**Blue Bunny
Homemade Turtle
Sundae** *(½ cup)*

180 calories
9 g fat
(5 g saturated)
19 g sugars

Eat This!

BEST YOGURT

**Chobani
Blueberry Nonfat
Greek Yogurt**

140 calories
0 g fat
20 g sugars

With other flavored yogurts, "strawberry" amounts to little more than corn sweeteners and red dye, but on Chobani's ingredient statement, fruit is second only to Greek yogurt —just as it should be. That fills your dessert out with more natural sugar and good stuff like vitamins C and A.

Not That!

**Yoplait Original
99% Fat Free
Strawberry**
(1 container)

170 calories
1.5 g fat
(1 g saturated)
27 g sugars

283

Lärabar Chocolate Jocalat
(1 bar)

200 calories
10 g fat (2 g saturated)
21 g sugars

Edy's Slow Churned Rocky Road
(½ cup)

120 calories
4 g fat (2 g saturated)
14 g sugars

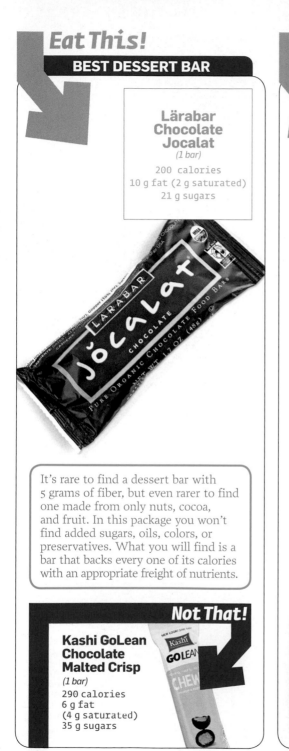

It's rare to find a dessert bar with 5 grams of fiber, but even rarer to find one made from only nuts, cocoa, and fruit. In this package you won't find added sugars, oils, colors, or preservatives. What you will find is a bar that backs every one of its calories with an appropriate freight of nutrients.

The secret to constructing a rich flavor like Rocky Road without breaking past 120 calories is to push fat-free milk up to the first ingredient in the recipe, which is exactly what Edy's has done. Oh, that and they put in a sugar-ceiling lower than what you'd find in one Pull 'n' Peel Twizzler.

Not That!

Kashi GoLean Chocolate Malted Crisp
(1 bar)

290 calories
6 g fat
(4 g saturated)
35 g sugars

Not That!

Häagen-Dazs Chocolate Peanut Butter Ice Cream
(½ cup)

360 calories
24 g fat
(11 g saturated)
24 g sugars

Eat This!

BEST ICE CREAM SANDWICH

**Klondike
Slim-A-Bear
No Sugar Added
Vanilla Ice Cream
Sandwich** *(1 bar)*

100 calories
2 g fat (1 g saturated)
3 g sugars

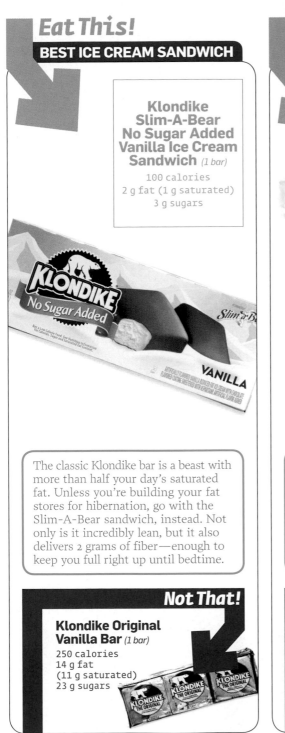

The classic Klondike bar is a beast with more than half your day's saturated fat. Unless you're building your fat stores for hibernation, go with the Slim-A-Bear sandwich, instead. Not only is it incredibly lean, but it also delivers 2 grams of fiber—enough to keep you full right up until bedtime.

Not That!

**Klondike Original
Vanilla Bar** *(1 bar)*

250 calories
14 g fat
(11 g saturated)
23 g sugars

Eat This!

BEST SORBET

**Ben & Jerry's
Berried Treasure
Sorbet** *(½ cup)*

110 calories
0 g fat
25 g sugars

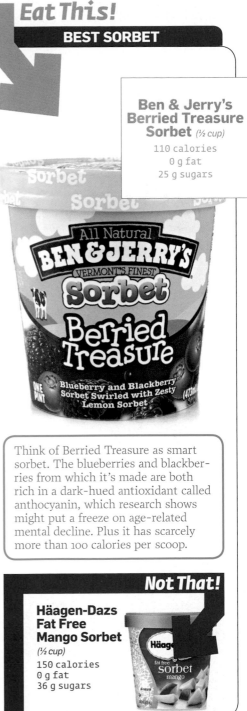

Think of Berried Treasure as smart sorbet. The blueberries and blackberries from which it's made are both rich in a dark-hued antioxidant called anthocyanin, which research shows might put a freeze on age-related mental decline. Plus it has scarcely more than 100 calories per scoop.

Not That!

**Häagen-Dazs
Fat Free
Mango Sorbet**
(½ cup)

150 calories
0 g fat
36 g sugars

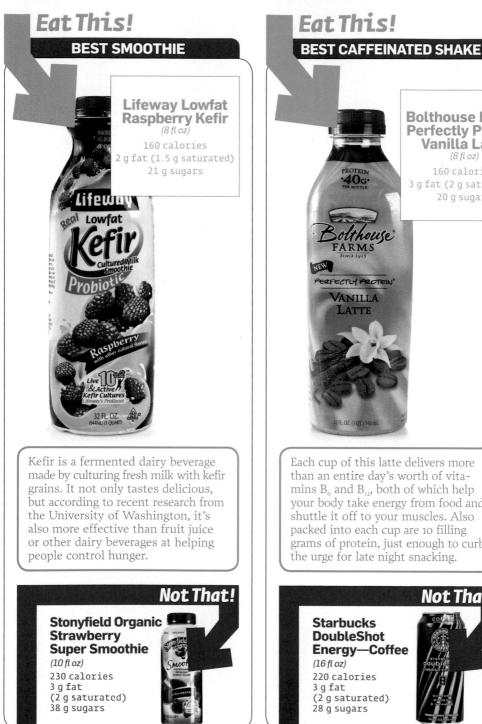

Eat This!

BEST SMOOTHIE

Lifeway Lowfat Raspberry Kefir
(8 fl oz)

160 calories
2 g fat (1.5 g saturated)
21 g sugars

Kefir is a fermented dairy beverage made by culturing fresh milk with kefir grains. It not only tastes delicious, but according to recent research from the University of Washington, it's also more effective than fruit juice or other dairy beverages at helping people control hunger.

Not That!

Stonyfield Organic Strawberry Super Smoothie
(10 fl oz)

230 calories
3 g fat
(2 g saturated)
38 g sugars

Eat This!

BEST CAFFEINATED SHAKE

Bolthouse Farms Perfectly Protein Vanilla Latte
(8 fl oz)

160 calories
3 g fat (2 saturated)
20 g sugars

Each cup of this latte delivers more than an entire day's worth of vitamins B_6 and B_{12}, both of which help your body take energy from food and shuttle it off to your muscles. Also packed into each cup are 10 filling grams of protein, just enough to curb the urge for late night snacking.

Not That!

Starbucks DoubleShot Energy—Coffee
(16 fl oz)

220 calories
3 g fat
(2 g saturated)
28 g sugars

Eat This!

BEST CHOCOLATE MILK

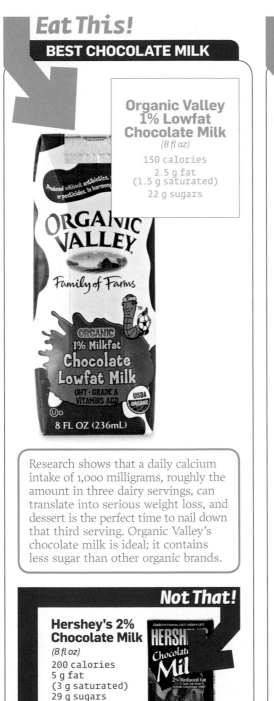

**Organic Valley
1% Lowfat
Chocolate Milk**
(8 fl oz)

150 calories
2.5 g fat
(1.5 g saturated)
22 g sugars

Research shows that a daily calcium intake of 1,000 milligrams, roughly the amount in three dairy servings, can translate into serious weight loss, and dessert is the perfect time to nail down that third serving. Organic Valley's chocolate milk is ideal; it contains less sugar than other organic brands.

Not That!

**Hershey's 2%
Chocolate Milk**
(8 fl oz)
200 calories
5 g fat
(3 g saturated)
29 g sugars

Eat This!

BEST FRUIT BAR

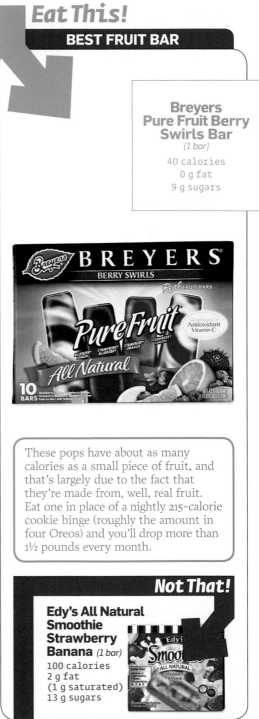

**Breyers
Pure Fruit Berry
Swirls Bar**
(1 bar)

40 calories
0 g fat
9 g sugars

These pops have about as many calories as a small piece of fruit, and that's largely due to the fact that they're made from, well, real fruit. Eat one in place of a nightly 215-calorie cookie binge (roughly the amount in four Oreos) and you'll drop more than 1½ pounds every month.

Not That!

**Edy's All Natural
Smoothie
Strawberry
Banana** *(1 bar)*
100 calories
2 g fat
(1 g saturated)
13 g sugars

BEST COOKIES

Newman-O's Mint Crème Filled Chocolate Cookies *(2)*

130 calories
4.5 g fat
(1.5 g saturated)
10 g sugars

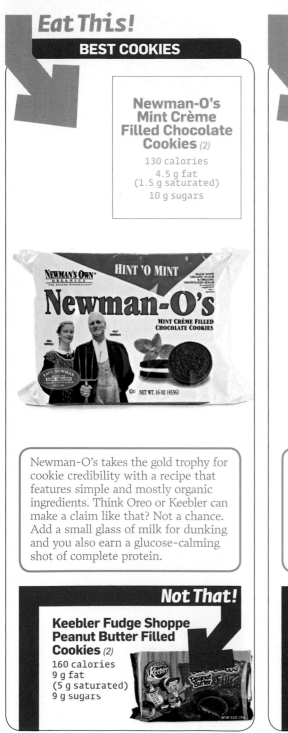

HINT 'O MINT

Newman-O's
MINT CRÈME FILLED
CHOCOLATE COOKIES

NEWMAN'S OWN ORGANICS
The Second Generation

PAUL NEWMAN
$300 MILLION

NET WT. 16 OZ (453G)

Newman-O's takes the gold trophy for cookie credibility with a recipe that features simple and mostly organic ingredients. Think Oreo or Keebler can make a claim like that? Not a chance. Add a small glass of milk for dunking and you also earn a glucose-calming shot of complete protein.

Not That!

Keebler Fudge Shoppe Peanut Butter Filled Cookies *(2)*

160 calories
9 g fat
(5 g saturated)
9 g sugars

NET WT. 9.5 OZ (269G)

Eat This!

BEST BROWNIE

No Pudge! Fat Free Original Fudge Brownie Mix

(¹⁄₁₂ package, prepared with ²⁄₃ cup fat-free vanilla yogurt)

110 calories
0 g fat
22 g sugars

Fat Free

No Pudge!

Fudge Brownie

Original

Single Serving in a Minute

serving suggestion

Just Add Yogurt

Net Wt. 13.7 OZ (388g)

Where most brownie mixes are prepared using cheap oils, No Pudge! brownies get their body from fat-free yogurt. The result is rich and chocolatey with about half as many calories as other low-cal brownies. Make it even tastier (and healthier!) by tossing chopped nuts into the batter.

Not That!

Betty Crocker Low-Fat Fudge Brownie Mix

(¹⁄₈ package, prepared)

140 calories
2 g fat
(0.5 g saturated)
20 g sugars

Low-Fat Fudge Brownie

Eat This!

BEST PUDDING

**Snack Pack
Sugar Free
Vanilla Pudding**
(1 container)
60 calories
3 g fat (1.5 g saturated)
0 g sugars

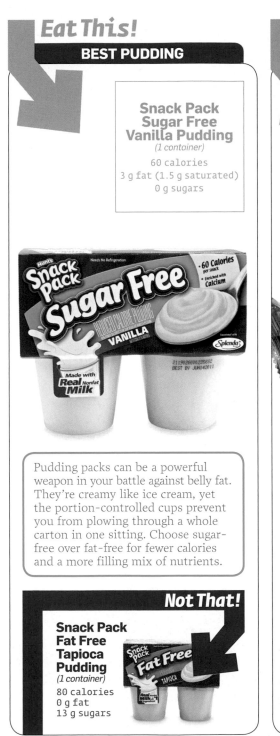

Pudding packs can be a powerful weapon in your battle against belly fat. They're creamy like ice cream, yet the portion-controlled cups prevent you from plowing through a whole carton in one sitting. Choose sugar-free over fat-free for fewer calories and a more filling mix of nutrients.

Not That!

**Snack Pack
Fat Free
Tapioca
Pudding**
(1 container)
80 calories
0 g fat
13 g sugars

Eat This!

BEST ON-THE-GO TREAT

**Rice Krispies
Treats
Strawberry**
(1 bar)
90 calories
2 g fat (0.5 g saturated)
8 g sugars

We've yet to discover a more indulgent bar with fewer grams of sugar. Granted, it consists of little more than fast-digesting carbohydrates, but if you eat it on the heels of a protein- or fiber-rich dinner, your body will have no trouble holding your blood sugar in a healthy range.

Not That!

**Honey Nut
Cheerios
Milk 'n Cereal
Bar** *(1 bar)*
160 calories
4 g fat
(2 g saturated)
14 g sugars

Chocolate Chip Cookies

190 calories
8 g fat (5 g saturated)
28 g carbohydrates
16 g sugars

No applesauce, protein powder, or Splenda—just good, honest, truly delicious chocolate chip cookies.

You'll Need:

8 tablespoons butter (1 stick), softened

½ cup packed brown sugar

½ cup granulated sugar

2 eggs

1 tsp vanilla extract

½ tsp baking soda

½ tsp salt

2 cups flour

½ cup dark chocolate chips

Sea salt flakes (optional)

How to Make It:

• Preheat the oven to 375°F.

• In a mixing bowl, thoroughly mix the butter, brown sugar, and granulated sugar until creamy. Stir in eggs and vanilla until well incorporated. Add the baking soda, salt, and flour and mix until the dough comes together, being careful not to overmix. Stir in the chocolate chips.

• Drop the dough onto a baking sheet in balls of about 3 tablespoons in size, leaving at least 3 inches between cookies.

• Bake until the edges are golden and the middles are just barely set. Remove from the sheet, sprinkle with a bit of sea salt (if using), and cool on a wire rack.

Makes about 12 cookies

Not That!

Atlanta Bread Company Chocolate Chunk Cookie

430 calories
21 g fat (10 g saturated)
58 g carbohydrates
35 g sugars

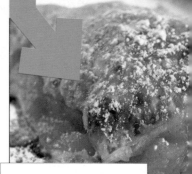

Crispy Apple Turnovers

200 calories
8 g fat (1 g saturated)
32 g carbohydrates
20 g sugars

You'll Need:

Flour

1 sheet puff pastry, defrosted

1 cup water

½ cup sugar

3 Granny Smith apples

¼ tsp ground cinnamon

⅛ tsp ground ginger

⅛ tsp ground nutmeg

Juice of 1 lemon

1 egg white, lightly beaten

How to Make It:

• Flour a work surface. Roll the puff pastry into a 9" x 15" rectangle. Cut the pastry into six equal squares.

Cheesecake Factory Warm Apple Crisp

1,420 calories
29 g saturated fat
193 g carbohydrates

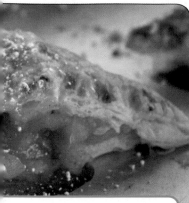

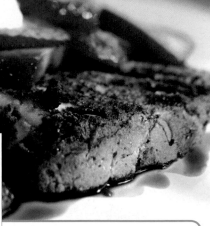

Eat This!

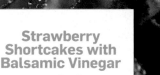

American as it may be, the caloric price of apple pie can be a steep one to pay. We've cut calories dramatically by packing all the appley goodness in a warm handheld vessel.

Strawberry Shortcakes with Balsamic Vinegar

160 calories
6 g fat (3.5 g saturated)
22 g carbohydrates
12 g sugars

To deliver flavor, restaurants rely on hulking scoops of ice cream, oversized brownies, and floods of molten chocolate. The home cook doesn't need such waist-expanding, palate-blunting effects to make dessert memorable. Here, low-calorie angel food cake picks up the smoke and char of the grill and is topped with strawberries soaked in balsamic vinegar and black pepper, an irresistible combination.

• Bring the water and sugar to a boil in a saucepan. Peel and core the apples; cut them into ½" chunks. Toss with the cinnamon, ginger, nutmeg, and lemon juice, then add to the water and simmer until the liquid thickens, 5 to 7 minutes. Set aside to cool.

• Preheat the oven to 425°F. Spoon 3 tablespoons of apples onto each of the puff pastry squares. Fold the pastry over the filling to make a triangle and seal by pinching the edges.

• Place the turnovers on a baking sheet and brush with the egg white. Bake until crispy and golden brown, 12 to 15 minutes.

Makes 6 servings

You'll Need:

2 cups sliced strawberries

¼ cup balsamic vinegar

Pinch of freshly cracked black pepper

4 wedges angel food cake, each 1" thick at the outside edge

Whipped cream

How to Make It:

• Mix the strawberries, vinegar, and pepper and marinate for 10 to 15 minutes.

• Heat a grill, stovetop grill pan, or nonstick sauté pan until hot. (If using a pan, add ½ tablespoon of butter.) Add the cake slices and cook on both

sides until caramelized and toasted. Transfer them to four dessert plates. Top each with a quarter of the strawberries and their liquid and a spoonful of whipped cream.

Makes 4 servings

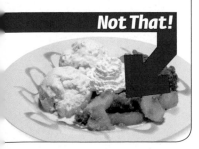

Not That!

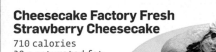

Not That!

Cheesecake Factory Fresh Strawberry Cheesecake

710 calories
30 g saturated fat
66 g carbohydrates

Grilled Apricots

170 calories
7 g fat (2 g saturated)
22.5 g carbohydrates
18 g sugars

Espresso Granitas

170 calories
8 g fat (5 g saturated)
33 g carbohydrates
28 g sugars

In many countries around the world, dessert is often as simple and satisfying as a single piece of perfect fruit. We've followed their lead but gussied it up a bit with yogurt, toasted nuts, and a bit of maple syrup. The result—a warm, cool, and crunchy treat filled with fiber, protein, and healthy fat—is about as good as dessert ever gets. (In fact, this is so healthy, we almost filed it in the breakfast chapter, which you can certainly do.)

A trip to the scoop shop may set you back half a day's worth of calories.

You'll Need:

2 apricots or peaches, halved and pitted

2 cups plain Greek-style yogurt (we like Fage Total 2%)

4 Tbsp chopped toasted walnuts

4 Tbsp maple syrup

The easiest way to toast nuts is to roast them in a dry pan set over medium heat for about 5 minutes, stirring once or twice as they toast.

How to Make It:

• Heat a grill, stovetop grill pan, or broiler until hot. Cook the fruits until nicely caramelized on the outside, about 5 minutes. They should be softened but still maintain their shape. Top each fruit half with ½ cup yogurt, 1 tablespoon walnuts, and 1 table-spoon maple syrup.

Makes 4 servings

You'll Need:

2 cups espresso or very strong brewed coffee, warmed

½ cup sugar

Light whipped topping

½ cup shaved dark chocolate

If you have the time and don't mind the extra 50 calories, fresh whipped cream is best. Beat a cup of heavy cream in a cold metal mixing bowl with a tablespoon of sugar until soft peaks form.

How to Make It:

• Combine the espresso with the sugar and stir until the sugar dissolves. Pour the mix-ture into a shallow metal bak-

Not That!

Cold Stone Creamery Vanilla Bean Ice Cream

with Peach Pie Filling and Walnuts
(Love It size)
720 calories
44 g fat (20 g saturated, 1 g trans)
71 g carbohydrates
59 g sugars

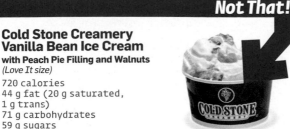

Cold Stone Creamery Coffee Ice Cream

with Chocolate Chips
(Gotta Have It size)
920 calories
54 g fat (34.5 g saturated, 1.5 g trans)
97 g carbohydrates
83 g sugars

Eat This!

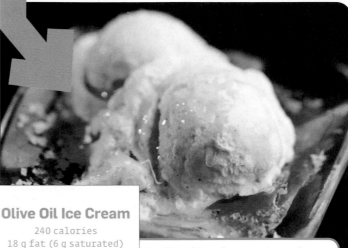

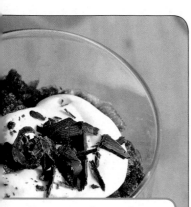

Learn to make granitas, frozen desserts that are every bit as satisfying as ice cream and easy enough for a 6-year-old to make, and you'll never need to go out again.

ing pan and place in the freezer.

• After 20 minutes, just as the mix has begun to freeze, remove the pan from the freezer and use a fork to scrape the ice crystals developing on the surface. Scraping will help you achieve a light, creamy granita rather than a chunky, icy one. Return the pan to the freezer and repeat this step every 30 minutes until the granita is entirely frozen.

• For each serving, place a small scoop of the granita in a chilled wine glass, top with a spoonful of whipped topping and a bit of the chocolate, then repeat with a second layer.

Makes 4 servings

Olive Oil Ice Cream

240 calories
18 g fat (6 g saturated)
20 g carbohydrates
15 g sugars

Studies show that a variety of taste sensations (salty, sweet, spicy) better satisfy the appetite than a single dominant flavor. Maybe that explains why it's so easy to spoon your way mindlessly through a pint of super-sweet Ben & Jerry's. This dish (inspired by Iron Chef Mario Batali and his New York restaurant Babbo) taps into that principle, contrasting the smooth sweetness of vanilla ice cream with the flaky crunch of sea salt and the rich, spicy notes of extra-virgin olive oil. The combination is elegant and strangely addictive—and a small bowl will quash your sweet tooth for less than 300 calories.

You'll Need:

4 large scoops vanilla ice cream (we like Breyers All Natural)

2 Tbsp extra-virgin olive oil

Sea salt flakes

Unsalted cashews (optional)

How to Make It:

• Divide the ice cream among four cold bowls. Drizzle with

the olive oil and a generous pinch of salt. Scatter a handful of cashews (if using) over the top.

Makes 4 servings

Not That!

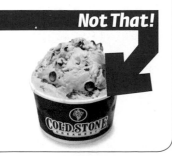

COLD STONE

Not That!

Ben & Jerry's Vanilla Ice Cream
(2 scoops)

380 calories
24 g fat (16 g saturated)
36 g carbohydrates
32 g sugars

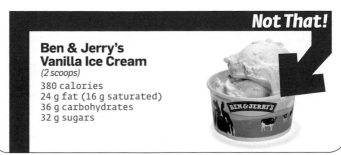

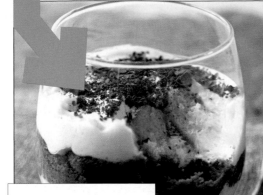

Tiramisu

260 calories
6 g fat (4 g saturated)
31 g carbohydrates
23 g sugars

We've traded egg yolks and mascarpone in favor of egg whites and whipped cream cheese, but you'll never know the difference.

You'll Need:

3 egg whites

¼ cup confectioners' sugar

½ cup whipped cream cheese, softened at room temperature

½ cup espresso (or 1 cup strong coffee)

½ cup coffee liqueur such as Kahlúa

½ package (7 oz) ladyfingers or 4 cups cubed angel food cake

1 oz dark chocolate, finely shaved

Espresso grounds or cocoa powder (optional)

How to Make It:

• Beat the egg whites until they form soft peaks. Add the sugar and lightly beat it into the whites. Place the cream cheese in a large bowl and fold in half of the whipped whites. Once fully incorporated, fold in the remaining whites.

• Combine the espresso and coffee liqueur in a small bowl. Place a layer of ladyfingers (or angel food cake, if using) in the bottom of four wine or martini glasses. Spoon enough of the coffee mixture over them to soak the ladyfingers. Divide the cream cheese mixture among the glasses, then top each with a goodly pile of chocolate shavings. Garnish with a dusting of espresso grounds if you like.

Makes 4 servings

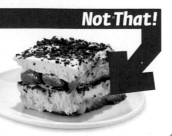

Not That!

Carrabba's Tiramisu

1,140 calories

°Carrabba's refuses to disclose anything beyond calorie counts.

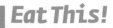

Mango-Chili Paletas

70 calories
0 g fat
17 g carbohydrates
16 g sugars

Beyond the fact that they pack nearly a full serving of fruit for just 70 calories, the best part about these fruit-based frozen treats, called paletas in Mexico, is the fact that you don't need

You'll Need:

1 mango, peeled, pitted, flesh roughly chopped

Juice of 1 lime

2 Tbsp agave syrup or sugar

Pinch of cayenne pepper

How to Make It:

• Place the mango, lime juice, agave syrup, and cayenne in a blender and puree, adding a bit of water if needed to help it.

Good Humor Strawberry Shortcake Bar

230 calories
12 g fat (5 g saturated)
31 g carbohydrates
17 g sugars

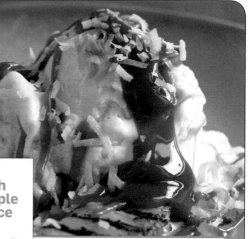

Eat This!

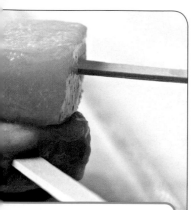

a recipe at all. Any pureed fresh or frozen fruit will do, whether you have a glut of bananas you're looking to get rid of, love blueberries more than your firstborn, or found a deal on honeydew at the supermarket. Just be sure to add a bit of sugar before blending.

Divide the mixture among four frozen pop molds and place them in the freezer for at least 3 hours. (Do not cheat by checking along the way, because the paletas won't freeze properly.) To easily release the paletas from the holders, briefly run warm water over the molds' bottoms.

Makes 4 servings

Sundaes with Grilled Pineapple and Rum Sauce

290 calories
11 g fat (7 g saturated)
42 g carbohydrates
35 g sugars

The banana may be the sundae fruit vessel of choice, but the standard split formula—one banana, three scoops ice cream—is a recipe for disaster. A ring of pineapple, on the other hand, holds one good scoop of ice cream perfectly, and when grilled, provides an irresistible counterpoint to the cold, rich vanilla. Throw in a rum drizzle and it's a serious party.

You'll Need:

4 slices (½" thick) fresh pineapple, cored

1 Tbsp butter

2 Tbsp brown sugar

2 Tbsp dark rum

1 tsp vanilla extract

2 cups vanilla ice cream

2 Tbsp shredded sweetened coconut, toasted

How to Make It:

• Heat a grill, grill pan, or large sauté pan over medium heat (adding a small pat of butter if using a sauté pan). Cook the pineapple rings for 3 to 4 minutes per side, until caramelized all over.

• Combine the butter, brown sugar, rum, and vanilla in a saucepan and cook over low heat, stirring occasionally, until the sugar fully melts and the sauce is a uniform dark brown. Keep it warm.

• Divide the pineapple among four bowls. Top each with a scoop of ice cream, a bit of rum sauce, and toasted coconut.

Makes 4 servings

Not That!

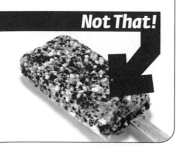

Not That!

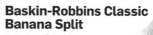

Baskin-Robbins Classic Banana Split

1,010 calories
34 g fat
(20 g saturated, 1 g trans)
173 g carbohydrates
125 g sugars

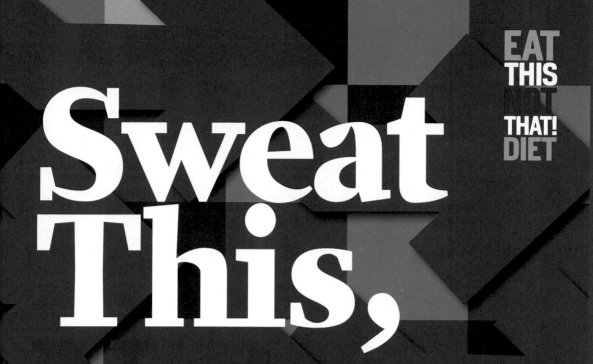

EAT
THIS
NOT
THAT!
DIET

Sweat This, Not That!

NO DIET!

CHAPTER 9

What if we could arrange it so that, starting tomorrow, you could go to the same job, do the same amount of work, and get paid twice as much for it?

Would you be likely to take an interest in such a deal? Or would you say, "Nah, fuggedaboutit, I'm good"?

Okay, well, it doesn't matter, because we can't do that. (We called your boss, but he was a total jerk about it. Go figure!) But we can do something almost as good: We can double the fitness payback you get for the same amount of work you put in on the bike, in the gym, or in your basement. Just as you can eat the same foods, but with fewer calories, by making a few simple swaps, so too can you perform the same exercises but burn more calories—and build more muscle—by swapping out less-effective variations for the top-of-the-line versions. Presto—you've just given yourself a fitness raise, and you didn't even have to ask your boss!

The World's Simplest, Most Effective Workout Ever!

This workout utilizes the latest research on resistance training to help you burn the most fat in the least amount of time possible. But first, you might be wondering: What is "resistance training," and how does it help you lose weight?

A) It's a boot camp program for guerillas—battling the occupying forces of socialism/fascism/capitalism/whaterism burns a ton of calories!

B) It's a sensory-deprivation plan that trains you to resist your favorite foods. They duct tape you to a chair with a Camelback of vegetable juice and make you watch an endless loop of Guy Fieri eating doughnuts.

C) It's a reverse-psychology trick in which you try to get a resistant 2-year-old to eat her vegetables, after which you're just too emotionally drained to eat anything yourself.

D) It's . . . something else.

It is something else. In fact, once you give it a try, you'll agree: Wow, this is something else! "Resistance training" is simply another term for weight-lifting, and it's just about the most surefire way to burn away fat, and keep it off forever. Not only will the workout itself burn calories, but, by putting your body into muscle-building mode, it will keep you burning additional calories for, literally, days afterward. And you don't need to spend hours in a gym—or any time at all in a gym, really—to make it work for you.

Turns out, just 15 minutes of resistance training can help flatten your belly, according to a study from Southern Illinois University at Edwardsville. Why? Because that's all it takes to turn on the hormones that rev up your metabolism. Use this super-simple, total-body workout to do just that. All you need is a light pair of dumbbells to burn calories, tone your muscles, and turn your body into a fat-burning machine.

HOW TO DO IT: Perform this workout as a circuit, completing the prescribed number of repetitions of each exercise without resting. Once you've done each exercise once, catch your breath, then repeat the entire circuit once or twice more. Try to do it 3 times a week—heck, that's still under an hour of exercise a week—which will help you keep your fat-burning furnace stoked 24 hours a day (even while you sleep).

Exercise 1:
Bodyweight Squat

What you'll work:
Your hips, thighs, calves, and abs

- Stand with your feet spread slightly wider than shoulder-width apart, and hold your arms straight out in front of your body at shoulder level.
- Then push your hips back, bend your knees, and lower your body as far as you can.
- Do 15 to 20 repetitions.

Exercise 2:
Incline Pushup

What you'll work:
Your chest, shoulders, arms, and abs

- Do a pushup, but with your hands on a raised surface—such as a bench, ottoman, or one of the steps of your stairs—instead of the floor.
- Simply bend your elbows and lower your body until your chest almost touches the surface of the bench. (The higher the surface on which you place your hands, the easier the exercise becomes—you can even lean against a wall if you need to.) If the incline pushup is too easy, do it the old-fashioned way, with your hands on the floor.
- Do 12 to 15 repetitions.

Exercise 3:
Reverse Lunge

What you'll work:
Your butt and thighs

- Grab a pair of dumbbells and stand with your feet shoulder-width apart.
- Now take a step back with your right leg and then lower your body until your front knee is bent at least 90 degrees.
- Push back to the start. That's 1 rep.
- Repeat by stepping back with your left leg, and alternate back and forth until you've done 16 to 20 repetitions.

Exercise 4:
Mountain Climber

What you'll work:
Your abs and lower back

- Assume a pushup position with your arms completely straight.
- Tighten your abs then slowly lift your left foot off the floor and raise your knee toward your chest (without allowing your lower back to round).
- Reverse the movement, and repeat with the other leg.
- Alternate back and forth for 30 to 60 seconds.

Exercise 5:
Dumbbell Row

What you'll work:
Your back and rear shoulders

- Grab a pair of dumbbells and bend at your hips and knees until your torso is almost parallel to the floor.
- Let your arms hang straight down from your shoulders.
- Without allowing your lower back to round, bend your elbows and pull the dumbbells to the sides of your torso.
- Pause, lower and repeat.
- Do 12 to 15 repetitions.

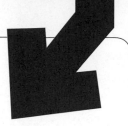

Sweat This!

Not That!

To torch the most calories...

**20 minutes on
the rowing machine**

**20 minutes on any
other cardio machine**

Rowing burns the most calories and works the most muscles, including
muscles in your back, and also improves posture. (Bump it up a notch:
In a Brazilian study, outdoor rowers burned 26 percent more calories during
a race than those on indoor rowing ergometers did.)

To build abs that show...

**The plank
for 1 minute**

**Roman chair
situps for 1 minute**

The crunching motion of a Roman chair situp puts stress on the lower back. (In general,
avoid machines and added weights when doing ab exercises, and focus on form.) The plank
is a body-weight exercise that works the abs and hip flexors, the glutes and lats. To do it,
get into a pushup position, but with your hands together and your weight resting on your
forearms, not your palms. Keeping your back straight, tighten your abs as though you are
about to be punched in the belly. Hold this position for 1 minute.

To build more muscle while weight-training...

**Compound exercises
(bench press, seated
row, squat, deadlift)**

**Isolation exercises
(chest flies, bicep curls,
calf raises, wrist curls)**

Isolation exercises focus on one muscle at a time, whereas compound exercises
engage multiple muscles with one exercise. The more muscle mass you call into play
with each exercise, the more human growth hormone your body unleashes, and the
bigger every muscle in your body will grow. The fastest way to build bigger biceps,
for example, is to do an exercise like the seated row that works not only the biceps, but
also the upper and lower back muscles. (You can always do a single-muscle exercise
afterward for added emphasis. But do the compound exercises first.)

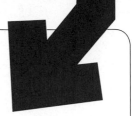

Sweat This!   Not That!

To burn more fat while weight-training...

**Higher weight,
fewer reps**   **Lower weight,
more reps**

The heavier you lift, the bigger the calorie burn. In one study, lifters torched nearly twice as many calories in the 2 hours after their workouts when they lifted 85 percent of their max load for 8 reps than when they did 15 reps at only 45 percent of their max.

To burn more fat while doing cardio...

**Short, high-intensity
cardio bursts**   **Steady-state
cardio**

In one Australian study, volunteers rode a stationary bike for either 40 minutes at a steady pace or 20 minutes of intervals, alternating 8 seconds of sprints with 12 seconds of easy pedaling. After 15 weeks, the sprinters had lost three times as much body fat—including thigh and core flab. Bursts of speed may stimulate a fat-burning response within the muscles, says lead researcher Ethlyn Gail Trapp, PhD.

To burn more fat while running...

Run outdoors   **Run on a treadmill**

Propelling yourself on land is more challenging than on an indoor treadmill, and it trains you better. In a Utah State study, habitual outdoor runners completed a 5K run 4 minutes faster than treadmill runners.

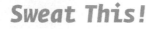

Sweat This!   ## Not That!

When you want to run indoors...

**30 minutes on
an elliptical machine**

**30 minutes
on a treadmill**

The elliptical burns the same number of calories, but puts less stress on your knees, shins, and ankles, according to researchers at the University of Mississippi.

If you absolutely insist upon the treadmill...

**Walk 3 mph on
a treadmill set at a
15 percent incline**

**Run 7 mph on
a treadmill set at a
0 percent incline**

Walking uphill on a treadmill is as challenging but easier on your knees than joint-pounding jogging, according to a study from A.T. Still University. Whenever you use a treadmill, use at least a slight incline—when your treadmill is set at zero, the belt is helping you move, and that means you're actually burning fewer calories than if you just went for a walk outside.

To maximize your exercise gains...

Find a workout buddy

Go solo

People exercise for an average of 34 minutes longer with a friend than they do alone, according to the American College of Sports Medicine.

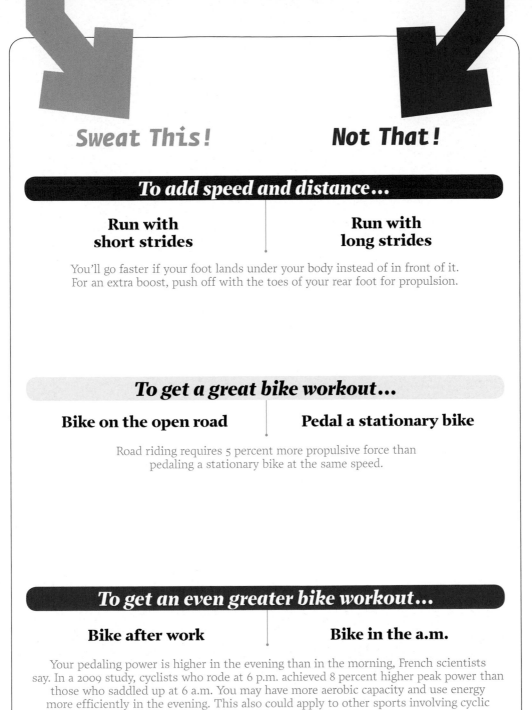

Sweat This!   Not That!

To add speed and distance...

**Run with
short strides**

**Run with
long strides**

You'll go faster if your foot lands under your body instead of in front of it.
For an extra boost, push off with the toes of your rear foot for propulsion.

To get a great bike workout...

Bike on the open road

Pedal a stationary bike

Road riding requires 5 percent more propulsive force than
pedaling a stationary bike at the same speed.

To get an even greater bike workout...

Bike after work

Bike in the a.m.

Your pedaling power is higher in the evening than in the morning, French scientists
say. In a 2009 study, cyclists who rode at 6 p.m. achieved 8 percent higher peak power than
those who saddled up at 6 a.m. You may have more aerobic capacity and use energy
more efficiently in the evening. This also could apply to other sports involving cyclic
patterns, such as swimming, running, and kayaking.

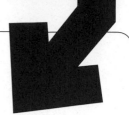

Sweat This!   ## Not That!

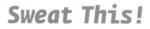

To burn an extra 840 calories in one round of golf...

**Carry your
own clubs**

Use a golf cart

Carrying your clubs burns 483 calories an hour, while golfing using a cart burns only 273 calories for a 175-pound man. In one study, guys walked an average of 4.6 miles during one round of golf. Carry your own clubs for 18 holes once a week and you'll burn off enough calories to lose 12.5 pounds of fat this year.

To lose weight in the water...

Swim freestyle

**Do the butterfly,
backstroke, or
breaststroke**

Butterfly is harder, but freestyle is the stroke recreational swimmers can execute for the longest with the most intensity, according to Emmett Hines, head coach of H₂Ouston Swims. "Unless you're a really adept and efficient swimmer, you'll lack the skills to swim the other strokes at a high enough level to get a good workout." Freestyle also works the largest amount of muscle mass while improving aerobic fitness.

To feel less tired during exercise...

**Rock out
with your iPod**

Sweat in silence

Your overall endurance improves by 15 percent when you exercise to music, according to a study in the *Journal of Sport and Exercise Psychology*.

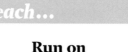

Sweat This!   ## Not That!

To burn fat on the beach...

Run on sand

Run on the boardwalk

Sand running is easier on the joints, builds more muscle, improves balance, and burns 60 percent more calories than running on a hard surface.

To burn fat while in the bedroom...

Have sex

Fool around

Intercourse burns three times as many calories as foreplay.

To burn fat while scoring brownie points...

Shovel snow

Go snowmobiling

Shoveling snow for 30 minutes burns nearly twice as many calories.

8 Exercise Machines You Must Avoid

Here's a secret the guys down at your fancy-pants gym will never tell you: No matter how cool, shiny, and high tech their weight machines may be, you are almost always going to get a better workout if you avoid them. And not just because of the sweaty fat guy who used the shoulder press before you and forgot to wipe it off.

First, studies show that you simply get a better workout using free weights. Take, for instance, the seated leg extension machine. University of Kentucky researchers studied 23 patients with knee pain to see which made them stronger—using a simple set of stairs or using one of these machines. They found that in every measure of leg strength, simple stepups using a flight of stairs built strength more effectively. The leg extension machine didn't make test subjects stronger at any tasks, except one: using the leg extension machine. It did nothing for how test subjects functioned in the real world. Another study, in the *Journal of*

SEATED LEG EXTENSION

What it's supposed to do: Train the quadriceps
What it actually does: It strengthens a motion your legs aren't actually designed to do, and can put undue strain on the ligaments and tendons surrounding the kneecaps.
A better exercise: One-legged body-weight squats. Lift one leg up in front of you and bend the opposite knee, dipping as far as you can with control by flexing at the hip, knee, and ankle. Use a rail for support until you develop the requisite leg strength and balance. Aim for 5 to 10 reps on each leg. (If you are susceptible to knee pain, do the Bulgarian split squat instead, resting the top of one foot on a bench positioned 2 to 3 feet behind you. Descend until the thigh of the other leg is parallel to the ground and then raise yourself back up. Do 5 to 10 reps per leg.)

SEATED MILITARY PRESS

What it's supposed to do: Train the shoulders and triceps
What it actually does: Overhead pressing can put shoulder joints in vulnerable biomechanical positions. It puts undue stress on the shoulders, and the movement doesn't let you use your hips to assist your shoulders, which is the natural way to push something overhead.
A better exercise: Medicine-ball throws. Stand 3 feet from a concrete wall. Bounce a rubber medicine ball off a spot on the wall 4 feet above your head, squatting to catch the ball and rising to throw it upward in one continuous motion. Aim for 15 to 20 reps.
Alternative: Standing alternate dumbbell presses. As you push the right dumbbell overhead, shift the right hip forward. Switch to the left side.

SEATED LAT PULL-DOWN

(BEHIND THE NECK)
What it's supposed to do: Train the lats, upper back, and biceps
What it actually does: Unless you have very flexible shoulders, it's difficult to do correctly, so it can cause pinching in the shoulder joint and damage the rotator cuff.
A better exercise: Incline pullups. Place a bar in the squat rack at waist height, grab the bar with both hands, and hang from the bar with your feet stretched out in front of you. Keep your torso stiff, and pull your chest to the bar 10 to 15 times. To make it harder, lower the bar; to make it easier, raise the bar.

SEATED PEC DECK

What it's supposed to do: Train the chest and shoulders
What it actually does: It can put the shoulder in an unstable position and place excessive stress on the shoulder joint and its connective tissues.
A better exercise: Incline pushups. Do a regular pushup, but instead of putting your hands on the floor, put them on a higher surface, like an exercise bench or step box. Aim for 15 to 20 reps. If this is too easy, progress to regular pushups and plyometric pushups (where you push up with enough force that your hands come off the floor), and aim for 5 to 8 reps.

Strength and Conditioning Research, found that men who did squats using free weights activated 43 percent more muscle than men performing squats on the Smith machine.

Second, machines may seem safer, but they can lead to injury, because they lock our bodies into planes of movement that aren't natural. For example, when you walk or climb a set of stairs or squat with a light weight, your thighbone rotates under your kneecap—the normal movement of your lower body. But on a leg extension machine, your kneecap rotates instead. That puts a lot of strain on the knee ligaments, patella, and the soft padding under the kneecap.

So if exercise machines are both ineffective and dangerous, why are gyms so packed with them? Simple: because they want you to think you can't get a great workout without all that fancy equipment, so you'll have to keep coming back to their sweat palaces! So before your next workout, take note of some equipment that's worth skipping altogether.

SEATED HIP ABDUCTOR MACHINE

What it's supposed to do: Train the outer thighs

What it actually does: Because you are seated, it trains a movement that has no functional use. If it's done with excessive weight and jerky technique, it can put undue pressure on the spine.

A better exercise: Place a heavy, short, looped resistance band around your legs at ankle height. Sidestep out 20 paces and back with control. This is much harder than it sounds.

SEATED LEG PRESS

What it's supposed to do: Train the quadriceps, glutes, and hamstrings

What it actually does: It often forces the spine to flex without engaging any of the necessary stabilization muscles in the hips, glutes, shoulders, and lower back.

A better exercise: Body-weight squats. Start at a standing position with either your arms out in front of you or your hands resting on your hips. Then bend slowly to a sitting position—the backs of your legs should form 90-degree angles. Focus on descending with control as far as you can without rounding your lower back. Aim for 15 to 20 for a set, and increase the number of sets as you develop strength.

SQUATS USING THE SMITH MACHINE

What it's supposed to do: Train the chest, biceps, and legs

What it actually does: The alignment of the machine—the bar is attached to a vertical sliding track—makes for linear, not natural, arched movements. This puts stress on the knees, shoulders, and lower back.

A better exercise: Body-weight squats. See "seated leg press" to the left.

ROMAN CHAIR BACK EXTENSION

What it's supposed to do: Train the spinal erectors

What it actually does: Repeatedly flexing the back while it's supporting weight places pressure on the spine and increases the risk of damaging your disks.

A better exercise: The bird dog. Crouch on all fours, extend your right arm forward, and extend your left leg backward. Hold for 7 seconds. Do 10 reps, and then switch to the opposite side.

The World's Most Dangerous Activity

IT'S NOT CAVE DIVING, IT'S NOT SWIMMING WITH SHARKS, IT'S NOT DATING LADY GAGA. IT'S SOMETHING YOU DO EVERY SINGLE DAY, OFTEN FOR HOURS AT A TIME, AND CHANCES ARE, YOU'RE DOING IT RIGHT NOW.

When someone delivers shocking news, they normally preface it with a warning: "You'd better sit down for this." In this case, let us tweak that advice:

You'd better stand up for this.

Why? Because new research shows that the more time you spend sitting on your tuckus, the sooner you're going to die.

In 2009, researchers at Pennington Biomedical Research Center, in Baton Rouge, Louisiana, studied the lifestyle habits of more than 17,000 men and women and found that the people who sat for most of the day were 54 percent more likely to end up clutching their chests than those who spent little time sitting.

That's no surprise, of course; spending all your time on your ass is the very definition of "sedentary." Except for one creepy additional finding: It didn't matter how much the sitters weighed, how fit they were, or how often they exercised. Lean, healthy, salad-bar-for-lunch, 4-times-a-week-at-the-gym types were just as likely to die of heart attacks as overweight, burger-snarfing, exercise-averse folks. Diet and exercise didn't

matter. What mattered was: How much do you sit?

Like we said, you'd better stand up for this.

Rubik's Cubicle

For a lot of Americans, getting an office job with a comfy desk chair is a sign that you've finally made it. Instead of spending your days walking the floor (like a waiter or a salesperson), digging in the dirt (like a landscaper or a roadworker), or tiptoeing across rooftops (like an HVAC installer or a building inspector or the Tooth Fairy), a coveted cubicle position means being able to relax for 8 hours a day. But it's a trap! Indeed, those of us whose jobs involve sitting—for example, guys who write books—have to puzzle out ways to spend less time doing so. Otherwise, we've got trouble. Because once you land a fancy desk job, even joining a fancy gym isn't going to save you.

Consider this: In a 2007 report, University of Missouri scientists said that the people with the highest levels of nonexercise activity—meaning people who just did things like walk-ing, digging, and tiptoeing across rooftops (but little to no so-called "exercise")—burned significantly more calories in a week than those who ran 35 miles a week but otherwise spent their time sitting. "It can be as simple as standing more," says Peter Katzmarzyk, PhD, a researcher at Pennington. For instance, a "standing" worker—say, a salesclerk—burns about 1,500 calories while on the job; a person behind a desk might expend only 1,000 calories. That's 500 calories a day, 5 days a week. It goes a long way toward explaining why people who get "promoted" to a cubicle gain 16 pounds, on average, within 8 months of starting sedentary office work, according to a study from the University of North Carolina at Wilmington.

Sixteen pounds in 8 months? Holy ham hocks!

That increase in weight and inactivity can result in a whole Chinese menu of trouble. Along with your promotion to a desk job you get:

A big, brand-new...belly!

In another study, researchers found that obese people remain seated for an average of 2 hours longer every day than skinny people do. As if the sudden and massive weight gain weren't enough, sitting all day will actually make you look fatter than you really are. That's because weak glutes, or butt muscles, as well as tight hip flexors (the muscles that connect your hips to the fronts of your thighs) cause your pelvis to tilt forward. This puts stress on your lumbar spine, resulting in lower-back pain. It also pushes your belly out, which gives you a protruding gut even if you don't have an ounce of fat. "The changes to your muscles and posture from sitting are so small that you won't notice them at first. But as you reach your 30s, 40s, 50s, and beyond, they'll gradually become worse," says Bill Hartman, PT, CSCS, a physical therapist and co-owner of Indianapolis Fitness and Sports Training. "And a lot harder to fix."

The keys to the executive coronary ward!

As we said above, research now shows that people who land desk jobs are 54 percent more likely to die of heart disease. According to Pennington researchers, the gene that's associated with heart disease simply doesn't respond to exercise, no matter how hard or how often you work out. (That's why famous athletes still die of heart attacks.) What it does respond to, in a negative way, is what researchers call "lack of contractile activity in your muscles." In other words, sitting and not moving. The more time you spend on your feet, the lower your heart disease risk, period.

Fast-tracked on the diabetes promotion plan!

A 2010 study in the *Journal of Applied Physiology* found that when healthy individuals limited the number of footsteps they took by 85 percent for 2 weeks, they experienced an average 17 percent decrease in insulin sensitivity, raising their diabetes risk. That's right: Just 2 weeks after your promotion to desk jockey, your blood sugar has risen significantly!

Declining jumping, running, and "having fun" skills!

"Your body adapts to what you do most often," says Hartman. "So if you sit in a chair all day, you'll essentially become better adapted to sitting in a chair." The trouble is, that makes you less adept at standing, walking, running, and jumping, all of which a truly healthy human should be able to do with proficiency. "Older folks have a harder time moving around than younger people do," says Hartman. "That's not simply because of age; it's because what you do consistently from day to day manifests itself over time, for both good and bad."

A shorter life—and you!

If you sit all day, you're courting muscle stiffness; poor balance and mobility; and lower-back, neck, and hip pain. This is because although fascia, the tough connective tissue that covers your muscles, is pliable, it tends to "set" in the position your muscles are in most often. Now think about where your hips and thighs are in relation to your torso while you're sitting. They're bent, which causes the muscles on the fronts of your thighs, known as hip flexors, to contract slightly, or shorten. The more you sit, the more the fascia will keep your hip flexors shortened. "If you've ever seen a guy walk with a forward lean, it's often because of shortened hip flexors," says Hartman. "The muscles don't stretch as they naturally should. As a result, he's not walking tall and straight because his fascia has adapted more to sitting than standing."

How to Solve The Puzzle

So, you've just been offered the job of your dreams (okay, let's be honest, a job, period). The only catch: your workspace looks an awful lot like Dwight Schrute's. How do you make sure your own personal Dunder Mifflin doesn't turn from a 40-hour-a-week gig into a ride in an extra-wide hearse?

Well, do what we do, and use this neat trick. Actually, it's a NEAT trick: "NEAT" stands for "non-exercise activity thermogenesis." Translated into words that make sense, it means stuff that burns calories when you're not intentionally trying to burn calories (by, say, hitting the weight room, sweating on a stairclimber, or training for a marathon). And as we said above, the real key to keeping weight off and reducing your risk of heart disease, diabetes, and all those other curses of modern life isn't going to the gym—it's simply spending less time in the dreaded Comfy Chair.

Goose yourself.

Write a sticky note and tack it above your desk. It should say, "Stand Up!"

Whenever you see it, stand up. On the phone? Stand up! Digging through the chaos of your files? Stand up! Googling your ex, whom you should really stop obsessing about, but you just know that he/she will come to his/her senses and soon be crawling back like a dog, at which point you'll just scoff—ha ha!—and be on your merry way? Stand up!

Consider a stand-up desk.

Several companies now sell them (one even makes a desk with a treadmill attached!). While it might seem odd at first, remember, Hemingway wrote entire books standing up. (He also drank too much and shot himself in the head, so make sure your emulation has limits, okay?)

Walk whenever, wherever.

When scientists at the Mayo Clinic studied how people burn calories, they discovered that the leanest folks burned 350 more calories every day than the heaviest ones (that's enough to lose, or gain, a pound of fat every 10 days!). But the scientists didn't look at what people did for exercise, only at what they did when they weren't exercising. A pound of flab gone every 10 days, without exercise! The researchers got so freaked out by these results that they started a new tradition: the "walking meeting." Whenever the team at the Mayo Clinic needs to compare notes, they do it while walking the halls instead of sitting in a conference room. Your takeaway: Never e-mail or call when you can walk down the hall. Never drive someplace you can walk to. Don't give up your seat just to little old ladies, give it up to everybody. If you can get there under your own power, do it. It will change everything.

Reward yourself with chores.
Maybe it goes back to Tom Sawyer tricking his little friends into painting his fence for him, but Americans are hardwired to think that getting out of

doing chores is a win. Wrong. If you can sweep the floor, vacuum the rug, do the dishes by hand, or tend the garden yourself instead of getting someone else to do it, then you're ahead of the game. In one study, people who burned 150 calories a day doing chores (that's about half an hour of raking leaves, 18 minutes of shoveling snow, or 24 minutes of puttering around the garden or painting Tom Sawyer's fence) reduced their blood pressure by an average of 13 points after just 2 days.

FINAL VERDICT:
Every moment you spend on your feet is helping you stay slim. Every moment you spend on your butt is helping you grow fat.

And that's the bottom line on your bottom line.

The Best Sources for 14 Vital Vitamins and Minerals

Sure you could just pop a multivitamin pill every day, but research shows that there is no better way to absorb the essential nutrients your body needs than by seeking them out from the fresh food sources that feature them most prominently. Here's a cheat sheet for some of the biggest nutritional players along with the recommended daily allowance (RDA) that you should consume every day.

VITAMIN A - *men: 900 mcg; women: 700 mcg*

What it is: A pale yellow crystalline compound also known as retinol.

Why you need it: It preserves and improves your eyesight as well as fights viral infections.

		SERVING SIZE	CALORIES	VITAMIN A
1.	Baked sweet potato	1 large	162	1,096
2.	Carrots	2 medium	50	1,019
3.	Cooked spinach	1 cup	41	943
4.	Baked winter squash	1 cup	76	877
5.	Cooked collard greens	1 cup	49	771
6.	Cooked greens	1 cup	28	549
7.	Romaine lettuce	2 cups	16	410
8.	Cantaloupe	1 cup	56	299
9.	Cooked broccoli	1 cup	55	120
10.	Cooked green peas	1 cup	134	64

VITAMIN B₁ - men: 1.2 mg; women: 1.1 mg

What it is: Also known as thiamin. Helps cells' enzyme systems convert oxygen into usable energy.

Why you need it: Maintains your energy, coordinates nerve and muscle activity, and keeps your heart healthy.

		SERVING SIZE	CALORIES	VITAMIN B₁
1.	Pork loin	3 oz	196	0.54
2.	Sunflower seeds	¼ cup	205	0.52
3.	Cooked black beans	1 cup	227	0.42
4.	Raw macadamia nuts	¼ cup	241	0.4
5.	Cooked asparagus	1 cup	43	0.29
6.	Sesame seeds	¼ cup	206	0.29
7.	Ground flaxseed	2 Tbsp	75	0.23
8.	Oatmeal	1 cup	145	0.18
9.	Cooked yellowfin tuna	4 oz	157	0.15
10.	Cooked corn	1 cup	177	0.14

VITAMIN B₆ - men/women: 1.3 mg

What it is: A vitamin involved in more than 100 enzyme reactions throughout the body.

Why you need it: Helps your nervous system, promotes proper breakdown of starch and sugar, and prevents amino acid buildup in your blood.

		SERVING SIZE	CALORIES	VITAMIN B₆
1.	Roasted chicken breast	4 oz	223	0.64
2.	Baked potato	1 medium	161	0.61
3.	Roasted turkey breast	4 oz	214	0.47
4.	Banana	1	108	0.43
5.	Garlic	1 oz	42	0.35
6.	Raw red pepper	1 cup	24	0.29
7.	Shelled pistachios	¼ cup	173	0.27
8.	Avocado	½ fruit	161	0.26
9.	Cooked cauliflower	1 cup	28	0.16
10.	Cooked cod	4 oz	120	0.15

VITAMIN D - *men/women: 15 mcg*

What it is: A vitamin present in just a few foods, but added to others. It's also produced when UV rays hit the skin.

Why you need it: Essential to calcium absorption—without it, bones become brittle. Also helps reduce inflammation.

		SERVING SIZE	CALORIES	VITAMIN D
1.	Cooked salmon	3 oz	121	11
2.	Cooked mackerel	3 oz	171	9.7
3.	Cooked halibut	3 oz	95	4.9
4.	Cooked shrimp	4 oz	112	4.1
5.	Vitamin D-fortified milk (reduced fat)	1 cup	125	2.5
6.	Canned sardines	½ can	96	2.2
7.	Cooked cod	4 oz	120	1.4
8.	Vitamin D-fortified cereal	1 cup	105	1.3
9.	Egg	1 medium	63	0.9
10.	Portabello mushrooms	1 cup	35	0.4

VITAMIN B$_{12}$ - *men/women: 2.4 mcg*

What it is: A vitamin formed by microorganisms like bacteria and yeast (and found in the various animals that ingest them).

Why you need it: Assists in processing protein and developing blood and nerve cells.

		SERVING SIZE	CALORIES	VITAMIN B$_{12}$
1.	Calf liver	3 oz	119	50.9
2.	Duck liver	3 oz	114	45.9
3.	Clams	3 oz	73	9.6
4.	Oysters	6	61	7.3
5.	Rainbow trout	3 oz	130	3.7
6.	Fat-free yogurt	1 cup	137	1.5
7.	Top sirloin	3 oz	160	1.5
8.	Low-fat milk	1 cup	121	1.1
9.	Swiss cheese	1 oz	108	0.95
10.	Lean cured ham	3 oz	130	0.6

FOLATE - *men/women: 400 mcg*

What it is: Also known as folic acid, a chemically complex vitamin that requires enzymes in the intestine to aid in its absorption.

Why you need it: Aids fetal development in pregnancy, prevents anemia, helps skin cells grow, aids nervous system function, prevents bone fractures, and lowers risk of dementia.

		SERVING SIZE	CALORIES	FOLATE
1.	Cooked lentils	1 cup	230	358
2.	Cooked navy beans	1 cup	258	255
3.	Cooked beets	1 cup	74	136
4.	Cooked split peas	1 cup	231	127
5.	Mustard greens	1 cup	21	102
6.	Papaya	1	118	99
7.	Enriched pasta noodles	¼ cup	212	98
8.	Raw peanuts	¼ cup	207	88
9.	Cooked quinoa	1 cup	222	78
10.	Orange	1	61	39

VITAMIN C - *men: 90 mg; women: 75 mg*

What it is: Also known as ascorbic acid, a water-soluble nutrient and antioxidant.

Why you need it: Regenerates vitamin E supplies and improves iron absorption. Plus it helps protect us from colds and infections, cardiovascular disease, cancer, and cataracts.

		SERVING SIZE	CALORIES	VITAMIN C
1.	Steamed broccoli	1 cup	55	101
2.	Strawberries	1 cup	43	85
3.	Pineapple	1 cup	76	79
4.	Cooked brussels sprouts	1 cup	60	71
5.	Orange	1	61	70
6.	Kiwi	1	46	64
7.	Cantaloupe	1 cup	56	59
8.	Grapefruit	½ fruit	36	44
9.	Cooked winter squash	1 cup	76	16
10.	Blueberries	1 cup	81	14

VITAMIN E - *men/women: 15 mg*

What it is: A group of fat-soluble vitamins found throughout the body.

Why you need it: Protects your skin from ultraviolet rays and lowers risk of prostate cancer and Alzheimer's disease.

		SERVING SIZE	CALORIES	VITAMIN E
1.	Sunflower seeds	¼ cup	205	12.3
2.	Roasted almonds	¼ cup	206	8.2
3.	Cooked spinach	1 cup	41	3.7
4.	Sweet potato chips	1 oz	139	2.8
5.	Olives	1 cup	154	2.3
6.	Peanut butter	2 Tbsp	190	2
7.	Cooked pinto beans	1 cup	235	1.6
8.	Cooked quinoa	1 cup	222	1.2
9.	Canned sardines	½ can	96	0.94
10.	Blueberries	1 cup	81	0.84

CALCIUM - *men/women: 1,000 mg*

What it is: A mineral found in bones and teeth.

Why you need it: It keeps your bones strong and healthy, promotes the efficient function of nerves and muscle fibers, and helps your blood clot.

		SERVING SIZE	CALORIES	CALCIUM
1.	Sesame seeds	¼ cup	206	351
2.	Low-fat yogurt	8 oz	155	345
3.	Calcium-fortified soy milk	1 cup	105	299
4.	2% milk	1 cup	121	293
5.	Cooked spinach	1 cup	41	245
6.	Tofu	4 oz	86	229
7.	Part-skim mozzarella cheese	1 oz	72	222
8.	Cooked kale	1 cup	39	179
9.	Cooked broccoli	1 cup	55	62

IRON - *men: 8 mg; women: 18 mg*

What it is: A common metal that's essential to nearly all life forms.
Why you need it: Key for cell growth, immunity, and oxygen transport throughout the body.

	SERVING SIZE	CALORIES	IRON
1. **Chicken liver**	3 oz	100	7.6
2. **Cooked spinach**	1 cup	41	6.4
3. **Sesame seeds**	¼ cup	206	5.2
4. **Soybeans**	½ cup	188	4.5
5. **Cooked lima beans**	1 cup	215	4.5
6. **Cooked kidney beans**	1 cup	225	3.9
7. **Venison**	4 oz	180	3.3
8. **Roasted turkey breast**	4 oz	214	2
9. **Beef tenderloin**	4 oz	240	2
10. **Tofu**	4 oz	86	1.8

MAGNESIUM - *men: 420 mg; women: 320 mg*

What it is: A mineral found mostly in our bones. The human body is unable to produce it, so it's vital to seek out foods that contain it.
Why you need it: Helps muscles and nerves relax, strengthens bones, and ensures healthy blood circulation.

	SERVING SIZE	CALORIES	MAGNESIUM
1. **Roasted pumpkin seeds**	¼ cup	169	162
1. **Prickly pear**	1 cup	61	127
2. **Sesame seeds**	¼ cup	206	126
3. **Cooked black beans**	1 cup	227	120
4. **Sunflower seeds**	¼ cup	205	114
5. **Roasted almonds**	¼ cup	206	97
6. **Cooked pinto beans**	1 cup	235	86
7. **Cooked brown rice**	1 cup	216	84
8. **Cooked summer squash**	1 cup	36	43
9. **Steamed scallops**	4 oz	127	42

SELENIUM - *men/women: 55 mcg*

What it is A mineral needed daily, but only in small amounts.

Why you need it: Protects cells from free radicals, allows the thyroid to produce hormones, and protects joints from inflammation.

		SERVING SIZE	CALORIES	SELENIUM
1.	Cooked shrimp	4 oz	112	56
2.	Canned white tuna (in water)	3 oz	109	55.8
3.	Cooked snapper	4 oz	145	55.4
4.	Cooked halibut	3 oz	95	47.1
5.	Roasted turkey breast	4 oz	214	33.2
6.	Beef tenderloin	4 oz	240	28.7
7.	Portabello mushrooms	1 cup	35	26.5
8.	Oysters	6	61	16.5
9.	Egg	1 medium	63	13.5
10.	Tofu	4 oz	86	11.3

POTASSIUM - *men/women: 4,700 mg*

What it is: Another mineral, stored within cells to regulate muscle contraction and nerve activity.

Why you need it: Keeps your muscles strong, balances electrolytes, and lowers risk of high blood pressure.

		SERVING SIZE	CALORIES	POTASSIUM
1.	Cooked pinto beans	1 cup	235	746
2.	Cooked lentils	1 cup	230	731
3.	Cooked beets	1 cup	74	518
4.	Baked winter squash	1 cup	76	494
5.	Avocado	½ fruit	161	487
6.	Cantaloupe	1 cup	56	473
7.	Figs	4 medium	148	464
8.	Cooked brussels sprouts	1 cup	60	450
9.	Tomato	1 cup	38	427
10.	Banana	1 medium	108	422

ZINC - *men: 11 mg; women: 8 mg*

What it is: A mineral that regulates carbohydrate metabolism and blood sugar.

Why you need it: Stabilizes metabolism and blood sugar, helps immune system when you're sick, and heightens your sense of smell and taste. Also plays an important role in male fertility.

		SERVING SIZE	CALORIES	ZINC
1.	Beef tenderloin	4 oz	240	5.6
2.	Venison	4 oz	180	4.1
3.	Wheat germ	1 oz	101	3.4
4.	Pastrami	2 slices	82	2.8
5.	Sesame seeds	¼ cup	206	2.8
6.	Roasted pumpkin seeds	¼ cup	169	2.3
7.	Roasted lamb (loin)	4 oz	230	2.1
8.	Cooked green peas	1 cup	134	1.9
9.	Cooked shrimp	4 oz	112	1.6
10.	Fat-free shredded mozzarella cheese	¼ cup	40	1.1

Your body is a living engine that runs on nutrients, and the world's highest-octane nutrients are found right in your supermarket.

Index

Boldface page references indicate photographs.
Underscored references indicate boxed text.

A

A1C test, 29
Add-meat meal, **228**, 228
Adipokines, xii
Agave syrup, 95
Alcohol, 203
Almonds, 21, 209
Applebee's food
 dinner, **182**, 182
 lunch, **108**, 108, **158**, 158, **169**, 169, **173**,
 173, **176**, 176
Apples, 29, 58
 Crispy Apple Turnovers, **290–91**, 290–91
 Oatmeal Pancakes with Cinnamon
 Apples, **96**, 96
 snacks, 256–57
Apricots
 Grilled Apricots, **292**, 292
Arby's food, **58**, 58, **183**, 183, **109**, 109
Arugula, 192
 Frittata with Arugula and Peppers, **97**, 97
 Italian Panini with Provolone, Peppers,
 and Arugula, **233**, 233
Asian Vinaigrette, 169
Asparagus
 Honey-Mustard Salmon with Parmesan
 Asparagus, **232**, 232
 parmesan, **232**, 232, 237
 Scrambled Eggs with Smoked Salmon,
 Asparagus, and Goat Cheese, **90**, 90
Atkins diet, 3
Atlanta Bread Company food, **59**, 59, **184**,
 184, **290**, 290
Au Bon Pain food
 breakfast, **60**, 60, **91**, 91
 dessert, **270**, 270
 dinner, **185**, 185
 lunch, **107**, 107, **162**, 162, **164**, 164
Avocados, 186, 205

B

Bacon, 121
 Breakfast Tacos with Bacon and Spinach,
 98, 98
 Turkey Sandwich with Guacamole and
 Bacon, **172**, 172
Bagels
 Atlanta Bread Company, **59**, 59
 Au Bon Pain, **60**, 60
 Dunkin' Donuts, **66**, 66
 supermarket, **78**, 78
Baja Fresh food
 dinner, **186**, 186
 lunch, **110**, 110
Baked goods, xvi, **76**, 76. See also specific
 type
Balsamic vinegar, 109
 Strawberry Shortcake with Balsamic
 Vinegar, **291**, 291

Bananas, 89
 Oatmeal with Peanut Butter and Banana,
 95, 95
Barbecue, **230**, 230
Bars, best snack, **260**, 260
Basal metabolism, 17
Baskin-Robbins food, **270**, 270, **295**, 295
Beans, 147, 181
 black bean chips, 256–57
 Roast Pork Loin Porchetta-Style with
 Lemony White Beans, **248**, 248
 Seared Scallops with White Beans and
 Spinach, **245**, 245
Beef. See also Burgers
 chain restaurant
 Applebee's, **108**, 108
 Boston Market, **190**, 190
 Chevys Fresh Mex, **246**, 246
 Chipotle, **196**, 196
 On the Border, **239**, 239
 Outback Steakhouse, **131**, 131, **206**,
 206, **244**, 244
 P.F. Chang's, **132**, 132
 Panda Express, **208**, 208
 Romano's Macaroni Grill, **214**, 214
 Ruby Tuesday, **215**, 215
 Taco Bell, **145**, 145
 Uno Chicago Grill, **220**, 220
 dietary fat in, 231
 flank steak, 239
 homemade
 Bloody Mary Skirt Steak, **244**, 244
 Coffee-Rubbed Steak, **239**, 239
 Grilled Steak Tacos, **246**, 246
 naturally raised, 118
 sandwiches
 Applebee's, **108**, 108
 Arby's, **109**, 109, **183**, 183
 Blimpie, **187**, 187
 Panera Bread, **134**, 134
 Quiznos, **137**, 137
 Subway, **143**, 143, **216**, 216
 supermarket, **154**, 154, **231**, 231
Bell peppers. See Peppers
Ben & Jerry's food, **271**, 271, **285**, 285
Beta-carotene, 188
Beta-glucan, 86
Beverages. See also specific type
 best snack, **261**, 261
 calories in, xvi
 Espresso Granitas, **292–93**, 292–93
 Starbucks, **286**, 286
Blimpie food, **111**, 111, **187**, 187
Blood pressure, 24–25, 32. See also High
 blood pressure
Blood sugar levels, 28–29, 33, 255. See also
 Diabetes
Blood tests, 29

Bob Evans food
 breakfast, **61**, 61, **94**, 94
 dessert, **271**, 271
 dinner, **188**, 188
 lunch, **113**, 113
Body fat, x, xii, 16–18
Body weight, xiv
Boston Market food, **177**, 177, **190**, 190
Breads, 60, **92**, 92, **262**, 262
Breakfast. See also specific food
 bowls, supermarket, **85**, 85
 calories, 6, 57
 chain restaurant, **58–77**, 58–77
 homemade, **90–101**, 90–101
 importance of, 56–57
 nutritious, 57
 organic, supermarket, **88**, 88
 sandwiches
 Arby's, **58**, 58
 Atlanta Bread Company, **59**, 59
 Burger King, **62**, 62
 Cheat Sheet, 73
 Cosí, **64**, 64
 Dunkin' Donuts, **66**, 66, **99**, 99
 Hardee's, **67**, 67, **101**, 101
 Jack in the Box, **69**, 69, **98**, 98
 McDonald's, **71**, 71
 Panera Bread, **72**, 72
 selecting, 71
 Sonic, **75**, 75
 Starbucks, **76**, 76
 Subway, **77**, 77
 supermarket, **89**, 89
 scenarios, 6, 8
 supermarket, **78–89**, 78–89
 weight gain and skipping, 66
 weight loss and, 6
Broccoli, 138, 250
 Orecchiette with Broccoli Rabe and
 Turkey Sausage, **250**, 250
Brownies, **271**, 271, **288**, 288
Brown rice, 132
Brussels sprouts, 238, 248
Burger King food
 breakfast, **62**, 62
 dessert, **272**, 272
 dinner, **191**, 191
 lunch, **114**, 114
Burgers
 Burger King, **114**, 114
 Carl Jr.'s, **241**, 241
 Cheat Sheet for fast-food, 127
 Chili's, 117
 Dairy Queen, **197**, 197
 MacDonald's, **128**, 128
 The Ultimate Burger, **241**, 241
 Wendy's, **147**, 147, **221**, 221
Burrito
 Baja Fresh, **110**, 110
 Breakfast Burrito, **101**, 101
 building, 10
 Chicken Fajita Burrito, **160**, 160
 Chipotle, **160**, 160, **196**, 196

Jack in the Box, **69**, 69
McDonald's, **71**, 71
supermarket, **87**, 87, **155**, 155
Taco Bell, **218**, 218
Butter, 131, 249
Blackened Tilapia with Garlic-Lime
Butter, **249**, 249
Butternut squash
Butternut Squash Soup, **168**, 168
Curry with Cauliflower and Butternut
Squash, **174**, 174

C

Cakes
Au Bon Pain, **270**, 270
Denny's, **274**, 274
Olive Garden, **277**, 277
Ruby Tuesday, **279**, 279
Starbucks, **280**, 280
Calcium, 67, 269, 320
California Pizza Kitchen food
dinner, **192**, 192, **232**, 232
lunch, **115**, 115, **165**, 165, **171**, 171
Calories
in beverages, xvi
breakfast meal, 6, 57
in buttermilk pancakes, 65
in chain restaurant food, 218
in Cheesecake Factory food, 63
consumption of, average daily, xiv, 14
dinner, 180–81
exercise in burning, 17, 302
in foods, traditional, xiv, xvi
in fries, 191
gender differences in burning, 16
lingo in cutting, 142
weight gain and, xiv
weight loss and deficit of, 3
Cancer prevention, 27
Carbohydrates, 105
Carl's Jr. food, **241**, 241
Carrabba's food, **294**, 294
Carrots, 256–57
Cauliflower
Curry with Cauliflower and Butternut
Squash, **174**, 174
Celery sticks, 256–57
Cereals, 79, 79, 86, 86, **262**, 262. *See also*
Oatmeal
Chain restaurant food. *See also specific
restaurant name*
breads, 60
breakfast, **58–77**, 58–77
calories in, 218
corn- and soy-based food in, xviii, 18
dessert, **270–81**, 270–81
dinner, **182–221**, 182–221
lunch, **107–47**, 107–47

Cheat Sheets
breakfast sandwiches, 73
burgers, fast-food, 127
chicken, 112, 219
fish and seafood, 189
fries, 140
pasta, 204
salads, 119
Cheese
Caprese Sandwich, **175**, 175
Cheesy Chicken-Sausage Waffles, 83
Chicken Parmesan, **237**, 237
Crispy Ham Omelette with Cheese and
Mushrooms, **100**, 100
Grilled Cheese with Sautéed Mushrooms,
234, 234
Honey-Mustard Salmon with Parmesan
Asparagus, **232**, 232
Italian Panini with Provolone, Peppers,
and Arugula, **233**, 233
Panera Bread, **175**, 175
parmesan asparagus, **232**, 232, 237
Scrambled Eggs with Smoked Salmon,
Asparagus, and Goat Cheese, **90**, 90
selecting, 175
in snack matrix, 256
Cheesecake, **275**, 275, **278**, 278, **291**, 291
Cheesecake Factory food
breakfast, **63**, 63
dessert, **272**, 272, **290–91**, 290–91
dinner, **234**, 234, **243**, 243
lunch, **166**, 166
Chevys Fresh Mex food, **193**, 193, **246**, 246
Chick-fil-A food
dessert, **273**, 273
dinner, **194**, 194
lunch, **116**, 116
Chicken
buffalo wings, 136
chain restaurant
Applebee's, **169**, 169, **173**, 173, **182**,
182
Baja Fresh, **110**, 110, **186**, 186
Bob Evans, **188**, 188
Boston Market, **177**, 177
Burger King, **191**, 191
California Pizza Kitchen, **165**, 165,
192, 192
Chevy's Fresh Mex, **193**, 193
Chick-fil-A, **194**, 194
Chili's, **117**, 117
Chipotle, **160**, 160, **196**, 196
Dairy Queen, **120**, 120, **197**, 197
Denny's, **198**, 198
IHOP, **200**, 200
Jamba Juice, **126**, 126
KFC, **125**, 125, **201**, 201
McDonald's, **202**, 202
Olive Garden, **129**, 129, **203**, 203
On the Border, **205**, 205
P.F. Chang's, **207**, 207
Panda Express, **133**, 133
Panera Bread, **134**, 134, **209**, 209

Romano's Macaroni Grill, **237**, 237,
238, 238
Ruby Tuesday, **250**, 250
T.G.I. Friday's, **217**, 217
Taco Bell, **218**, 218
Uno Chicago Grill, **220**, 220
Cheat Sheets, 112, 219
fried, **222**, 222
homemade
Breakfast Hash with Sweet Potatoes
and Chicken Sausage, **94**, 94
Cheesy Chicken-Sausage Waffles, 83
Chicken Fajita Burrito, **160**, 160
Chicken Marsala, **238**, 238
Chicken Parmesan, **237**, 237
Chicken Salad Sandwich with Curry
Raisins, **177**, 177
Chicken Tacos with Salsa Verde,
170, 170
Chili-Mango Chicken, **173**, 173
Chinese Chicken Salad, **169**, 169
Sesame Noodles with Chicken and
Peanuts, **165**, 165
sandwiches
Blimpie, **111**, 111, **187**, 187
Bob Evans, **113**, 113
Burger King, **114**, 114
Cheat Sheet, 112
Chick-fil-A, **116**, 116
Chicken Salad Sandwich with Curry
Raisins, **177**, 177
IHOP, **124**, 124
KFC, **125**, 125
McDonald's, **202**, 202
Quiznos, **212**, 212
Wendy's, **221**, 221
selecting, 125, 136
supermarket
frozen, **153**, 153
rotisserie, 170, **222**, 222
stir-fry, **225**, 225
tryptophan in, 220
Chickpeas, spicy, 247
Chili, **148**, 148, **195**, 195, **242**, 242
Chili peppers. *See* Peppers
Chili's food, **117**, 117, **170**, 170, **195**, 195
Chipotle food, **118**, 118, **160**, 160, **196**, 196
Chips, black bean, 256–57
Chocolate, dark, 257
Chocolate milk, **287**, 287
Cholesterol levels, 26–27, 33. *See also* High
cholesterol
Choline, 269
Cilantro, 110
Cinnamon
Oatmeal Pancakes with Cinnamon
Apples, **96**, 96
Coffee, 58
Coffee-Rubbed Steak, **239**, 239
Espresso Granitas, **292–93**, 292–93
Tiramisu, **294**, 294

Cold Stone Creamery food, **273**, 273, **292**, 292
Cookies
    Atlanta Bread Company, **290**, 290
    Au Bon Pain, **270**, 270
    Chocolate Chip Cookies, **290**, 290
    homemade, **290**, 290
    Red Lobster, **278**, 278
    Starbucks, **280**, 280
    Subway, **280**, 280
    supermarket, **288**, 288
Corn-based foods, xviii, 18
Così food, **64**, 64, **97**, 97, **161**, 161
Cottage cheese, low-fat, 257
Crackers, whole wheat, 256–57
Cranberries, 27, 111
Cravings, food, 4, 18
Cream cheese, 99
Croissants, **62**, 62, **75**, 75
Crunchy foods, **38–39**, 38–39
Curcumin, 177
Curry, 153
    Chicken Salad Sandwich with Curry
        Raisins, **177**, 177
    Curry with Cauliflower and Butternut
        Squash, **174**, 174
Cycling, 305

D

Dairy products, 57, **263–64**, 263–64. See
    also specific type
Dairy Queen food, **120**, 120, **197**, 197, **274**,
    274
Deli food, 46, **46–49**, 46–49, 78, 143
Denny's food
    breakfast, **65**, 65, **90**, 90
    dessert, **274**, 274
    dinner, **198**, 198, **249**, 249
    lunch, **121**, 121
Dessert. See also specific food
    chain restaurant, **270–81**, 270–81
    homemade, **290–95**, 290–95
    nutritious, 269
    questions to ask before indulging in, 269
    supermarket, **282–89**, 282–89
Dessert bars, **284**, 284
Diabetes, xii, 21–22, 27, 28–29, 29, 313
Diet, ix–x, 20–22, 29
Dietary fat
    in beef, 231
    fat cells and, xii
    healthy, 18
    omega-3 fatty acids, xviii, 130
    omega-6 fatty acids, xviii
    trans fats, xvi, 23
    vitamin A and, 205
Dieting, ix–x, 2–4

Dijon mustard
    Honey-Mustard Salmon, **232**, 232
Dinner. See also specific food
    calories, 180–81
    chain restaurant, **182–221**, 182–221
    homemade, **232–51**, 232–51
    nutritious, 181
    supermarket, **222–31**, 222–31
Dips, 135, **264**, 264
Doctor Decoder, 32, 32–33
Domino's food, **122**, 122, **159**, 159, **199**, 199
Doughnuts, **276**, 276
Dressings, 144
Dunkin' Donuts food, **66**, 66, **99**, 99, **123**,
    123

E

Eat This, Not That! No-Diet Diet. See also
        Cheat Sheets; Personal stories
    advantages of, 12–14, 16–18
    checklist, 15
    confusion about, x
    cost of eating and, reducing, 18
    creation of, ix–x, xi
    as defense against health problems,
        21–22
    design of, 2
    Doctor Decoder, 32, 32–33
    foods in, 4
    goal of, 13
    hunger prevention and, 13
    meals in, 13
    nutrients in, 14, 16, 18
    overview, xix
    premise of, 4, 6
    resources, 5
    revolution of, xviii, xx–xxi
    secret weapons
        deli salads, 46, **46–49**, 46–49
        fruit salad matrix, 41, **41**, 41
        homemade salad matrix, 42, **42–45**,
            42–45
        overview, 37
        smoothie matrix, 50, **50–53**, 50–53
        trail mix matrix, 38, **38–40**, 38–40
    snacks in, 13
    uniqueness of, 6
    weight loss and, 4
Eggs
    chain restaurant
        Arby's, **58**, 58
        Burger King, **62**, 62
        Cheesecake Factory, **63**, 63
        Così, **64**, 64, **97**, 97
        Denny's, **65**, 65, **90**, 90
        Dunkin' Donuts, **66**, 66
        Hardee's, **67**, 67
        IHOP, **68**, 68, **100**, 100
        Jack in the Box, **69**, 69
        McDonald's, **71**, 71
        Panera Bread, **72**, 72, **93**, 93
        perfect scrambled, 101

Sonic, **75**, 75
Subway, **77**, 77
homemade
    Baked Egg with Mushrooms and
        Spinach, **93**, 93
    Crispy Ham Omelette with Cheese
        and Mushrooms, **100**, 100
    Frittata with Arugula and Peppers,
        97, 97
    Scrambled Eggs with Smoked
        Salmon, Asparagus, and Goat
        Cheese, **90**, 90
Energy, x, xii, 18, 255
English muffins, **71**, 71, **80**, 80
Exercise
    ab-building, 302
    body-fat burning, **303**, 307
    calorie-burning, 17, 302
    cycling, 305
    for distance, 305
    fatigue-preventing, 306
    golf, 306
    HDL increase and, 27
    in high blood pressure prevention, 24
    indoor running, 304
    machines to avoid, 308–9, 308–9
    muscle-building, 302
    partner, 304
    resistance training, 300–301
    running, indoor, 304
    for speed, 305

F

Fascia, 313
Fasting glucose test, 29
Fat cells, xii
Fiber, 57, 58, 62, 181
Fish and seafood. See also Tuna
    breaded, **223**, 223
    broccoli in, 138
    chain restaurant
        Bob Evans, **188**, 188
        California Pizza Kitchen, **232**, 232
        Cheesecake Factory, **243**, 243
        Denny's, **198**, 198, **249**, 249
        On the Border, **130**, 130
        Outback Steakhouse, **206**, 206
        P.F. Chang's, **245**, 245
        Red Lobster, **138**, 138, **213**, 213
        Ruby Tuesday, **141**, 141
        Uno Chicago Grill, **167**, 167
    Cheat Sheet, 189
    cooking tip, 232
    in high blood pressure prevention, 24
    homemade
        Blackened Tilapia with Garlic-Lime
            Butter, **249**, 249
        Grilled Mahi Mahi, **243**, 243

Honey-Mustard Salmon with
Parmesan Asparagus, **232**, 232
Scrambled Eggs with smoked
Salmon, Asparagus, and Goat
Cheese, **90**, 90
Seared Scallops with White Beans
and Spinach, **245**, 245
Shrimp Roll, **167**, 167
Smoked Salmon Sandwich, **99**, 99
omega-3 fatty acids in, 130
sandwiches, Burger King, **191**, 191
searing, 245
supermarket
bagged meal, **229**, 229
best, **223**, 223
quick dinner, **227**, 227
Five Guys food, **251**, 251
Flavor enhancers, **46–47**, 46–47
Folate, 18, 319
Foods. See also specific type
alcohol and, 203
calories in traditional, xiv, xvi
corn-based, xviii, 18
cravings, 4, 18
crunchy, **38–39**, 38–39
as defense against health problems,
20–22
in Eat This, Not That! No-Diet Diet, 4
organic, 53, 157
plant-based, 213
searing, 245
sodium in, 23
soy-based, xviii, 18
supersized, xvi
swapping, 299
sweetener, **38–39**, 38–39
thermic effect of, 16
Fries, 140, 191
Fruit bars, **287**, 287
Fruits. See also specific type
colors of, 41
organic, 53
salad matrix, 41, **41**, 41, 75
smoothie matrix, **50–51**, 50–51
snacks, **265**, 265
Funnel cake, **272**, 272

G

Genetics and health problems, 21
Ginger, 153
Glucose levels, 28–29. See also Diabetes
Golf, 306
Grains. See Breads; Whole grains
Grapefruit, 85
Guacamole, 256
Turkey Sandwich with Guacamole and
Bacon, **172**, 172

H

Häagen-Dazs food, **275**, 275, **282**, 282,
284–85, 284–85
Ham
Crispy Ham Omelette with Cheese and
Mushrooms, **100**, 100
sandwiches
Atlanta Bread Company, **184**, 184
Subway, **216**, 216
Hardee's food, **67**, 67, **101**, 101
HDL, 26–27, 27
Health problems, 20–22. See also specific
type
Heart disease, xii, 21–22, 312–13
HFCS, xiv, xvi, xviii
High-density lipoprotein (HDL), 26–27, 27
High-fructose corn syrup (HFCS), xiv, xvi,
xviii
High blood pressure, xii, 23–25, 24, 25, 32,
147
High blood sugar, 28–29, 29
High cholesterol, 26–27, 27
Homemade food. See also specific ingredient
breakfast, **90–101**, 90–101
dessert, **290–95**, 290–95
dinner, **232–51**, 232–51
lunch, **158–77**, 158–77
salads, 42, **42–45**, 42–45
Hot dogs, **150**, 150, **251**, 251
Houlihan's food, **174**, 174
Hummus, 78, 257
Hunger, preventing, 13, 255, 258–59
Hypertension, xii, 23–25, 24, 25

I

Ice cream
Baskin-Robbins, **270**, 270, **295**, 295
Ben & Jerry's, **271**, 271, **293**, 293
Bob Evans, **271**, 271
Breyers, **282–83**, 282–83, **287**, 287
Burger King, **272**, 272
Chick-fil-A, **273**, 273
Cold Stone Creamery, **273**, 273, **292–93**,
292–93
Dairy Queen, **274**, 274
Denny's, **274**, 274
Edy's, **284**, 284, **287**, 287
Good Humor, **294–95**, 294–95
Häagen-Dazs, **275**, 275
homemade
Olive Oil Ice Cream, **293**, 293
Sundaes with Grilled Pineapple and
Rum Sauce, **295**, 295
IHOP, **275**, 275
KFC, **276**, 276
McDonald's, **277**, 277
nutrients in, 269
Red Lobster, **278**, 278
Sonic, **279**, 279
supermarket, **282–84**, 282–84
Uno Chicago Grill, **281**, 281

Wendy's, **281**, 281
Ice cream bars, **282**, 282
Ice cream sandwiches, **285**, 285
IHOP food
breads, **92**, 92
breakfast, **68**, 68, **92**, 92, **96**, 96, **100**, 100
dessert, **275**, 275
dinner, **200**, 200, **248**, 248
lunch, **124**, 124
Inflammation, xii
Insulin levels, 28
Iron, 64, 321

J

Jack in the Box food, **69**, 69, **98**, 98
Jalapeño peppers. See Peppers
Jamba Juice food, **70**, 70, **95**, 95, **126**, 126

K

KFC food, **125**, 125, **201**, 201, **276**, 276

L

Lamb
Lamb with Tzatziki, **247**, 247
Outback Steakhouse, **247**, 247
Laughter in diabetes management, 27
LDL, 26–27
Lettuce, **42–43**, 42–43. See also Salads
Longevity, 21
Low-density lipoprotein (LDL), 26–27
Lunch. See also specific food
chain restaurant, **107–47**, 107–47
homemade, **158–77**, 158–77
lean, guidelines for, 106
nutritious, 105
supermarket, **148–57**, 148–57
typical, 104–5

M

Magnesium, 321
Mangos, 70
Chili-Mango Chicken, **173**, 173
Mango-Chili Paletas, **294–95**, 294–95
Marsala wine
Chicken Marsala, 155, **238**, 238
McDonald's food
breakfast, **71**, 71
dessert, **277**, 277
dinner, **202**, 202
lunch, **128**, 128
Meals, 13, 23. See also specific type
Meat, 257. See also specific type
Meat substitute, **152**, 152
Medical care, 22
Mediterranean-style diet, 29
Metabolic syndrome, 21
Metabolism, 16–17

Milk, 88, **287**, 287
Minerals, 18, 57, 316. *See also specific type*
Muscles, building, 16–18, **302**
Mushrooms
　Baked Egg with Mushrooms and Spinach, **93**, 93
　Cheesecake Factory, **166**, 166
　Crispy Ham Omelette with Cheese and Mushrooms, **100**, 100
　Grilled Cheese with Sautéed Mushrooms, **234**, 234
　Mushroom Melt, 166
　Shiitake, 63

N

Niacin, 222
Nutrients
　in arugula, 192
　in bananas, 89
　in coffee, 58
　in cranberries, 111
　in curry, 153
　in Eat This, Not That! No-Diet Diet, 14, 16, 18
　in ice cream, 269
　in mangos, 70
　in roasted peppers, 233
Nuts. *See also specific type*
　heart disease prevention and, 21–22
　longevity and, 21
　snacks, **265**, 265
　spice-roasted, 40
　in trail mix, **38–39**, 38–39

O

Oatmeal
　Au Bon Pain, **60**, 60
　Denny's, **65**, 65
　in diabetes prevention, 29
　Oatmeal Pancakes with Cinnamon Apples, **96**, 96
　Oatmeal with Peanut Butter and Banana, **95**, 95
　supermarket, **86**, 86
Obesity, x, 18
Oils, 111. *See also specific type*
Olive Garden food, **129**, 129, **203**, 203, **277**, 277
Olive oil, 109
　Olive Oil Ice Cream, **293**, 293
Olive oil mayonnaise, 167
Olives, 210
Omega-3 fatty acids, xviii, 130
Omega-6 fatty acids, xviii
On the Border food, **130**, 130, **205**, 205, **239**, 239, **240**, 240
Onions, caramelized, 241
Organic foods, 53, 157

P

P.F. Chang food, **132**, 132, **207**, 207, **245**, 245, **278**, 278
Pancakes
　Bob Evans, **61**, 61
　buttermilk, 65
　IHOP, 68, **96**, 96
　Oatmeal Pancakes with Cinnamon Apples, **96**, 96
　supermarket, **82**, 82
Panda Express food, **133**, 133, **208**, 208
Panera Bread food
　breakfast, **72**, 72, **93**, 93
　dinner, **209**, 209, **233**, 233
　lunch, **134**, 134, **168**, 168, **175**, 175
Pantry snacks, **262–63**, 262–63
Papa John's food, **135**, 135, **210**, 210
Pasta
　chain restaurant
　　California Pizza Kitchen, **115**, 115, **165**, 165
　　Olive Garden, **129**, 129
　　Red Lobster, **213**, 213
　　Romano Macaroni and Grill, **139**, 139
　　Ruby Tuesday, **250**, 250
　Cheat Sheet, 204
　homemade
　　Orecchiette with Broccoli Rabe and Turkey Sausage, **250**, 250
　　Sesame Noodles with Chicken and Peanuts, **165**, 165
　protein in, 156
　Ronzini Smart Taste, 165
　supermarket, **156**, 156
Pastrami, prime, 176
Peanut butter, 257
　Oatmeal with Peanut Butter and Banana, **95**, 95
Peanuts
　Sesame Noodles with Chicken and Peanuts, **165**, 165
Pears, 256–57
Pepperoni, 236
Peppers
　bell, 211, 224
　chili, 196
　Frittata with Arugula and Peppers, **97**, 97
　Grilled Chili Relleno, **240**, 240
　Italian Panini with Provolone, Peppers, and Arugula, **233**, 233
　jalapeño, pickled, 172
　On the Border, **240**, 240
　roasted, 233
　Sausage Sandwich with Peppers, **159**, 159
　swaps, 240

Personal stories
　Boyd, Dave, **xv**, xv
　Clark, Michael, **7**, 7
　Cuartero, James, **9**, 9
　Guerrero, Raul, **xiii**, xiii
　Holden, Allison, **xvii**, xvii
　Phillips, Del, **19**, 19
　Starn, Danielle, **31**, 31
　Thorpe, Marcus, **30**, 30
Pesto
　Minestrone with Pesto, **171**, 171
Physician's care, 22
Pies, **276**, 276, **290–91**, 290–91
Pineapple
　Sundaes with Grilled Pineapple and Rum Sauce, **295**, 295
Pita, whole wheat, 256–57
Pizza
　California Pizza Kitchen, **115**, 115
　Domino's, **122**, 122, **199**, 199
　Loaded Pizza, **236**, 236
　Papa John's, **135**, 135, **210**, 210
　Pizza Hut, **136**, 136, **211**, 211, **236**, 236
　supermarket frozen, **226**, 226
　toppings, selecting, 122
　Uno Chicago Grill, **146**, 146
Pizza Hut food, **136**, 136, **211**, 211, **236**, 236
Plant-based foods, 213
Plaque, arterial, 26
Pork
　IHOP, **248**, 248
　Roast Pork Loin Porchetta-Style with Lemony White Beans, **248**, 248
Portions, xvi, 72
Posture, 312
Potassium, **24**, 139, 158, 322
Potatoes
　Baked Potato Soup, **158**, 158
　Bob Evans, **94**, 94
　Breakfast Hash with Sweet Potatoes and Chicken Sausage, **94**, 94
　fries, **140**, 191
　herb-roasted, 244
　KFC, **201**, 201
Pot pies, avoiding, 113
Poultry. *See* Chicken; Turkey
Prehypertension, 25
Probiotics, 61
Produce, **42–43**, 42–43. *See also* Fruits; Salads; Vegetables
Protein
　for breakfast, nutritious, 57
　in deli salad matrix, **46–47**, 46–47, 81
　for dinner, nutritious, 181
　in homemade salad matrix, **42–43**, 42–43
　for lunch, nutritious, 105
　Marsala wine, 155, 238
　in pasta, 156
　snacks, **265**, 265
　weight loss and, 6, 48
Puddings, supermarket, **289**, 289

Q

Quercetin, 72
Quiznos food, **137**, 137, **163**, 163, **172**, 172, **212**, 212

R

Raisins
Chicken Salad Sandwich with Curry Raisins, **177**, 177
Red Lobster food, **138**, 138, **213**, 213, **278**, 278
Red Robin food, **242**, 242
Resistance training, 300–301
Reuben sandwiches, **176**, 176
Roasted peppers. *See* Peppers
Romano's Macaroni Grill food, 139, 139, **214**, 214, **237**, 237
Ruby Tuesday food, **141**, 141, **215**, 215, **250**, 250, **279**, 279
Running, indoor, 304

S

Salads
chain restaurant
Applebee's, **169**, 169
Au Bon Pain, **107**, 107
Baja Fresh, **186**, 186
Chevy's Fresh Mex, **193**, 193
Chipotle, **118**, 118
Cosí, **161**, 161
Dairy Queen, **120**, 120
On the Border, **205**, 205
Panera Bread, **209**, 209
T.G.I. Friday's, **144**, 144, **217**, 217
Taco Bell, **145**, 145
Cheat Sheets, 119
deli matrix, 46, **46–49**, 46–49
dressings for, 144
fruit matrix, 41, **41**, 41, 75
homemade
add-ons for, **42–43**, 42–43
Chinese Chicken Salad, **169**, 169
Greek Salad, **161**, 161
matrix, 42, **42–45**, 42–45
side, simple, **45**, 45
rules of, 44, 49
standout, **48–49**, 48–49
super, **44–45**, 44–45
Salsa, 257
Chicken Tacos with Salsa Verde, **170**, 170
Salt, 23, 139, 216
Sandwiches. *See also specific type*
Applebee's, **108**, 108
Arby's, **109**, 109
Atlanta Bread Company, **184**, 184
Au Bon Pain, **185**, 185
Blimpie, **111**, 111
Cheesecake Factory, **234**, 234

Denny's, **121**, 121
Dunkin' Donuts, **123**, 123
Grilled Cheese with Sautéed Mushrooms, **234**, 234
Italian Panini with Provolone, Peppers, and Arugula, **233**, 233
Panera Bread, **134**, 134, **233**, 233
Quiznos, **137**, 137, **212**, 212
selecting, 184
soups and, 149
Starbucks, **142**, 142
Subway, **143**, 143, **216**, 216, **235**, 235
Turkey Sloppy Joes, **235**, 235
Sausage
Al Fresco Chicken Sausages, 159
Breakfast Hash with Sweet Potatoes and Chicken Sausage, **94**, 94
Cheesy Chicken-Sausage Waffles, 83
Domino's, **159**, 159
Sausage Sandwich with Peppers, **159**, 159
Searing foods, 245
Seeds in trail mix, **38–39**, 38–39
Selenium, 198, 322
Serving sizes, xvi, 72
Sex in high blood pressure prevention, 24
Shakes, **273**, 273, **279**, 279, **281**, 281, **286**, 286
Shortcake
Strawberry Shortcakes with Balsamic Vinegar, **291**, 291
Sitting, 310–13
Smoothie King food, **74**, 74
Smoothies
Jamba Juice, **70**, 70, **126**, 126
making, 50
matrix, 50, **50–51**, 50–51
organic fruit in, 53
rules of, 53
Smoothie King, **74**, 74
Super, **52–53**, 52–53
supermarket, **286**, 286
Snacks. *See also specific type*
advantages of, 255
bars, **260–61**, 260–61
best, 260, **260–65**, 260–65
beverages, **261**, 261
canned, **261–62**, 261–62
dairy, **263–64**, 263–64
dips, **264**, 264
in Eat This, Not That! No-Diet Diet, 13
frozen, **261–62**, 261–62
fruits, **265**, 265
hunger prevention and, 255, **258–59**, 258–59
matrix, 256, **256–57**, 256–57
nuts, **265**, 265
on-the-go, **289**, 289
pantry, **262–63**, 262–63
protein, **265**, 265
spreads, **264**, 264
two-piece, 256, **256–57**, 256–57
weight gain and, 255
Sodium, 23, 139, 216
Sonic food, **75**, 75, **279**, 279

Sorbet, **275**, 275, **285**, 285
Soups
Au Bon Pain, **164**, 164
Baked Potato Soup, **158**, 158
Butternut Squash Soup, **168**, 168
California Pizza Kitchen, **171**, 171
Gazpacho, **164**, 164
improvising, 171
Minestrone with Pesto, **171**, 171
Panera Bread, **168**, 168
sandwiches and, 149
selecting, 134
supermarket, **149**, 149
Soy-based foods, xviii, 18
Spinach, 93, 243
Baked Egg with Mushrooms and Spinach, **93**, 93
Breakfast Tacos with Bacon and Spinach, **98**, 98
Seared Scallops with White Beans and Spinach, **245**, 245
Spreads, **264**, 264
Spring rolls, **207**, 207
Stage 1 and 2 hypertension, 25
Standing, 313–15
Starbucks food, **76**, 76, **142**, 142, **280**, 280, **286**, 286
Starch, 133
Strawberries
French Toast Stuffed with Strawberries, **92**, 92
Strawberry Shortcake with Balsamic Vinegar, **291**, 291
Stress and high blood pressure, 23–24
Stroke, 21–22
Subway food
breakfast, **77**, 77
dessert, **280**, 280
dinner, **216**, 216, **235**, 235
lunch, **143**, 143
Sugar crashes, preventing, 13
Sundaes. *See* Ice cream
Supermarket food. *See also specific type*
breakfast, **78–89**, 78–89
dessert, **282–89**, 282–89
dinner, **222–31**, 222–31
lunch, **148–57**, 148–57
Supersized food, xvi
Sweetener food, **38–39**, 38–39

T

T.G.I. Friday's food, **144**, 144, **217**, 217
Taco
Baja Fresh, **110**, 110
Breakfast Tacos with Bacon and Spinach, **98**, 98
Chevys Fresh Mex, **193**, 193
Chicken Tacos with Salsa Verde, **170**, 170
Chili's, **170**, 170
Chipotle, **196**, 196

Grilled Steak Tacos, **246**, 246
On the Border, **205**, 205
Taco Bell, **145**, 145, **218**, 218
Taco Bell food, **145**, 145, **218**, 218
Tex-Mex meal, **224**, 224
Thermic effect of eating, 16
Thickener enhancers, **50–51**, 50–51
Tiramisu, **272**, 272, **278**, 278, **294**, 294
Toaster pastry, supermarket, **81**, 81
Tomatoes, 121, 235
  Au Bon Pain, **185**, 185
  Caprese Sandwich, **175**, 175
  Panera Bread, **175**, 175
  Romano Macaroni and Grill, **139**, 139
Trail mix matrix, 38, **38–40**, 38–40, 62
Trans fats, xvi, 23
Triglycerides, 27
Tryptophan, 220
Tuna
  Au Bon Pain, **107**, 107, **185**, 185
  canned, 257
  Dunkin' Donuts, **123**, 123
  Italian Tuna Melt, **163**, 163
  premium, 163
  Quiznos, **163**, 163
  supermarket, **151**, 151
Turbinado, 74
Turkey
  Au Bon Pain, **107**, 107
  Orecchiette with Broccoli Rabe and
    Turkey Sausage, **250**, 250
  Quiznos, **17**, **137**, 137, 172
  Ruby Tuesday, **141**, 141
  sandwiches
    Arby's, **183**, 183
    Atlanta Bread Company, **184**, 184
    Au Bon Pain, **107**, 107
    Blimpie, **111**, 111

Panera Bread, **209**, 209
Ruby Tuesday, **215**, 215
Subway, **216**, 216
Turkey Reuben, **176**, 176
Turkey Sandwich with Guacamole
  and Bacon, **172**, 172
Turkey Sloppy Joes, **235**, 235
tryptophan in, 220
Turkey Chili, **242**, 242
Turmeric, 153
Type 1 and 2 diabetes, 27, 28–29, 29

U

Uno Chicago Grill food, **146**, 146, **167**, 167,
  220, 220, **281**, 281

V

Vegetables. *See also specific type*
  Curry with Cauliflower and Butternut
    Squash, **174**, 174
  for dinner, nutritious, 181
  Grilled Vegetable Wrap, **162**, 162
  Houlihan's, **174**, 174
  for lunch, nutritious, 105
  P.F. Chang's, **132**, 132
Vegetarian entrées, frozen supermarket,
  157, 157
Vitamin A, 107, 205, 316
Vitamin B_1, 317
Vitamin B_6, 207, 317
Vitamin B_{12}, 318
Vitamin C, 64, 319
Vitamin D, 67, 318
Vitamin E, 320
Vitamins, 18, 57, 316. *See also specific type*

W

Waffles, **83**, 83
Water intake, 27, 61, 200
Watermelon, 185
Weight gain, ix, xiv, 3, 23, 66, 255
Weight loss, 3–4, 6, 48, 61
Weight Watchers plan, 3
Wendy's food, **147**, 147, **221**, 221, **281**, 281
Whole grains, 27, 79, 181, 256–57
Workout, 300–301
Wraps
  Arby's, **58**, 58
  Au Bon Pain, **162**, 162
  Chick-fil-A, **194**, 194
  Grilled Vegetable Wrap, **162**, 162

Y

Yogurt
  Au Bon Pain, **91**, 91
  Baskin-Robbins, **270**, 270
  Bob Evans, **61**, 61
  Cold Stone Creamery, **273**, 273
  Greek Parfait, 84
  Ruby Tuesday, **279**, 279
  supermarket, **84**, 84, **283**, 283
  Yogurt Parfait, **91**, 91

Z

Zinc, 323